Birth Control in China 1949–2000

This comprehensive volume analyses Chinese birth policies and population developments from the founding of the People's Republic to the 2000 census. The main emphasis is on China's 'Hardship Number One Under Heaven': the highly controversial one-child campaign, and the violent clash between family strategies and government policies it entails.

Birth Control in China 1949–2000 documents an agonizing search for a way out of the predicament and a protracted inner Party struggle, a massive effort at social engineering and grinding problems of implementation. It reveals how birth control in China is shaped by political, economic and social interests, bureaucratic structures and financial concerns. Based on own interviews and a wealth of new statistics, surveys and documents, Thomas Scharping also analyses how the demographics of China have changed due to birth control policies, and what the future is likely to hold.

This book will be of interest to students and scholars of modern China, Asian studies and the social sciences.

Thomas Scharping is Chair for Modern Chinese Studies at the University of Cologne, Germany. He has published widely on modern China, including *Floating Population and Migration in China: The Impact of Economic Reforms* (Hamburg: 1997) and the documentary collection, *The Evolution of Regional Birth Planning Norms in China 1954–97* (for the journal *Chinese Sociology and Anthropology*, Armonk: 2000).

Chinese Worlds

Chinese Worlds publishes high-quality scholarship, research monographs, and source collections on Chinese history and society from 1900 to the present.

'Worlds' signals the ethnic, cultural, and political multiformity and regional diversity of China, the cycles of unity and division through which China's modem history has passed, and recent research trends toward regional studies and local issues. It also signals that Chineseness is not contained within territorial borders – some migrant communities overseas are also 'Chinese worlds.' Other ethnic Chinese communities throughout the world have evolved new identities that transcend Chineseness in its established senses. They too are covered by this series. The editors see them as part of a political, economic, social and cultural continuum that spans the Chinese mainland, Taiwan, Hong Kong, Macau, South East Asia, and the world.

The focus of Chinese Worlds is on modern politics and society and history. It includes both history in its broader sweep and specialist monographs on Chinese politics, anthropology, political economy, sociology education, and the social-science aspects of culture and religions.

The Literary Fields of Twentieth-Century China
Edited by *Michel Hockx*

Chinese Business in Malaysia
Accumulation, Ascendance, Accommodation
Edmund Terence Gomez

Internal and International Migration
Chinese Perspectives
Edited by *Frank N. Pieke* and *Hein Mallee*

Village Inc.
Chinese Rural Society in the 1990s
Edited by *Flemming Christiansen*
and *Zhang Junzuo*

Chen Duxiu's Last Articles and Letters, 1937–1942
Edited and translated by *Gregor Benton*

Encyclopedia of the Chinese Overseas
Edited by *Lynn Pan*

Chinatown, Europe
Flemming Christiansen

New Fourth Army
Communist Resistance along the Yangtze and the Huai, 1938–1941
Gregor Benton

A Road is Made
Communism in Shanghai 1920–1927
Steve Smith

The Bolsheviks and the Chinese Revolution 1919–1927
Alexander Pantsov

Chinas Unlimited
Gregory Lee

Friend of China – The Myth of Rewi Alley
Anne-Marie Brady

Birth Control in China 1949–2000
Population Policy and Demographic Development
Thomas Scharping

Birth Control in China 1949–2000

Population policy and demographic development

Thomas Scharping

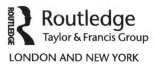
Routledge
Taylor & Francis Group

LONDON AND NEW YORK

First published 2003 by Routledge
2 Park Square, Milton Park, Abingdon, Oxon, OX14 4RN

Simultaneously published in the USA and Canada
by Routledge
605 Third Avenue, New York, NY 10017

Routledge is an imprint of the Taylor & Francis Group, an informa business

Copyright © 2003 Thomas Scharping

Typeset in Goudy by LaserScript Ltd, Mitcham, Surrey

British Library Cataloguing in Publication Data
A catalogue record for this book is available from the British Library

Library of Congress Cataloging in Publication Data
A catalog record for this book has been requested

ISBN 13: 978-0-415-96817-1 (hbk)
ISBN 13: 978-0-415-38604-3 (pbk)

Contents

List of tables		ix
List of charts		xi
Preface		xiii

Part I
Introduction — 1

1 Levels of understanding — 3

2 Moral and cultural dimensions — 7

3 Information and sources — 13

Part II
Policy formulation — 27

4 Motives and goals of Chinese birth control — 29
   4.1 Leadership perceptions — 29
   4.2 Defining population targets — 38

5 Phases of the one-child policy and its forerunners — 43
   5.1 Stir and hush: the muddle 1949 to 1978 — 43
   5.2 Drums and gongs: the campaign 1979 to 1983 — 50
   5.3 Small holes and big gaps: the relaxation 1984 to 1985 — 58
   5.4 Tit for tat: the controversy 1986 to 1989 — 63
   5.5 Law and order: the administration 1990 to 1999 — 74

Part III
Bureaucratic implementation — 81

6 Legal norms and practice in flux — 83
   6.1 Channels, types and rhythm of birth-control norms — 83
   6.2 Late marriage, late birth and birth spacing — 91
   6.3 Procedures for birth permits — 94

6.4 Second-child permits 96

6.5 Contraceptive measures 105

6.6 Abortions 117

6.7 Material incentives 125

6.8 Economic and disciplinary sanctions 136

6.9 Special group rules 150

    6.9.1 National minorities 150

    6.9.2 Others 155

7 Problems of organization 159

7.1 Institutions 159

    7.1.1 The role of the Party 159

    7.1.2 Birth-planning commissions 160

    7.1.3 Coordination with other government organs 165

    7.1.4 Grass-roots organization 169

    7.1.5 Medical network 176

    7.1.6 Production and supply of contraceptives 181

    7.1.7 Academic bodies and mass organizations 184

7.2 Personnel and remuneration 185

7.3 Budget and financing 189

8 Planning and evaluation 197

8.1 The planning process 197

8.2 Statistical controls 202

8.3 Other information systems 207

Part IV

Popular response 211

9 Gender roles, family size and sex preferences 213

10 Strategies and evidences of non-compliance 224

Part V

Demographic results 237

11 Female marriage trends 239

11.1 Marriage rates and marital status 239

11.2 Average age at marriage 241

11.3 Early- and late-marriage rates 244

12 Fertility levels 249

12.1 Absolute numbers, birth rates and proportions of birth orders 249

12.2 Age-specific, duration-specific and total fertility rates 253

12.3 Fertility by parity progression and sex of previous children 261

12.4 Birth spacing   263
12.5 Provincial differentials   265
12.6 Urban and rural fertility levels   270
12.7 Fertility by social characteristics   274
12.8 Fertility by ethnic group   283

13 Changes in sex and age structure   288
13.1 Sex at birth and in age groups 0–4   288
13.2 Age structure   298

Part VI
Conclusions and future perspectives   305

14 Looking back: causal structures and policy impact   307

15 Looking forward: demographic projections and their implications   318

16 Weighing the options: past experience and new ideas   330

Epilogue: The population census of November 2000   343

Notes   346
Bibliography   372
Index   396

List of tables

1 Beginning of provincial birth-planning activities: year of earliest reference   46
2 Provincial birth-planning rules: conditions for second-child permits 1979–99 and implied total fertility rate (children per woman) 1990   98
3 Contraceptive rates by methods and provinces 1981, 1999   110
4 Contraceptive rates by methods, age groups and residence 1982, 1988, 1992   114
5 Motives of women for final acceptance of sterilization: survey from Fengyang County, Anhui, 1992   115
6 Reasons for no contraceptive use 1982, 1988, 1992   116
7 Contraceptive prevalence, operations, and abortions 1963–99   121
8 Abortion rate by provinces 1965–96   124
9 Rate of one-child certificates by provinces 1979–99   127
10 Provincial birth-planning rules: one-child incentives 1979–99   130
11 Provincial birth-planning rules: economic and disciplinary sanctions 1979–99   138
12 Birth-planning evaluation form for townships and towns 1992   173
13 Institutions and personnel for maternity and child care 1949–99   177
14 Birth-planning stations in townships/towns and villages 1991–95   180
15 Personnel of birth-planning commissions 1979–95   186
16 Birth planning expenditures 1963–98   190
17 Birth-planning budget allocations per capita by provinces 1965–94   192
18 Birth-planning budget allocations by expenditure items 1980–96   194
19 Surveys on family-size preferences 1980–97   215
20 Advantages and disadvantages of more children: survey from Danjiang County, Hubei, 1986   219
21 Percentage of births outside plan by provinces 1979–97   234
22 First-marriage rates of women of reproductive age by generations 1930–73   239
23 Marital status of women of reproductive age 1982, 1990, 1995   240
24 Average first-marriage age of women by provinces and place of residence 1978–92   243
25 Early-marriage rate and age-specific marriage rate 1978–97   244

26 Early-marriage rate by provinces 1980–99   246
27 Late-marriage rate by provinces 1980–99   247
28 Average birth intervals 1950–92   265
29 Total fertility rate by provinces 1957–95   267
30 Total fertility rate for educational level by place of residence 1989   278
31 Minority population and total fertility rate by ethnic group
    1981/82, 1989/90   285
32 Sex ratio of births and cohorts ages 0–4: national totals 1953–95   290
33 Sex ratio of cohorts age 0 by provinces, 1953–90   293
34 Projections of age structure 2000–50   327
35 Major results of the November 2000 census and the preceding
    counts   344

List of charts

1   Percentage of births outside plan by birth order 1979–99   232
2   Average age of women at first marriage 1949–98   242
3   Absolute birth numbers and crude birth rates: original and
    revised figures 1978–99   250
4   Proportions of second and higher-order births 1980–99   252
5   Age-specific fertility rates 1957–99   254
6   Crude birth rate and total fertility rates 1949–90   257
7   Total fertility rates 1978–99: a comparison of survey and
    census figures   259
8   Period parity progression ratios 1955–95   262
9   Urban and rural total fertility rates 1949–99   271
10   Total fertility rates for urban and rural areas by component
    age groups 1978–95   273
11   Total fertility rates for urban and rural areas by component
    birth orders 1978–95   274
12   Total fertility rates for educational levels by birth order 1989   276
13   Total fertility rates for occupational groups by birth order 1989   279
14   Sex ratio by birth order and registration status 1989   291
15   Sex ratio by birth order and existence of son, agricultural
    population 1989   292
16   Age pyramids 1982, 1990   300
17   Women of reproductive age 1982, 1990, 1995   301
18   Age structure of total population 1953, 1964, 1982, 1990, 1995   303
19a   Past Chinese projections of total population 1990–2050   324
19b   New projections of total population 1990–2050   324

Preface

This book is based on many years of studying Chinese population problems. It incorporates the results of numerous visits to China to research social developments and population policy in that country. This field research has greatly enhanced my knowledge of normative issues, procedural questions, and problems of implementation in the course of China's one-child campaign. All information in the study that is not backed up by references is based on it. The Deutsche Forschungsgemeinschaft (DFG) supported three of these research stays in 1986, 1990 and 1992, during which half-structured in-depth interviews with about 140 Chinese demographers, sociologists, statisticians, birth-control cadres and civil servants were conducted. I am deeply indebted to the Deutsche Forschungsgemeinschaft for this support. The University of Cologne, Germany, relieved me of my teaching duties during a sabbatical leave.

Within China the research was conducted with the friendly assistance of many colleagues from academies, universities and other research institutes, and the cooperation of various state agencies. They are so numerous that I can thank them only collectively here. In particular, the following research institutions have extended their hospitality and provided valuable information: the Population Institutes of the Chinese Academy for Social Sciences and the provincial academies of Shanghai, Sichuan and Yunnan; the Population Institutes of Beijing University, People's University and Beijing College of Economics, Fudan University and East China Normal University in Shanghai, Sichuan University, Southwest China College for Finance and Economics and Yunnan University; the National Library in Beijing, the Shanghai Library, and the Provincial Libraries of Sichuan and Yunnan. Much patience in suffering my endless questions has been shown by the State Birth-Planning Commission and the Birth-Planning Commissions of the provinces mentioned above; the State Statistical Bureau and the Statistical Bureaux of Beijing, Shanghai, Sichuan and Yunnan; the Ministry of Labour and the Labour Departments of all three provinces. Discussions with various administrations, academies and university institutes of Guangdong, Fujian and Hainan provinces which I had in the course of a different project during 1993 and 1994 have also enriched the work. Attending the Conference of the International Union for the Scientific Study of Population in Beijing during October 1997 offered me yet another chance to meet and exchange views.

As always, Kuan Hsin Chi from the Universities Service Centre, Chinese University of Hongkong, provided superb working conditions. The same applies to Andrew Mason from the Population Program of the East-West Center in Honolulu, where discussions with Griffith Feeney, Wang Feng, Minja Kim Choe and other colleagues have given me much stimulation during two stays in 1992 and 1994. I am also grateful to Judith Banister, formerly with the US Bureau of the Census, and Susan Greenhalgh, formerly with the Population Council in New York and currently with the University of California at Irvine, for help and information. James Lee from the California Institute of Technology and Wang Feng were kind enough to send me an advance copy of their important study on *One Quarter of Humanity*. Yves Blayo from the Institut National d'Etudes Démographiques in Paris provided me with his new and competent outline of Chinese population policies since the 1950s.

An earlier German version of this study was published in 1995 by the Institut für Asienkunde in Hamburg as a contribution to a collection of materials on Chinese birth control, which I edited together with my colleague Robert Heuser. The material used for it was mainly limited to the period 1978 to 1992. Thanks are due to the Institut für Asienkunde for almost three decades of good cooperation and for transferring the copyright of my part of the study to me. I have translated, revised and enlarged it for this book.

This English version is more than double the size of the earlier German edition and effectively supersedes it. While it still concentrates on the one-child campaign from 1979 to the present, it also gives a broad overview of Chinese population policy during the past fifty years. After the publication of many hitherto classified materials on the earlier period, this has become a topic worthy to be reworked again. All chapters on special aspects of birth control therefore contain condensed reviews of pertinent measures in the pre-reform period. A summary of earlier birth policies between the founding of the People's Republic in 1949 and the beginning of economic reforms in 1978 has been added in Chapter 5.1.

In addition, all chapters have been updated to include a discussion of developments from 1992 up to 2001. For this purpose, new and extensive materials on organizational arrangements, procedures and information systems, as well as survey data on peasant fertility behavior, have been checked and incorporated. Further additions relate to a new round of birth-control norms from the 1990s and to the new Law on Population and Birth Planning from 2001. These new norms were not available for the earlier German version. I wish to thank Eric Florence (Liège), Robert Heuser (Cologne) and Thomas Hoppe (Lübeck) for providing some of them. Many other new material and interview notes from China were also scrutinized. This led to a large number of additions and revisions, some of which also refer to the record of policies in the 1980s. In the process, passages of the German edition which contained inaccurate information were corrected.

The English version contains additional chapters on the Chinese demographic record, on the assessment of policy impact and the projection of future population trends. The chapters on contraception and abortion have likewise become enlarged by demographic analysis. All demographic sections integrate past demographic figures with findings from the 1990 population count, the 1992 national fertility survey, the 1995 microcensus and the latest annual sample surveys. Detailed figures from the 1997 survey on population and reproductive health were not yet published; thus only the summary findings could be used. Nor were detailed data available from the fifth national census in November 2000. Preliminary results are given in the Epilogue.

The demographic sections concentrate on providing a condensed, up-to-date and integrative review of major marital and fertility trends of the twentieth century. For this purpose easy-to-digest charts have been combined with tables giving the exact figures necessary for further research. In many cases, tables and charts have to be confined to the more documented period of the one-child policy. They then range from 1978/79, a point of reference for the period of two-child policies, to the latest year for which relevant data are available. The text also contains brief summaries of prior developments starting in the first half of the twentieth century. An effort has been made to capture the essence from a wealth of demographic data and to make the text readable for non-specialists. While various analyses of the demographic materials are based on my own work, the chapters on the demographic record would have been impossible without the sustained efforts of many colleagues from China, the USA and Europe, who have continuously sifted through the flood of population statistics from China.

Finally, the bibliography and the review of the literature have also grown. They will hopefully serve as a guide to an interdisciplinary subject of key importance, which has developed into a highly specialized field with sometimes arcane conventions. Materials and studies on China's population are meanwhile reaching awesome dimensions. Since the beginning of the one-child campaign they have turned China from a white spot into one of the most studied areas on the world population map.

Has all this new information altered the conclusions of the study's earlier version on the state of affairs in the 1980s? After examining the additional material on birth control in the 1990s, I am impressed by the thoroughness of the attempts to address the host of implementation problems that surfaced in the preceding decade. Many deficiencies in organizational, technical and financial matters have been amended. This has stretched human and financial resources to the limit. In addition, the leadership has been uncompromising in its drive to perfect legal stipulations and administrative procedures. Some of its most sweeping measures have revived ingredients of campaign politics discarded after the early 1980s. They have erected a tight system of control and surveillance in the service of birth planning. It is indicative of the torments of present-day China that such revivals none the less coexist with slow progress for citizens' rights.

The Chinese leadership has scored undeniable successes in its stubborn determination to close all loopholes for births outside plan. However, I am not convinced that this has changed the fundamental conflict between state policies and family interest with its ensuing dilemma of spiraling sanctions against massive evasions. Watching this persisting antagonism and noting the many irregularities that show up in the analysis of fertility data, I also uphold my earlier scepticism in regard to some spectacularly low fertility numbers of recent years. Meanwhile, it is also openly voiced by Chinese specialists. Both population statistics and policies will only improve if socio-economic developments lead to greater self-assuredness and produce a demographic transition working on its own. This will happen sooner or later. For the Chinese people one can only wish that it will be sooner.

I am indebted to my secretary Susanne Grimm for her painstaking work with the manuscript and for diligent proof-reading. Karin Färber and Liliane Kreider helped me in combing Chinese journals and press reports of the last three years. Björn Alpermann assisted in the compilation of an index. Last but not least, I want to thank my wife Anne and my two daughters Franziska and Julia, three beautiful women who supported me during my long pregnancy with this book, even though they wished more than once that I would have practised some birth control before.

Cologne, April 2001
Thomas Scharping

Part I

Introduction

1 Levels of understanding

On his tour through Liaoning province in 1987, a Chinese magazine reporter met a vice-mayor. The following conversation ensued:

'Which work is giving you most headaches?'
'Birth planning.'
'How big are your headaches?'
'I never suffered from insomnia. But each time I hear birth-planning reports from below I cannot close my eyes at night any more.'

The cadre continues to describe a mass meeting, with pointed criticism of a peasant couple who refused sterilization even after their sixth child. Incensed at the criticism, the peasant left 'an eternal memory' on the face of the cadre. When the reporter toured another province and posed the same question as to what was the most awkward type of work, he received the following response:

You do not need to guess for long, the whole world knows about it. Birth planning is the Hardship Number One Under Heaven! One month ago I did inspection work in the countryside. We had not even entered the village, when a voice started yelling: 'The devils are coming!' When the women with unauthorized pregnancies heard this, they immediately made for the hills and woods. We searched the whole day long, but we did not even discover a shadow of the 'village guerrilla troops'.[1]

Such unabashed reports about implementation problems of China's one-child policy are rare. There are good reasons for the dearth of reports, since birth planning is one of the most sensitive issues of Chinese policy both at international and national level. It has evoked highly diverse reactions, ranging from a medal for meritorious work granted by the UN to the Chinese Birth-Planning Commission in 1983 to repeated accusations against violations of human rights. These have served as an argument for the refusal of the USA to pay arrears in UN dues, and led to the highly publicized US withdrawal of financial support for UN population programmes under the Reagan and Bush administrations.[2] Even today, the world continues to be deeply divided in regard to Chinese birth-control policies, and a revival of fundamentalist policies in the

USA is in the cards. The polemic has a long line of antecedents, as the pros and cons of birth planning in China have been debated since the 1920s, both inside and outside the country. The discourse on Chinese population problems in a wider sense has an even longer history and stretches back to the eighteenth century. While in Europe it came to serve as a topic in the polemics of enlightenment, political economy and revolutionary thinking, in China it is closely intertwined with the nation's quest for modernization and the re-attainment of wealth and power.

Population policy in the People's Republic thus has a long and tortuous history. Its most extreme expression, the one-child policy pursued since 1979, has evolved through decades of searching and feuding that first saw violent rejection of birth planning, then cautious experimentation with voluntary contraception, and finally ever wider inroads of state intervention into fertility matters. Despite arduous propaganda, it continues to be a sensitive subject within China. This is not only because the one-child policy squarely contradicts the traditional pro-natalist ideals of the country, but it also mercilessly lays bare other problems, foremost among which is the basic conflict of the reform period between liberalizing the economy and maintaining tight control of the political and social sphere. In spite of the repeated veerings of high politics to the left and right, Chinese society continues its march to emancipation from direct state control. At the same time, however, the state effects one of the strongest interventions in family life ever proposed by a government. In consequence, even Peng Peiyun, the former minister for birth control, has deemed it necessary to comment a prevalent question within China: 'Why is everything liberalized except birth planning?'[3]

The conflict between liberalization and control approaches has been repeatedly waged within the leading bodies of the country. In contrast to the facade of unity and the urge to present birth control as an unflinching long-term concern, many years of controversy within the Party leadership can be documented. In this controversy pragmatists pleading for a flexible accom-modation of social concerns have been poised against hard-line proponents of the one-child policy who dismiss conditional permissions for second children by invoking the risks for the country's future. On a more general level, such controversies mirror the different approaches of politicians who continue to believe in their ability to steer social and economic policy according to professed laws of development, and power holders who, just like many people in authority in other parts of the world, restrict themselves to mediating the present while refraining from moulding the future.

This can be precarious in China's case, since, in view of the high base numbers, minimal discrepancies of growth rates can entail maximum long-term consequences. In this way, differences in total population numbers that seem to be negligible in the mid-term can expand to differences in the range of hundreds of millions of people decades later. The high degree of inertia in demographic processes also produces age structures, which generations later result in population dynamics not prone to outside intervention. If these structures are radically breached, inertia occurs again. Population ageing offers a good example: only decades later a dramatic decline in birth numbers may lead to an equally dramatic problem of old-age support – which thereby can be put aside for some time. Under these circumstances, the controversy over liberalizing or controlling China's present has always been waged by invoking different perspectives of the country's future. There are those who fear gambling away this future here and now, and there are others who reply:

> China's population cannot be but controlled. But if one generation must swallow everything that has been heaped up by decades and centuries of mistakes, then the following generation will only suffer from new misery.[4]

Such problems of perspective may also be discerned at academic level. Here the controversy recurs in different analyses of causal relations in population matters, in a conflict about culpabilities for the manifest failure of some one-child policies, and in debates about advice for future action. In these debates China's demographers display the age-old ambiguity of the Chinese intelligentsia: Should it articulate social concerns, in particular peasant interests, against government policy? Or should it make its know-how available for use by the government in order to effect better policy implementation? In this classical conflict of roles, large parts of the intellectual elite identify themselves as spokesmen for government interests. At the same time, they evince a deep-felt inner detachment from the peasant majority of the population.

However, the advocates of tight population control have also come to recognise the limits of government intervention. The compromises they have been forced to accept are telling for the political culture of China: the gap between hard-line declarations and lagging implementation; the facade of outside unanimity concealing a highly diverse range of opinions; the mental and verbal sophistication in reinterpreting policy guidelines; the ramification of bureaucratic hierarchies compensating for their control deficits by a continuous delegation of tasks to lower levels; the brutality born of helplessness and the passiveness of calculation prevalent at the grass roots; the cycle of directives from above, evasion from below, new measures and new countermeasures, which continues until new rules of the game are devised.

China is not a straight society. Centuries of bureaucratic experience have bred a rich tradition of administrative refinement struggling with popular evasion, and this tradition is resurfacing with the progressive collapse of both socialist systems and socialist morals. It is a long, drawn-out collapse as the leadership tries to stem the tide and prevent the danger of total disintegration. In its wake a classical structural problem of the Chinese polity re-emerges: extreme normative centralization coexisting with extreme factual decentralization. At times, it entails evolution in the forms of government coupled with involution of their substance.[5] But in spite of much red tape and blockages from within, the system has demonstrated remarkable capacities for learning and innovation. On the other hand, it can also practise self-deception on a grand scale, as is documented by Chinese birth-control reports. One of the findings of this study is a continuous backsliding of quality standards in current population statistics. This has reached such high proportions that it is beginning to affect economic planning, and to render dubious many per-capita indicators from running statistics.

In this way, a study of Chinese birth planning tells many stories at the same time: the story of China's demographic problems and their reflection in political thought, as well as the country's agonizing search for a way out of its predicament. It can also be read as a paradigm for the hardships of policy implementation in China and the failure of planning systems, which are eroded from within once they transgress popular interests too severely. Other questions of general importance are also involved. There are few policy arenas that provide as many vivid examples of China's internal information problems as population policy. The multiple and elaborate channels for retrieving demographic information are testimony to the internal checks and balances of the system; at the same time, they clearly demonstrate the problems of staying within its confines. Chinese approaches to law, administration and central–regional relations are further leitmotivs contained in the account of birth planning. Finally, there is the story of the one-child policy as a mobilization issue. Later historians may evaluate it as the last mass campaign and the last large-scale attempt at social engineering in China.

It is not only China's political system and culture which are mirrored in the implementation problems of birth control. The successes and failures of the government's population policy also reflect the profound transformations of Chinese society in recent times. Following the violent upheavals and mass campaigns of the Mao era, economic reforms have left Chinese society breathless. There are few nations which have undergone as rapid a change as China in the 1980s and 1990s. In only a few years the country has been catapulted into modern times and into the world market from the partly self-imposed and partly enforced isolation of the former period. Old fissures of Chinese society have been deepening ever since. Whereas industrialization and urbanization, the rising level of education, new consumer habits and ideals of life leave their marks in the reproductive behaviour of China's urban population, the fertility record of large parts of the rural population continues to be highly traditional. Apart from the glaring urban–rural gap, the increasing diversification within China and the growing tendencies for decentralization are also mirrored in the different regional fertility records. The consequences of birth planning transcend the political realm as they sever a core element of Chinese culture: the traditional family with its religious, social and economic foundations. Within this context, the issues involved are inseparable from the subject of gender roles and women's emancipation in China.

All these processes may be clearly discerned in the various aspects of birth planning. On another level, social, economic and political developments are always closely linked to changing values and ideals. But values also guide any empirical analysis of China's one-child policy and should therefore be discussed explicitly.

2 Moral and cultural dimensions

The introduction of birth planning in China and its successive tightening until the start of the one-child policy has evoked heated debates. In most of its statements on population policy directed at foreign audiences, the Chinese leadership has tried hard to gloss over the toughness of its measures. A typical example are remarks by former Party leader Zhao Ziyang, who in July 1987, in a television spot sponsored by the UN to commemorate the 'Day of 5 Billion People', declared categorically: 'Birth planning in China is practiced on a voluntary basis.'[1]

On the eve of the 1994 World Population Conference in Cairo, China again summed up her point of view for the foreign community. She stressed the economic and ecological motivations of birth control, and supported the UN principles of voluntariness, education and gradual change, the emancipation of women and the fight against poverty. An outline on population policy published at the same time stated that in China, medical personnel and family planning propagandists 'offer' services for abortion, sterilization and contraceptive advice to couples of reproductive age. According to the outline, personnel also 'provide' medical devices and 'help families that practice family planning', respecting the principle that 'whether or not a pregnant woman has a sterilization or abortion depends totally on her own wish'. The statement continued:

> The Chinese government promotes voluntary adoption of birth control on the basis of extensive education, and opposes forced imposition of it. However, we don't deny that shortcomings and mistakes occur. China is very vast, with over 3,000 counties, and the standards of officials vary. In some areas, coercion may happen in the initial phases of family planning activity. On finding such actions, we resolve them resolutely.[2]

Such formulations and similar statements ever since are an indirect reply to the criticism of Chinese birth planning, which has become vociferous in the USA and other Western countries. One of the most influential critics has been former China population specialist John S. Aird from the US Bureau of the Census, who had been warning for years against unabated population growth in China. In 1990, however, he registered a strong protest against China's birth-control programme, which according to him has been 'the most draconian since King Herod's slaughter of the innocents'. Aird argued: 'The Chinese program remains highly coercive not because of local deviations from central policies but as a direct, inevitable, and intentional consequence of those policies.'[3]

Aird's conclusions have been taken up by numerous politicians, journalists and human rights groups. They cannot be simply dismissed – the evidence collected by him for coercive abortion and sterilization in China is too overwhelming. This study will also confirm it. Apart from violating general human rights, Chinese birth planning is also provoking public ire because many critics discern violations of women's special rights. Among them are the right of inviolability of the body, the right to self-determine fertility, and the option to choose from a range of different contraceptives. All these rights have been successfully claimed by feminist groups at the most recent World Population Conference.

These are justified objections against Chinese practices and should be taken seriously. To them could be added the well-known and principally correct argument that development is the best pill, because raising economic and cultural standards of life entails a spontaneous reduction of fertility. Nevertheless, the objections refer only to one side of the coin. They are one-sided because other important aspects of the problem are neglected and because different forms of coercion are not clearly differentiated.

Chinese practices of birth planning mostly do not imply the use of direct physical force. It has been proven that such force has been applied during early phases of the one-child policy in different regions of the country, when it was tacitly condoned by the Chinese leadership. Even today it is not far-fetched to assume that it has not vanished completely. However, since the mid-1980s we are mainly facing an increasingly sophisticated system of normative, remunerative and administrative coercion. Within this system, China's leadership utilizes its legislative monopoly to decree highly restrictive birth-control regulations. In cases of non-compliance these spell out tough sanctions, ranging up to well-nigh obliteration of a family's economic existence. Second, the leadership has designed increasingly tight procedures for population planning and birth rationing. Third, it has further enhanced this system of structural coercion by calling lower cadres to account once demographic targets are not met.

In this way, the spontaneous fertility behaviour of the population has increasingly come under state control. This has grave consequences for the individual which should not be extenuated. For even if procedures become more calculable and civilized in time, the final effect for the victims can remain the same. In former times it may have been zealots demolishing the houses of pregnant women and their families – today it may be the marshal who, if everything works out according to the will of the state, will knock politely yet commandingly at the door to present a writ of execution and to confiscate personal belongings of families violating birth-control norms.

Such ideas are shocking. Nevertheless, we accept fines and sentences if, for instance, they serve to punish non-compliance with state schooling or quarantine regulations. This is because of our understanding that self-determination in the private family sphere ends where the needs of a new generation and responsibilities towards society at large are not respected. It is an understanding which, because of its general validity, has been invoked in UN population documents. The Teheran Declaration on Human Rights of 1968 therefore has good reason to urge couples to use their right to decide the number of children they want freely but responsibly. Responsibility primarily means that the number of children born should not exceed the number who can be supported. While it would be fairly easy to reach agreement on this principle, the judgement becomes more complicated if economically viable family-size preferences on the private level conflict with the concerns of society at large. This happens in a situation of paradox, where a large population excess on the macro level is coexisting with simultaneous manpower demand on the micro level.

It is exactly this collision of private and collective interests that is shaping the population problems of China. A taboo of state intervention in reproductive behaviour seems to be out of place if the outlook of future generations is severely constrained by dramatically rising population numbers over the past 200 years. In recent years, the most populous nation of the world has been growing annually by net nearly 15 million people. Without birth planning it would be nearly 30 million. Quite rightly, Chinese statements in defence of birth control have repeatedly pointed out that this increase in population is equal to the annual creation of a new medium-sized country. On a corresponding scale are the labour, nutrition and housing problems, as well as the difficulties in the health and education sectors induced by China's population growth. The world must also face the ecological problems of China's natural environment, which permits the cultivation of only 14 per cent of the nation's territory. There is a need for action, even if it has to be admitted that technological change and constant remodelling of economic organization do not permit a final judgement as to the question of maximum carrying capacities. The fact that population developments cannot be isolated from other agents of change and that multiple interdependencies prevail translates into sharply differing outlooks for China and into controversies that are as old as the debate on population issues between Robert Malthus, William Godwin and Karl Marx in the late eighteenth and early nineteenth centuries.[4]

Whoever has personally experienced the hard struggle for space, jobs and life chances waged in China knows that such points are anything but theoretical. The permanent need to take into consideration large masses of people constitutes one of the basic facts of life in China. It effectively limits the options for state and society in economics and in many other spheres of life. Some arguments in China's White Book on human rights should therefore be taken seriously. In this document of 1991, the Chinese government declares its inability to wait for a spontaneous decline of birth rates in the wake of economic growth. In contrast, it reaffirms its responsibility for future generations by promoting birth planning now.[5]

But even if such a position is accepted, the reasonableness of policy measures for birth planning must be periodically judged anew. The same applies to complicated issues that arise if conflicts of goals occur between birth planning, economics and social welfare. An example is the rapid ageing of the population and the ensuing problems of old-age support which are looming on the horizon as a consequence of the one-child policy. These are extremely difficult problems, which give rise to heated discussions within the country. There are no comprehensive and satisfactory solutions at hand, and this is why the one-child policy has encountered many qualifications and reservations. Yet it has been reaffirmed time and again, at least in principle. The most basic reason for such reaffirmations has been the unquenchable urge to reach a standard of living comparable to industrialized countries within the not too distant future. This is an understandable and legitimate wish and should be respected by those who all too often regard their own well-being without further reflection as a self-evident right. Usually, human rights protests wither away on the lips of Western societies once they confront the world's population problems by facing poverty migration.

But discussions of Chinese birth planning restricting themselves to normative principles not only have to face moral problems on their own side of the fence. Since they also tend to abstract from social and cultural realities in China, they sometimes carry signs of the unreal. It is, for instance, not persuasive to discuss the reasonableness of policies without considering the reasons behind them. Conditions in China's countryside simply do not square with the propaganda suggestion of intensive educational efforts and a consequential voluntary reduction in birth numbers. It is against the background of stubborn resistance that China's politicians propagated the one-child family, reckoned with an average fertility rate of 1.5 to 1.7 children per woman in their internal calculations for the 1980s, and finally reached a figure of 2.3 during the population census of 1990.[6] This sobering result was attained in spite of tough regulations and draconian policies. It should be permitted to pose the question: What would have been the result without these sanctions?

Large parts of the Chinese population also think of birth planning as 'inhumane', a reproach that has even prompted a commentary by the official Party paper.[7] In particular, it is the peasantry that is voicing this opinion. Cultural, social and economic factors compel it to fight for more children, specifically for the right to have sons. It would be a grave error, however, to conclude that this opposition is in harmony with Western ideas about human rights. Human rights activists and women's lib proponents from the West would have a hard time in China should they try to defend the private sphere against the ubiquity of state power, for it is not the individual but the institution of the family, in a broad sense also society at large, that opposes the government's birth-planning efforts. In their analysis of peasant behaviour in contemporary China, the American anthropologists Sulamith and Jack Potter have pinpointed the values playing a role in this regard:

> An emotional rationale for marrying or having children would strike the villagers as flimsy and insubstantial at best, indecent at worst. . . . Valuing a child as 'human life' in isolation from its significance to the family and to society, is a senseless abstraction.[8]

Traditional family ethics keep prevailing in many Chinese villages, where they have been both subtly changed by political influences and restrengthened by the return to household farming. They exert a dominant influence in mate selection, perceive marriage primarily as an instrument for reproduction, the perpetuation of the family line and the attainment of prosperity. Single people beyond a certain age develop into an embarrassing problem for friends and relations, who move heaven and earth to arrange a marriage. Family ethics also enforce prompt childbearing after wedlock. The enduring dominance of traditional gender roles, especially in the countryside, continues to turn the birth of a male child into the major responsibility and *raison-d'être* of daughters-in-law. If couples, and particularly women, do not perform in this vital sphere of life, the ridicule of society and perhaps even suicide threats from reproachful parents set in. Time and again, Chinese birth-control cadres and propaganda media have battled with one of the most widely quoted dictums of the Confucian philosopher Mencius from the fourth century BC, a maxim that has become proverbial and deeply internalized in Chinese culture: 'There are three things which are unfilial, and to have no posterity is the greatest of them.'[9]

The concept of posterity here refers to male progeny only – a self-evident fact for the Chinese reader that may be lost in the English translation. 'Many sons bring much riches' is another of the time-honoured proverbial expressions extolling the bearing of male progeny. Ancestor worship and Chinese family dynamics, as well as the traditional name, inheritance and hierarchy rules based on them, are at the root of such admonitions. Operating in a secular civilization with fragile links to transcendency and weak clerical organization, they define identities and unite individuals with eternity by way of the family line. Functioning in a cultural setting with strong foundations of profit-oriented behaviour but feeble protection of individual rights, they turn family-based strategies into a prime mechanism for realizing economic and social advancement. Honouring the principle of patrilineal descent and patrilocal residence, excluding unmarried daughters from ancestral ritual and married ones from agnate family obligations, they promote a marked son preference and sex-specific discrimination. Recognizing a wide gap between elite and mass persuasions, with the idea of the latter one that new-born children have not yet fully joined the human community, they also seem to lower barriers against predominantly female infanticide and abortion.

A cultural environment as such strongly favours male offspring. Its overall role for fertility dynamics is hard to assess. On the one hand, evidence is accumulating that it may further a disposition for intervention in natural fertility. Recent advances in the historical microdemography of China document the prevalence of traditional techniques of population control such as delayed marriage of males, abstention, infanticide or fatal neglect. On the other hand, the fostering of births until a sufficient number of children, primarily sons, are born works against strict birth control. This cultural setting is reinforced by powerful social and economic forces. Most important among these are the absence of social security for the majority of the population, the resulting principle of family-based old-age support, and the economic logic of petty-peasant manual labour.[10]

In this way, pregnancies, which at the outset of the one-child policy were experienced by 80 per cent of all women within one year after marriage, continue until a son is born. This moral obligation is deeply ingrained in the mind. If it is not met, it can be enforced by all kinds of means ranging from social pressure to physical assault. Both in past and present times, women have been threatened with divorce should male offspring fail to materialize. The pressures are such that in extreme cases a husband may murder his 'failing' wife, or one of the spouses commits suicide. Until recently such cases have been brought to Chinese courts. The catastrophe that people try to avoid with such extreme action is not the personal misfortune of individuals but rather the ritual, social and economic disintegration of the family line by extinction of ancestor worship, outmarriage of daughters and lack of manpower.

Such conditions of predominant human obligations are hard to reconcile with our ideas about individual human rights. Chinese ethics transfigure the subordination rather than the triumph of the individual, be it the traditional subordination towards the family or the modern one towards the state and the Party. It is less private emotion that is guiding people in reproductive behaviour but rather the consideration of group interests fostered over the centuries. In Europe, the bourgeois family revolution, giving rise to the ideals of romantic love and a nuclear family centred on precious children, has been a recent development of the late eighteenth and early nineteenth centuries. In China, it has hardly taken place outside the cities, and even there it is anything but complete. A revolution of sexual behaviour or of gender roles is just beginning.[11]

Because these elements of social change are still largely lacking, because popular medical knowledge continuously pre-dating the beginning of life is unknown, because modern psychology bestowing a soul to infants has not entered the peasant mind and because basic religious ideas are different, the question of abortion in China does not lend itself to the passionate pro and con arguments we witness in Western discussions. Perhaps a brief glance at the high abortion rates prevailing in other parts of the world will help to dispel some of the revulsion that reports on abortion in China provoke. Besides, remembering pre-modern family life in Europe could also serve as a useful corrective against taking present-day Western ethics as the sole point of reference. In some cases it is not even necessary to look back over centuries when decades are sufficient.

Moral values cannot be refuted by citing empirical evidence or claiming universal relativism. Opinions on China's birth planning will therefore continue to be divided. But if the inevitable discussion of its moral and cultural dimensions allows for a conclusion at all, then perhaps it is this one: population development and birth planning in China constitute an extremely complicated and many-faceted policy arena as they touch on the very nerves of Chinese society, Chinese economics and the Chinese state. Many students of China have looked for some of the biggest and most basic problems of the country in this field. It is unsuitable for intervention from outside.

3 Information and sources

The scale of the problems mentioned above, the coyness of demographic data and the lack of publicity for many aspects of Chinese birth planning have all combined to produce some noticeable gaps in scholarly literature. Earlier studies on Chinese population problems after 1949 did not enjoy access to the wide array of sources existing today. Written in an environment hostile to balanced academic work but eager for impassioned ideological debate, they were all too often limited to theoretical discussion or had to pursue an art that has been aptly described as a blend of social science and archaeology. Similar to other economic and social policy arenas, the few available population figures had to be stretched to the utmost in order to derive projections for the many gaps in the record. Information on the political process in birth planning remained patchy, too. With the exception of lengthy Marxist critiques of Malthusianism, not one major book on demographic issues was published in China. Among the better Western works from that period are Chandrasekhar (1959), Aird (1961, 1968), Orleans (1972, 1979) and Tien (1973, 1980). Focusing on the first Chinese birth-control efforts from 1954 to 1978, they had to ply the difficult trade of collecting the refuse from heated internal debates smothered in terse Party pronouncements. The gap between the state of knowledge then and our information now may be measured by comparing these works with White (1994), a first reworking of Chinese population policy in the 1950s.

It was only with the end of the Cultural Revolution, the beginning of economic reforms and the restoration of statistical work that Chinese population studies were revived. The most important role was played by the introduction of the one-child policy in 1979 and the holding of a new census in 1982, which received international support and wide publicity abroad. Monographic treatment of the one-child policy by Western authors starts with the pioneering study of Croll et al. (1985). Because this work had to rely on the very unsatisfactory information available during the early 1980s, it had to restrict itself to a rough outline of macro-relationships, a presentation of local reports, and a review of birth planning in the period 1949 to 1981. The short article by Kallgren (1985) goes further by sketching rural one-child policies up to 1983. Although it also suffers from a general lack of information, it already takes note of second-child permits granted in reaction to popular dissatisfaction with government policy goals.

Incorporating the results of the 1982 census and the national fertility survey staged in the same year, Banister (1987) is a standard work on Chinese population developments since 1949. The book also traces the one-child campaign up until 1983/84. It discusses guidelines, incentives and sanctions, contraceptive usage, ethical problems and international implications of the Chinese programme as far as could be discerned from contemporary Chinese press reports and patchy statistics published at the time. The work contains an excellent discussion of the Chinese fertility record and an independent reconstruction of vitality rates for the period 1949 to 1981. It is complemented by Lee and Wang Feng (1999), a thought-provoking *tour de force* through the last 300 years of Chinese population history. Kane (1987) is largely a restatement of existing Western literature. Nevertheless, the work offers a good overview of Chinese population policy until the early 1980s. However, changes in the one-child campaign that begun in 1982 are not mentioned.

With his long statements of 1986 and 1990, John S. Aird has exerted a great influence on Western perceptions of Chinese population policies. Both works contain pointed criticism of coercive measures, the main emphasis being on human rights problems and normative questions. Although both studies offer a rather detailed description of political developments up until 1988 and draw on a large source base, they display a lack of empathy for the implementation problems of Chinese birth planning and the discrepancy between norm and reality. The conclusions drawn tend to be one-sided.

Peng Xizhe (1991) and the preprinted article published as Peng Xizhe (1989) are studies of one of China's bright young demographers and are the very opposite of Aird. These are competent and highly technical analyses of changes in fertility levels between 1949 and 1981, as far as they could be reconstructed by China's national fertility survey of 1982. The political aspects and concrete policy measures of birth planning are largely ignored, however, while the demographic material is no longer up-to-date. Similar deficits are evident in the Sino-Australian coproduction by Wang Jiye and Hull (1991). Demographic and economic data in this work are analysed up until 1987. But critical points in the political sphere such as conceptional disputes, legal changes, coercive measures and passive resistance are avoided, and the discussion is limited exclusively to the macro level.

The best monographic treatment of population policy until 1989 is given in Tien (1991). This book briefly sketches long-term trends of marriage and fertility since 1929 and discusses the basic issues in Chinese population policies. As its most important thesis it reflects on a never completely resolved conflict between one-child and two-child policies in China since 1979. Policy analysis for the early 1980s is dense, whereas the picture becomes blurred after 1986. Regional variations in population policy, the evolution of legal norms and the problems of bureaucratic implementation are neglected, the demographic data largely pertaining to the early 1980s only. This also tends to be the situation for the comprehensive outline in Blayo (1997). It is strong on birth-control guidelines, contraceptive use, and marriage and fertility trends in the 1970s and 1980s, but does not pursue subsequent developments.

Whereas monographic treatment of Chinese birth planning remains unsatisfactory, the subject has been widely debated in scholarly journals and collections, among the latter the very useful volume by Poston and Yaukey (1992). Chen and Tyler (1982) and Wong Siulin (1984) have described the one-child campaign during the early 1980s and its possible demographic and social repercussions in the future. Still worth a look is the article by Bianco and Hua Chang-ming (1988). Making use of vivid press reports, it succeeds in illustrating the collision of interests and the problems of implementation met by the one-child policy. These problems also come out clearly in Croll (1991), which succinctly summarizes one-child policies up until 1988.

The highly technical character of population studies and the opaque nature of internal developments in China, however, have created problems of communication between various scholarly communities. Large gaps are often visible between those stressing statistical significance, representative figures and the universalism of social science on the one hand, and those emphasizing historical meaning, cultural setting and political context on the other. Synthesis of historical, demographic, economic, sociological and political science approaches could therefore be improved. It is indicative that some aspects of Chinese birth control are more or less confined to discussion in journals of Chinese studies, while other important debates have been taking place only in demographic periodicals.

One of the first demographic contributions has been the highly influential work of Bongaarts and Greenhalgh (1985), which presented an alternative to China's one-child policy. This article, which has also been widely debated in Chinese demographic circles, pleaded for a two-child policy governed by late-birth requirements and extended spacing intervals. Wolf (1986) has underlined the dominant role of political interventions in Chinese fertility levels. His article, which also draws on personal fieldwork in China, is largely restricted to the period 1949 to 1979. Hardee-Cleaveland and Banister (1988) have followed up this theme up until 1988. They have outlined a pattern of recurrent policy cycles, and they have reported on the hardening of the one-child policy in 1986. Exploring China's problematic sex ratio at birth, Arnold and Liu Zhaoxiang (1986), Hull (1990), Johansson and Nygren (1991), Johansson (1995), and Johnson *et al.* (1998) brought increasing variation into the former mono-causal impressions of large-scale infanticide. Still, Coale and Banister (1994) insist on the impact of increased mortality for infant girls.

Quite different conclusions from the authors reporting on a tightening of birth-control policies have been reached by Greenhalgh (1986) and Zeng Yi (1988). In these studies, Chinese birth planning is described as a continuous process of learning furthered by irreversible social and economic changes. Both Greenhalgh and Zeng see a long-term trend in a relaxation of strict one-child norms. In contrast to Aird, their main emphasis is on an increasing number of second-child permits and on flexible implementation of birth planning at the grass-roots level. A heated reply to these arguments may be found in Aird (1990).

The Western studies cited so far have largely been limited to secondary analysis of Chinese data and to a reading of both press reports and studies emanating from China. They are augmented by a small number of case studies drawing on work in the field in an attempt to gain more direct access to Chinese realities. Sample surveying by Western scholars, however, continues to be a sensitive affair. If such attempts occasionally succeed, many spoken and unspoken reservations remain *vis-à-vis* delicate issues contained in the questionnaire. The extremely small number of sample studies therefore remains restricted both in depth and scope. This gives rise to the problem of generalizing from limited case studies, whose results can differ widely.

It is against this background that all studies, including this one, wrestle with the problem that analysis of Chinese birth planning can generally be performed better at macro level than at micro level. There are good reasons for this state of affairs, since birth planning is enacted as a programme from above, taking popular wishes into only limited consideration. For many years, Chinese scholarship, too, faced a situation where studying such wishes was not exactly a welcome approach. Yet during recent times, family-size preferences, which are indispensable in an understanding of birth-planning performance, have won more recognition as a subject worthy of further study. This may be taken as a further indicator of the continuing process of social emancipation in China. In Western literature, more recent contributions on this subject have been submitted by Whyte and Gu (1987), Gates (1993) and Milwertz (1997). While the first study is a reworking of the limited Chinese sample research on family size preferences, the latter two are based on interviews with city women in Chengdu, Beijing and Shenyang during 1988 and 1992. Greenhalgh (1988) provides a well-wrought discussion of Chinese fertility decisions within the context of cultural and socioeconomic changes in modern Chinese history.

One of the earliest case studies has been Saith (1981), a report on birth-planning regulations and practices in a people's commune near Suzhou, Jiangsu province, during the years 1979 to 1980. The works by Steven Mosher published in 1982 and 1983 have been highly influential. These are dense eyewitness reports on the birth-control campaign in the Guangdong Pearl River delta during 1979 and 1980. The documentation of coercive measures, social pressures and psycho-terror in a Chinese village produced a crisis in Sino–American academic exchanges during 1983. Ever since, Mosher has been cited as a chief witness to the violation of human rights in China. In 1993 he continued his battle against Chinese birth planning by publishing the biography of a Chinese nurse, which contains startling information about compulsory abortions in Chinese hospitals.

Whereas Mosher and Aird view Chinese birth planning through the eyes of its victims, other field studies try to adopt the perspective of the birth-planning bureaucracy. The first researches in this direction were submitted in White (1985 and 1987). These are descriptions of birth planning on the basis of interviews conducted with responsible cadres in urban and rural areas of Wuhan city, Hubei province, during 1984. They offer a good overview of organizational and financial arrangements for birth planning and the function of birth-planning bureaux in that province. Since it was not possible to conduct interviews among relevant sections of the population, important aspects of popular response had to be analysed by documentary study. In spite of this limitation, White's work exposed grave problems of implementation and gaps in the enforcement of birth-planning regulations.

Huang Shu-min (1989) in many respects enlarges on the work of White. In this personal account of a cadre from Xiamen region, Fujian province, the toughness of one-child policies and their coercive enforcement are not glossed over. However, the emphasis is on mediation by local cadres which eventually results in grumbling acceptance of birth planning by the peasants. The report refers mainly to the situation up to November 1984.

Kaufman *et al.* (1989) continue along these lines. They submit the results of a 1987 sample survey of 318 married women of reproductive age, conducted in two counties of Heilongjiang and Fujian provinces, respectively. This survey yielded higher rates for second and third children than were reported in official statistics. It also supplied information about delayed collection or even a complete waive of birth-control fines and an irregular distribution of sterilizations and abortions peaking after contraceptive failures. Later studies on regional policy implementation (e.g. Li Jiali (1995) and Zhang Weiguo (1999)) reached basically parallel conclusions.

Greenhalgh (1990 and 1993) strike similar chords. The author, who was working with the Population Council in New York, based her conclusions on field research conducted in a medium-sized city of Shaanxi province in 1988. She researched local and regional birth-control regulations from the 1979–86 period and conducted interviews with cadres and 550 heads of households. Before she reversed her position after another field trip to the same area in 1993 (Greenhalgh *et al.* 1994), Greenhalgh's main thesis was a linear relaxation of the one-child policy since 1981. She discerned both constant improvement in birth-planning rules, as well as the failure of erstwhile sanctions in the wake of decollectivization. Greenhalgh also reported on largely defunct rules on late marriage, late birth and birth spacing.

Potter and Potter (1990) is an indirect reply to Steven Mosher. This work on the cultural dimensions of peasant behaviour by two American anthropologists was produced in the same region in which Mosher collected his shocking reports from the early 1980s. Potter and Potter sum up their various interviews with grass-roots cadres and peasants in a Pearl River delta village during repeated research stays between 1981 and 1985. In comparing their description of birth planning with the Mosher reports, they expose wide differences in implementation between counties of the same region. Overall, Potter and Potter present a markedly milder version of birth planning than that outlined by Mosher. The Potter and Potter volume also describes a trend to greater popular liberties, mainly as a result of decollectivization in the countryside. However, after checking internal birth-control regulations, the comments on the discretionary powers of local cadres seem somehow to be overdrawn.

There are other controversial problems in secondary literature. Besides the coercion issue, the related question as to the degree of acceptance or resistance to birth-planning policy is answered quite differently. Because the available studies only offer glimpses of birth-control practices limited in time and space, there is great uncertainty as to the general trend of developments. Differences between central and regional policies, as well as variations within provinces, are largely unknown. This lack of information pertains both to differences in norms and differences in implementation. Because these areas have been charted in rough outline only, the judgement on the character of birth-planning processes also differs. We meet both the picture of highly centralized planning from the top down as well as the counter-picture of flexible planning from the bottom up, with large discretionary liberties for the lower echelons. Since there is no precise information on concrete methods of birth planning, this tends to be only a competition of images. Finally, opinions on the intermediate balance sheet of birth planning also differ. While some deem it to have been an almost complete failure, others attest remarkable successes to it. There is disagreement among the latter to what extent political or socioeconomic factors have been responsible for the lowering of fertility levels.

This is the situation as far as Western literature on the subject is concerned. If the above works by Western authors are augmented by Chinese studies of birth planning, the picture both gains and loses depth. The Chinese studies make it possible to draw a much more detailed picture of formal structures and normative guidelines governing the population policies of the country. However, they almost completely ignore the empirical analysis of implementation problems or of popular response. Of course, this reflects the political constraints faced by the authors.

Liu Zheng *et al.* (1981) is directed at foreign audiences. It offers a good overview of the aims and motives giving rise to the one-child policy at the outset. Many of the social scientists writing in this volume participated in the drafting of the policy. Song Jian *et al.* (1985) continue the argument. Their work, published in English, is based on a number of previous publications in Chinese language (Song Jian and Li Guangyuan 1980; Song Jian *et al.* 1982; Song Jian and Yu Jingyuan 1985). It contains theoretical groundwork for Chinese birth planning and a mathematical modelling of desirable demographic targets. The authors are among the influential advocates of hard-line one-child policies. Liang Jimin (1986) and Liu Hongkang (1988) offer popular handbooks for propaganda usage and cadre support. They introduce contraceptive techniques, basic medical knowledge, outlines of population policy, demographic terminology and simple statistical methods. While these books and a host of similar works can be used for reference, they do not contain any new information.

Descriptive histories of population policies are supplied by Shi Chengli (1980, 1988), and Sun Muhan (1987). Both authors hail from the Birth-Planning Commissions. Their work is typical of the cadre outlook since it is limited to the reproduction of relevant Party documents, the paraphrasing of official press reports and the bureaucratic perspective from above. On this level, the works contain a detailed description of past policy. It should be noted, however, that policy disputes in leadership organs are largely glossed over, and a wealth of internal materials on policy implementation is ignored. The works are also weak in demographic analysis as they are restricted to reproducing success figures that are largely devoid of content. While Sun Muhan (1987) offers quite an interesting description of organizational aspects in addition to the historical outline, Shi Chengli (1988) contains the more detailed chronology.

The works by Chen Shengli and Zhao Shi (1991) and Li Jifeng (1992), as well as the manual published as *Jihua shengyu guanlixue* (1992), also stand out from the great mass of popularized and propagandist literature. All these publications have been issued by the State Birth-Planning Commission for cadre training purposes. While the first volume includes a concise overview of technical questions of birth planning and population statistics, the other two concentrate on management, organization and evaluation issues in birth control. In contrast, Chang Chongxuan (1992) serves as a semi-official presentation of Chinese birth planning edited by a vice-minister of the State Birth-Planning Commission. It contains a much more diffuse and markedly shorter historical outline of past population policy than is available from either Sun Muhan or Shi Chengli. The chapters on various aspects of birth planning are largely confined to the world as it ought to be, and it, too, glosses over many controversial or sensitive questions. A glimpse of these discussions may be caught by reading the increasingly diverse contributions to specialist periodicals from China or juridical works on birth control such as Zou Ping (1993) and Yang Zhuquan (1995).

Although the big national dailies and political journals of the People's Republic supply very little demographic information, they have documented the leadership dispute on population policy with remarkable candour. During the period 1986 to 1989, centrally supervised publications, such as the Party organ '*Renmin ribao* (People's Daily)', the cultural gazette '*Guangming ribao* (Enlightenment)', or the political journal '*Liaowang* (Outlook)', carried a number of articles that clearly delineated the different points of view.

Apart from the works mentioned above, this study uses a number of Chinese projections of either desirable or expected future population numbers. In some cases, these projections also include detailed structures of the future population by age and sex. Because such projections require methodological stringency, precise quantification of constant parameters and critical variables, they unreservedly lay bare the problems of birth planning. Used together with the proper qualitative interpretation, they may thus help to draw a clearer picture than lengthy descriptive narratives.

Apart from the works of Song Jian and his co-authors mentioned above, the most important sources are the projections of the former director of the Population Institute of the Academy of Social Sciences, published in Tian Xueyuan (1984), and the data published in Ma Hong (1989), an influential study on 'China in the Year 2000' that was edited by the State Council's Research Center for Technical, Economic and Social Development. Other, less elaborate projections have been published in article form; examples are Hu Baosheng *et al.* (1981), Song Duanyu *et al.* (1981), Zhou Shujun (1984), Xiao Jiabao 1989, and He Bochuan (1990). More recent projections are available via the alternative scenarios of seven Chinese research institutes published in ZJSN (1990). Calculations of future population developments in

Kua shiji de zhongguo renkou (1994) already incorporated inferences from the 1990 census results. The most elaborate methodology is employed in the latest projections of several research institutes (Zeng Yi 1994; Chen Wei 1995; Zha Ruichuan *et al.* 1996; Lin Fude and Zhai Zhenwu 1996; Yuan Yongxi 1996; ZRTN 1997; Li Jianxin 1997). Based on the 1990 census, they apply multiregional or stratified analysis.

Important articles on birth planning have been published in the demographic journals of the PRC. Among them, the most important ones are '*Renkou yanjiu* (Demographic Research)' published by People's University, '*Zhongguo renkou kexue* (Chinese Population Science)' by the Academy of Social Sciences, '*Renkou yu jingji* (Population and Economics)' from the Beijing College of Economics, the journal '*Renkou* (Population)' by Fudan-University in Shanghai, '*Renkou xuekan* (Journal for Population Science)' by Jilin University, '*Renkou zhanxian* (Demographic Front)' by Sichuan University, as well as '*Xibei renkou* (Northwest China's Population)'. Apart from these journals, the approximately forty other demographic periodicals from China were also checked. In general, their additional information is limited to regional matters only.

The articles by Guo Shenyang (1985), Liu Xian (1985), Feng Litian *et al.* (1987), Lu Li (1990), Feng Xiaotian (1991) and Lü Hongping (1991) are particularly noteworthy as they fell outside the mainstream of Chinese demography. These were first attempts at studying family-size preferences of the urban and rural population in the context of cost–benefit analysis. Although sample size, sampling and questionnaire design were unsatisfactory, they nevertheless gave new impetus to researching hitherto neglected questions. The same applies to the study on family-size preferences of Beijing and Sichuan youth published by Zhang Ziyi *et al.* in monographic form in 1982. Recent years have seen much improvement in research along these lines. Peng Xizhe and Dai Xingyi (1996), as well as Wei Jinsheng and Wang Shengling (1996), have been major achievements in studying the cultural, social and economic background of peasant fertility behavior and in bringing more contours into the picture.

An important topic that cannot be pursued in this book are the consequences of the one-child policy in terms of childrearing practices, socialization in primary groups and adolescent behaviour. Time and money spent on the education of children has risen markedly – a trend that is in accord with population economics. But at the same time, egocentric single children have developed into a problem for the collective group values of Chinese civil culture. Relying on a survey of elementary students in four provinces of China, a Sino-American investigation of physical, social and psychological characteristics of single children (Falbo 1996) breaks new ground in this largely unexplored field.

Another subject that documents the positive development of Chinese academic work is the sex ratio at birth and the sensitive issue of the missing girls connected with it. After some initial pooh-poohing, Chinese demographers now squarely recognize the problem. The assessment of the dominant reasons for sex imbalances among infants and young children differs from some Western evaluations, yet is nuanced enough in itself. Major contributions may be found in Zeng Yi *et al.* (1993), Tu Ping (1993), Gao Ling (1995), Gu Baochang and Roy (1996), as well as State Family Planning Commission (1997). While, at first sight, gender issues are submerged in the demographic details of these studies, the problems are there for all to see.

Regular documentation, reports and statistical data are contained in various yearbooks published by government research institutes, state agencies and ministries. Among the most important ones are the yearbooks published by the State Birth-Planning Commission and its subordinate organs (ZJSN, ZRZS), the Ministry of Health (ZWN), the State Statistical Bureau (ZTN, ZRTN) and the Population Institute of the Academy of Social Sciences (ZRN). A close reading of these volumes provides a highly diverse picture not available in the historical outlines of birth planning mentioned above. For a discussion of bureaucratic problems of implementation, the yearbooks are an indispensable source.

In addition to these generally available materials, this study also draws on reports and evaluations written for the UN Population Fund (UNFPA). These were prepared for China-related country reports and internationally funded projects (UNFPA 1984a, 1984b, 1989, 1997). Both for political and technical reasons, such reports consciously limit themselves to a discussion of UN-sponsored population activities, and largely refrain from commenting on sensitive issues.

A further group of primary sources is partly published and partly internal materials documenting Chinese birth-planning procedures. These comprise approximately 200 provincial documents from the period 1979 to 1999, which are systematically analysed here for the first time. Amongst them are about 130 birth-planning regulations or rules from all provinces of China, estimated to account for three-quarters of all relevant province-level norms during that period. The most recent amendments to these texts were passed between 1989 and 1999. All thirty-one provincial birth-planning regulations in force today have been compared with each other and with preceding versions. Furthermore, a large number of relevant circulars, directives, proposals, reports, supplementary regulations and explanations have been analysed. These have been drawn up for provincial Party organs, government agencies and people's congresses, and hail from different sources. Annotated selections of some of these materials are available in Scharping and Heuser 1995 (with German translations of ten documents from the period 1980 to 1990), Scharping (2000a, 2000b) (with English translations of forty-four other documents from the period 1954 to 1997).

On the national level, major collections of birth-planning documents are contained in internal compendiums, such as the one from 1989 that was partially translated in White (1992), or the more recent Guojia jihua shengyu weiyuanhui (1992). Provincial birth-planning regulations were long treated as internal documents and only began to be publicized in the late 1980s. In 1997 the Birth-Planning Commission undertook a major step forward by openly publishing the massive '*Zhongguo jihua shengyu quanshu* (ZJSQ 1997, Encyclopedia of Birth Planning in China)'. This is an unrivalled source of information on organizational arrangements and written norms governing birth control at the national level since 1950. It reproduces nearly 900 directives and regulations, pronouncements and commentaries on birth planning by central Party and government organs, the State Birth-Planning Commission, and the various departments and organizations subordinate to it, by Party leaders, national dailies and leading experts. Although the collection is still selective and a number of documents are suppressed, many formerly classified materials on formal norms, structures and procedures have been made available. This pertains both to past decades and the present. Notable exceptions to the new candour still involve information on the decision-making process in population policy, internal implementation reports, and statements deviating too overtly from the present political line. More precise information on sensitive issues such as unauthorized births and open resistance to birth-control measures, abortions, infanticide, eugenics and fatal accidents in birth-control surgery, corruption cases and other violations of norms, fine collection and prosecution of birth-control offences also continues to be restricted.

The above materials allow for a much more detailed analysis of implementation problems, developments over time and regional differences than is possible by using only the hitherto available case studies. Even if the new materials largely consist of normative documents that should not be confounded with uncensored factual reports, they still mirror indirectly the manifold problems of putting birth control into practice. As far as the internal documents contain investigation reports, these reports tend to cling to the official line both in style and content. In most cases, evidences of non-compliance that explode public propaganda tend to be phrased in such a way that the detonating power contained within them is barely recognizable.

Because censorship and biased reporting continue to cloud many issues, secondary analysis of demographic mass statistics from China is an indispensable instrument for evaluating the success of birth-control measures. It serves to check and augment descriptive literature, normative regulations and summary pronouncements. It also gives further clues as to the acceptance or rejection of birth-control measures by the populace. For this purpose, the following national surveys and regular compilations were used:

- The annual statistics of the State Birth-Planning Commission, the Ministry of Public Security, the Ministry of Civil Administration and the Ministry of Health, which are aggregated from the regular statistical reports of lower-level organs and published in various official yearbooks (ZJSN, ZTN, ZWN, ZSTZ).
- The population censuses of July 1954, July 1964, July 1982, July 1990 (Zhongguo 1982 nian renkou pucha ziliao, Guowuyuan renkou pucha bangongshi (1987), Sheng renkou pucha bangongshi (1992–93), Zhongguo 1990 nian renkou pucha ziliao, Wang Ming (1996)), as well as the first preliminary results of the population census of November 2000.

- The micro-censuses of July 1987 and October 1995 (Zhongguo 1987 nian 1% renkou chouyang diaocha ziliao, 1995 nian quanguo 1% chouyang diaocha ziliao).
- The annual sample surveys of the State Statistical Bureau on regional population numbers and vitality rates, which have been conducted at the end of each year since 1982 (ZRTN; '98 zhongguo renkou 1999).
- The National Fertility Sample Surveys conducted by the State Birth-Planning Commission in September 1982, July 1988, September and October 1992 (Quanguo 1% renkou shengyulü chouyang diaocha fenxi 1983; ZJSN 1986; Coale and Chen Shengli 1987; Li Honggui and Zhao Shi 1990; Peng Xizhe 1991; ZRTN 1989; Liang Jimin and Chen Shengli 1993; Chen Shengli and Coale 1993; ZJSN 1993–94; Jiang Zhenghua 1995; Zeng Yi 1995; State Family Planning Commission 1997).
- The national in-depth fertility surveys conducted in April 1985 and April 1987 by the State Statistical Bureau in collaboration with the International Statistical Institute (State Statistical Bureau 1986 and 1989; International Statistical Institute 1991).
- A large-scale sample survey on contraceptive use, conducted in the rural areas of Jiangsu province in 1986 (Qiu Shuhua *et al.* 1994).

There are a number of demographic analyses which have broken ground in charting this daunting mass of statistics and checking its internal consistency. Apart from the commentary contained in some of the statistical sources and their analytical companion volumes mentioned above, a number of Chinese studies have presented their findings from analysis of these mass statistics. In addition to numerous articles in the demographic journals of the country, encyclopedic publications such as the thirty-two volumes of '*Zhongguo renkou congshu* (Encyclopedia of Chinese Population)', published between 1987 and 1993, the English-language synopsis of this series issued by China Financial and Economic Publishing House in 1988, the thirty-three volumes of '*Kua shiji de Zhongguo renkou* (China's Population at the Turn of the Century)' issued in 1994, the voluminous collection of figures from the last two censuses edited by Yuan Yongxi in 1996, or the work of Zha Ruichuan *et al.* (1996) in the series '*Zhuanbian zhong de Zhongguo renkou yu fanzhan* (Chinese Population and Development in Flux)' have contained such analyses in condensed form. An important collection of studies based on the 1988 fertility survey is submitted in Chang Chongxuan (1991).

Studies that link such demographic figures to social and economic trends at the macro level have been rather uneven. Painstaking work on the basis of national, provincial and county data may be found in Jiang Zhenghua (1986), Poston and Gu Baochang (1987), Jiang Zhenghua and Chen Songbao (1988), Poston and Jia Zhongke (1989), Peng Xizhe and Huang Juan (1993), and, above all, Zhang Fengyu (1997). Testifying to the fast assimilation of international research standards, Wei Jinsheng and Wang Shengling (1996) is an impressive attempt at quantitative evaluation of birth-control performance. But the genre also includes many other contributions indulging in number-crunching without sufficient attention to significance, both in the statistical and the substantive sense.

A specialized subfield that has started from scratch and seen rapid development in recent years is the ethno-demography of China. Chinese academic work on the topic started in the 1980s with comparisons of minority population totals, vitality rates and the usual set of socioeconomic background figures. Better specimens of this type of work are based on ethno-specific census materials, more superficial ones confining themselves largely to juxtaposing macro-indicators for administrative regions from the statistical report system. These voluminous studies include research on individual nationalities (Yang Kuifu 1995), bigger minority regions (Yunnan sheng renkou xuehui 1984; Qinghai sheng renkou xuehui 1984; Xu Xifa 1995; Yan Tianhua 1996), or local communities (Zhongguo renkou qingbao yanjiu zhongxin 1989; Zhang Tianlu 1993). More detailed investigations are available on the large, populous nationalities (Zhang Tianlu and Huang Rongqing 1996) or on the Tibetan population (Sun Jingxin 1993). In some cases work has progressed to the stage of integrative approaches (Yang Yixing *et al.* 1988; Zhang Tianlu 1989; Zhang Tianlu and Huang Rongqing 1996; Deng Hongbi 1998) and deeper analysis of ethno-specific data from the fertility survey (Gao Ersheng and Yuan Wei 1997). In contrast to the maturing of ethno-demography, specialist literature on the fertility of other newly rising segments of the population such as migrants, rich peasants and private entrepreneurs is underdeveloped. This is a consequence of the strong government pressures for birth control among these strata, which hampers independent verification of fertility levels. It shows the considerable problems encountered in studying the behaviour of groups living on the borderline of the socialist state and a slowly emancipating society.

Apart from the monographic studies cited above, some of the most important Western-language studies on macro-level trends have emanated from the East-West Center in Honolulu, where Griffith Feeney and other population specialists have published a number of collaborative research papers with demographers from China. The work done in Honolulu is noteworthy for its innovative use of period parity progression ratios, more refined indicators which augment the conventional vitality rates and fertility measures. An early example may be found in Feeney and Yu Jingyuan (1987), which reworked the 1982 national fertility survey. This survey, together with the 1982 population census, has likewise been used for the different adjustments of official vital rates offered in Coale (1984) and Banister (1987). Important retrospective studies making use of the 1982 fertility survey are Lavely and Freedman (1990) on the link between education and fertility rates, and Zhao Zhongwei (1997) on the relationship between the sex ratio of children and parity progression.

Period parity progression ratios have also been employed in Feeney *et al.* (1989), Luther *et al.* (1990), which started from the 1987 micro-census, and Feeney and Wang Feng (1993), which took the 1988 national fertility survey as its baseline. In a similar way, the 1990 census results and the 1992 fertility survey have been analysed in Feeney *et al.* (1992), Nygren and Hoem (1993), and Feeney and Yuan Jianhua (1994). While these studies concentrate on national aggregate numbers, regional variation in fertility levels has been studied in Coale and Chen Shengli (1987), Zeng Yi *et al.* (1991), Kim Choe *et al.* (1992), Feeney *et al.* (1993), and Chen Shengli and Coale (1993). The latter volume makes use of total duration-specific fertility rates, another instrument for tackling the considerable difficulties in measuring the impact of the Chinese birth-planning programme. These alternative measures are also used in Coale *et al.* (1991), which discusses national trends and makes an important methodological contribution.

This present study tries to incorporate findings from these various studies. Besides making use of primary documents, statistical data and the existing secondary literature in Western and Chinese languages, it is based on more than 200 interview notes and a continuous dialogue with Chinese population experts during numerous research stays in that country. In addition to the regular discussion of current demographic problems, half-structured in-depth interviews were conducted in universities, academies, statistical bureaux and Birth-Planning Commissions of Beijing, Shanghai, Sichuan and Yunnan in 1986, 1990 and 1992. Further interviews were held in Guangdong, Hainan and Fujian provinces during 1993 and in Beijing in 1997. They have provided valuable insights into the context of various population policies, the functioning of birth planning and its problems of implementation.

Part II
Policy formulation

4 Motives and goals of Chinese birth control

4.1 Leadership perceptions

Like the great majority of other policy arenas, Chinese birth control has been overshadowed by the personal beliefs and interventions of Mao Zedong during the first three decades of the People's Republic. In September 1949, on the eve of the founding of the new state, Mao declared:

> Each time the Chinese overthrew a feudal dynasty it was because of the oppression and exploitation of the people by the feudal dynasty, and not because of any overpopulation. ... It is a very good thing that China has a big population. Even if China's population multiplies many times, she is fully capable of finding a solution; the solution is production. The absurd argument of Western bourgeois economists like Malthus that increases in food cannot keep pace with increases in population was not only thoroughly refuted in theory by Marxists long ago but has also been completely exploded by the realities in the Soviet Union and the Liberated Areas of China after their liberation. ... Revolution plus production can solve the problem of feeding the population.[1]

The Chairman's verdict was in rebuttal of an American White Book on relations with China published shortly before which cited demographic evidence for explaining the Guomindang debacle on the mainland. Issued as the last text in the official canon of his selected writings, Mao's vehement criticism fully conformed with Stalin's views and the reasoning of Soviet theoreticians. It was long treated as a beacon light guiding all Chinese population policies. In 1952, it led the Party organ to spread the diatribes against proponents of birth control with articles proclaiming the thesis: birth control can ruin China; it means murder without shedding blood.[2] The denunciations came at a time of intensifying 'thought reform' among non-Communist intellectuals and the abolishment of all university programmes in the 'bourgeois' social sciences.

Seen from the historical perspective, however, some strange affinities emerge from the battle lines of ideological class struggle. For the American White Book of August 1949 had based its assessment on the analyses of Frank Notestein, the noted American demographer, who was to become one of the fathers of the international family-planning movement and a source of inspiration for Chinese birth control in later years. Mao Zedong in turn shared basic perceptions of his political opponents, the Guomindang leaders from the preceding republican period. Bemoaning high population losses since the mid-nineteenth century and stressing the need to combat foreign encroachments, both Sun Yatsen and Chiang Kaishek had urged high demographic growth for safeguarding national independence. Whether consciously or subconsciously, the men at the helm of the Chinese Republic inherited the traditional ideas of Chinese emperors, who cherished high population numbers since these bolstered tax revenues and strengthened military manpower against hostile barbarian tribes.

The pro-natalist stand of China's leaders was not uncontroversial, however. Starting in the early years of the Republic, a growing number of social scientists had come to view China's population more as a liability than an asset. They believed the poverty and economic backwardness, the low standards of health and education, as well as the prevalent food problems of the country, were all intimately connected with the problem of overpopulation. Amid the ranks of sociologists and among a minority of politicians, birth control had already become a catchword in the 1930s.[3]

Arguments between proponents and opponents of birth control continued to surge back and forth during the 1950s. Public pronouncements were dominated by constant reference to Mao's dictum of 1949 and by Marxist criticism of Malthusian thought. This criticism was bolstered by reliance on the Soviet Union, where Stalin's policy reversal of 1936 had led to the reinstatement of pre-revolutionary family norms, the promotion of childbearing, and a ban of the abortions that had been permitted by Lenin. Soviet policies under Stalin agreed with the 1935 Criminal Code from Guomindang China that had penalized abortion, permitting it only in case of danger to the mother's life. Again there existed a basic unity of outlook between the adversaries of the Chinese civil war: despite experimentation with extremely liberal marriage laws, all punitive codes in the revolutionary base areas of the Communist Party had penalized abortion between 1931 and 1948. The central Party organ *People's Daily* summed it up neatly in 1951: while imperialist and capitalist states furthered birth control, socialist and democratic states promoted childbearing.[4]

The convictions of Chinese modernism met with the traditions of Chinese familism, which continued to permeate wide segments of society despite growing fissures in the old family system. It contained the pro-natalist ideals of an elite culture, which honoured early marriage and abundant offspring. In Chinese public discourse during the first half of the twentieth century, abortion and birth control continued to be largely taboo subjects. The continuing depth of social censure may be gleaned from the fact that in April 1950 rules for army and government personnel in the Beijing region made abortion contingent on medical indications, plus the written consent of husbands, superiors and doctors. Given the strong patrilineal hierarchy in Chinese families, in real life the husband's parents would have to be added to the list. Moreover, all cadres in central government and Party organs had to obtain the personal endorsement of the Minister of Health himself.[5]

When second thoughts about the burden of a huge population resurfaced in 1953/54, they focused on the difficulty of providing universal education for the ever-growing number of school-age children and the need to protect the health of mothers. The re-emergence of food and employment problems over subsequent years prompted additional concerns about the adequacy of food supplies, land resources, investment and employment for the rapidly growing population. At the height of the Hundred-Flowers campaign, even Mao Zedong registered his support for cautious moves towards birth control in February 1957. Relevant passages are contained in the internal version of his pioneering speech 'On the correct handling of contradictions among the people'. Still, the subject was considered sensitive enough to expurgate his commentary from the published version and to permit only intermittent signs of a policy change in contemporaneous sources. Likewise, another Mao speech before a Central Committee meeting of October 1957, in which he alluded positively to the need for birth planning, was published after a delay of twenty years.[6]

Mao's remarks were made in the midst of a debate on population issues raging both inside and outside the Party. It saw adherents of birth control such as Party Vice-Chairman Liu Shaoqi, Premier Zhou Enlai, his deputies Li Xiannian and Deng Xiaoping pitched against more radical followers of Mao such as his personal secretary, Party theoretician and Politburo candidate Chen Boda. Although the latter voiced the opinion that 'there is no sign of overpopulation … and China can provide room for at least another 600 million people', his master admitted the necessity of introducing some birth-control measures once a limit of 800 million had been reached in the future.

Ultimately, however, the Chairman's belief in revolutionary transformation, rapid economic growth and the positive role of population growth prevailed. In January 1958, it led him to announce his belief in an uninterrupted revolution, to urge a general raising of plan targets, and to state bluntly that 'a large population is a good thing'. In the Great Leap Forward of 1958 to 1960, these convictions caused the termination of all birth-control propaganda. Conversely, China's press began to praise the invincible force of human endeavour, enlarging on Mao's complaints about 'a climate of pessimism in population matters' and his quip of March 1958 that at present the nation was under- instead of overpopulated. Many articles propounded the idea that more people mean more producers, enlarging the country's resources instead of draining them. Liu Shaoqi, the second-in-command of the Party, also became an adherent of this position. In an internal talk of June 1958, he joined the general chorus about the approach of the ideal communist society with astonishing asides typical of his collectivist outlook, his perennial preoccupation with organization and a new lust for record numbers:

> Do not assume that under communism there will be all that individual freedom! In a certain sense, there will be a lot less freedom. When China's population has reached 6 billion, I am afraid not everyone will be able to

have his own private single bed; it would not surprise me if people will have to sleep in shifts. No more of this chaotic way of walking in the streets either![7]

It was only after the crisis following the Great Leap that birth control was once again put on the political agenda in 1962. In his long-term role as the discreet yet influential opponent of Mao Zedong in birth-control matters, Premier Zhou Enlai had to shoulder the thankless task of reconciling the Chairman's views with the emergency measures provoked by the situation. As he phrased it delicately in a speech of February 1963, 'a large population is a good thing, but as we are the most populous country in the world, we already have plenty of this good thing, and if we still let the population grow rapidly in an unplanned manner, it won't be a good thing any more.' One year later Zhou still had to defend family planning against ideological objections within the Politburo. Typically enough, it continued to be relegated to the status of health work, and earned just one line in the government reports presented to sessions of the National People's Congress in 1963 and 1964.[8]

In the Cultural Revolution, political mass campaigns again took precedence over birth-control efforts. Just as during the Great Leap Forward, the belief in the unlimited potential of New Man proved incompatible with notions of Malthusian predicament. It was only after Communist utopia once again vanished behind the grinding problems of economic construction that another change set in. Again, Zhou Enlai acted as the main promoter of renewed birth-control activities. In January 1970, the Politburo, including Mao Zedong, at long last endorsed his proposal to cease treating birth control as an aspect of health work and to deal with it instead in the context of food and economic policies. Henceforth, birth control occupied an increasingly important place in government policy.

Nevertheless, Mao Zedong's ideological qualms remained and circumscribed all activities. In December 1974 he finally attached the urgently requested directive 'There is no way around control of population growth!' to an economic report of the Planning Commission. It was due to his overpowering presence and the influence of the left-wing ideologues, however, that the Party carefully refrained from including population growth among the causes of economic problems until his death in 1976. It rather side-stepped the issue by noting that human reproduction should follow the example of economic development and also be subjected to planning. But planning and the demographic research necessary for it were again highly suspect topics, struggling with political prejudice, years of neglect, and a consequent paucity of reliable planning data. Only occasional glimpses of internal discussions permit the conclusion that old worries about the employment of the growing population prevailed among the leadership. An example are remarks of Zhang Chunqiao, a left-wing member of the Standing Committee of the Politburo, later to be purged as one of the Gang of Four, who foresaw an end to the compulsory rustication of unemployed Shanghai youth after 1980, should birth planning be carried out satisfactorily.[9]

The uneasiness of the Chinese leadership concerning the country's huge population in the 1970s is a well-established fact. In 1971, the numbers used by various ministries for internal calculations differed by 80 million; the difference between the assumed population total and later numbers based on a new population census ranged to more than 100 million. Even in 1977, Chinese politicians calculated a population total that was 50 million less than the real number.[10] When the State Statistical Bureau began to tabulate more precise data in 1978, it turned out that at the end of the Cultural Revolution China not only faced huge economic deficits but also high population growth, the dimensions of which confirmed the misgivings of all sceptics. Essentially, the nation's population total was again underestimated in the same way and in the same range as twenty-five years before.

Ever since, various Chinese politicians have termed the neglect of birth control in former decades a 'hard to correct, historical mistake'.[11] Former Vice-Premier and Central Committee Secretary Wang Renzhong outlined the gravity of the mistake during a birth-planning conference in January 1981. He compared the negligent population policy of former years with the Great Leap Forward and the Cultural Revolution, thereby bracketing it among the greatest disasters in the history of the People's Republic.[12] And the alarm of Chinese politicians about the legacy of former policies continued to increase. Although Mao's successor Hua Guofeng in February 1978 believed in the possibility of lowering annual population growth to 1 per cent within three years, the new census of July 1982 forced the leadership to recognize the inertia of demographic processes. 'Mistakes of population policy can be only corrected within twenty to thirty years' concluded Qian Xinzhong, the then Minister of the Birth-Planning Commission, in May 1982.[13]

In addition to the sudden confrontation with the impact of formerly underestimated population developments, China's economic crisis at the end of the 1970s contributed to the design of the one-child campaign.[14] It lent a sense of urgency to radical policy changes and added an undercurrent of hidden pessimism to the overt optimism of the modernization programme and, just as in the parallel economic debates, it led the political elite to pick up lost threads. In many respects, proponents of the one-child policy have been resuming their old arguments of the 1950s and 1960s that were silenced in the intervening years of the Maoist mass campaigns.

It was with a degree of embarrassment that the Politburo took note of the fact that after thirty years of revolution, begging for food still prevailed in many places and raising standards of living for the huge population continued to be a major stumbling-block.[15] References to the weak economic base and the high population as major constraints of China's modernization persisted as one of the most important themes of Chinese politicians between 1979 and 1981. In March 1979, Deng Xiaoping himself saw 'unbearable burdens for the state' should the country fail to halve population growth within the next five years.[16] Meeting a Nigerian delegation two years later, he confessed his fear that without birth planning 'economic growth would be consumed by population growth.'[17]

Calculations on the development of private consumption in the period 1952 to 1978 confirm a somewhat milder version of this assessment. They result in 49 per cent of real growth in consumption being absorbed by population increase.[18] Figures as such carry an ambivalent message with them. On the one hand, they indicate not total stagnation but rather economic growth in spite of population increase. On the other hand, they demonstrate a highly unsatisfactory commitment of resources that could have been better used for productive investments and for financing modernization measures. China's government has thus been continuously facing a sharp conflict between welfare objectives and economic growth.

All economic planning has therefore presupposed a success in limiting population increase after 1979. In particular, this was implicit in Deng Xiaoping's goal of quadrupling social product and reaching a moderate standard of living with a gross national product of US$ 1,000 per capita until the turn of the century. Up to the end of the 1980s, all projections for reaching this goal have worked under the premise that the country's population will not exceed 1.2 billion in the year 2000. This has been reflected in the multi-volume study *China in the Year 2000*, which contained the most detailed projections from China, as well as in concurrent foreign studies, the most voluminous of which was a World Bank investigation in 1985.[19]

Among the various symptoms of crises provoked by excessive population growth, the food situation in particular has worried Chinese politicians. Innumerable speeches and written pronouncements document their preoccupation with securing food for the nation. Their fear of a new famine clearly mirrors the experiences of a generation of revolutionaries who personally endured privation and hunger in the first half of the twentieth century. Food problems combined with the constant need to mediate in conflicts between peasants keen on raising grain prices and urban dwellers looking for cheap food supplies have occupied China's leaders for decades – if not for centuries.[20] With memories of the experience of food crises in Guomindang China still fresh, they were one of the core issues in social and economic policies of the early 1950s, when they were closely linked with the politics of rural collectivization.

China's last mass starvation was provoked by the Great Leap Forward between 1959 and 1961. According to different calculations, 16 to 27 million people died from malnutrition at that time. Even from Chinese dimensions and for the historical experience of a country suffering from recurrent food problems heightened by natural catastrophes, such numbers are huge. Although no food crisis on the scale of the Leap Forward has since recurred, in 1978 approximately 200 million Chinese still lived in grain-deficit regions providing under 80 per cent of minimum food consumption. These regions are mostly located in the Northwest and Southwest of China. Higher death rates and a clearly divergent morbidity pattern continue to be marked characteristics of these areas, with long-term malnutrition being one of the principle causes of death.[21] The number of people living beneath the poverty line has certainly decreased since the 1980s. But in the face of high population growth, decreasing acreage and limited agrarian investments, raising grain production levels per capita remains a major challenge for the future.[22]

It is therefore understandable that continuing nutrition problems have been one of the major motives for tightening birth planning. Both Deng Xiaoping and Hu Qiaomu, the then chief ideologue of the CCP, stated in 1978 that 'China's food problem has not been really solved'. The realization that per-capita grain production in 1977 stagnated at the level of 1955 upset both politicians and was a major theme of a birth-planning conference in October 1978.[23] Speaking before a national grain conference in November 1977, Li Xiannian, another member of the top leadership, had already set the tone by mentioning the 'explosive problem' of excess population growth.[24] Three months later, he took a position that sounded like a verbatim replay of a similar statement he made more than twenty years before: 'We now face an annual increase of about 12 million people. If grain production rises by 5 million tons annually, it just suffices for feeding the additional population.'[25] The influential late Vice-Chairman of the Central Committee, veteran politician and economic expert Chen Yun, backed him up in 1981: 'If we only have to care for enough food and everything is consumed, there will be no hope for the country.'[26]

In September 1985, in the face of new crop failures and a significant lapse of per-capita grain production, Chen Yun again used the food argument in order to warn the CCP National Conference of Delegates against the unsecured provision of basic needs for the population, to justify his calls for economic planning within a socialist system and to register his open opposition to the Party's reform course.[27] He based his argument on the earlier report of a national birth-planning conference, which had highlighted sufficient food production as the most important parameter for setting future population targets.[28]

China's small area of cultivated land has always constituted a particularly important aspect of the food problem. At the end of the 1970s, the cultivated area amounted to no more than 130 million hectares, equivalent to only 14 per cent of Chinese territory. Until the late 1950s, land reclamation continued to be a major device for raising grain production, but industrialization, urbanization, as well as shrinking land reserves, have since produced an irreversible decline of cultivated area. Constraints as such resulted in a dramatic decrease of the man–land ratio since 1949. While at the time of the founding of the People's Republic cultivated area per capita was estimated at 0.22 hectares, it was reported to have shrunk by more than one half to 0.08 hectares in 1979. Although the latter figure has since been proven to be distinctly higher, an adjusted 1979 value of 0.14 is still low by world standards. The alarm triggered by such figures has been intensified by the fact that approximately half of the acreage consists of low-yield areas, endangered by erosion, salinization or desertification.[29] All Party leaders have therefore constantly underlined their worry about China's food supply. Balances comparing China's minuscule per-capita figures for cultivated land, forests and grassland with the considerably higher world averages have been a constant feature of both internal Party discourse and external propaganda.[30]

Securing work for China's population has been another leitmotiv in all discussions of population policy. In March 1979, Deng Xiaoping restated earlier concern that in view of the high number of births the country would 'face the social problem of lack of employment for a long time to come'. At the same time, Chen Yun emphasized that the rationalization of work would aggravate employment problems in the course of modernization.[31] At the end of the 1970s, unemployment rose further due to the termination of forced rustication for city youth, used by Mao Zedong in the 1960s and 1970s for rerouting urban unemployment to the countryside.[32]

Politburo member Wang Zhen summed up the situation in January 1980: 'With great efforts we created 7 million additional jobs last year, but more than 10 million new infants have been added at the same time.'[33] This echoed earlier complaints of 1957, when school graduates vainly looking for urban jobs took to the streets, and participants in the birth-control debate bemoaned a growing gap between limited job creation and high birth numbers. The discrepancy between the growth of the working-age population and the creation of new employment has been a long-term structural problem for China. It has always produced high labour redundancy in the cities, which after 1949 became disguised by the employment guarantees of the socialist state. The price paid by the country for such guarantees was bureaucratization and overstaffing in all employment sectors, leading to low productivity everywhere. Job allocation replaced the labour market, forced rustication of urbanites, migration controls for peasants, and a general restriction of the freedom of movement set in. Preventing the imminent danger of mass unemployment thus entailed severe constraints on personal liberty and sacrifices in the standard of living.[34]

The message of Chinese statistics for the period 1952 to 1978 is clear. While the working population aged 15–64 grew by an annual average of 7.5 million, new urban employment for only 2.7 million people on average per year was created. As was customary, the agricultural sector had to absorb the bulk of additional manpower.[35] China's third population count of 1982 provided the basis for more precise projections for the rest of the century. It resulted in a total of 237 million people added to the working-age population between 1983 and 2000. The problems of employment creation indicated by this huge number were further aggravated by a rising rural exodus in the wake of decollectivization.[36] In the mid-1980s, up to 150 million peasants, or about 30 per cent of the rural labor force, and approximately 25 million city dwellers, or 20 per cent of urban workers and staff, were affected by underemployment. In the 1990s, peasant underemployment has been combated by shifting surplus labour to other sectors, while retrenchment of state industries has brought disguised urban unemployment into the open. Rural–urban migration remains an urgent social problem, the future dimensions of which depend on the extension of non-agricultural employment in the countryside and patterns of co-migration of family members.[37]

These difficulties do not exhaust the number of social problems created by the population increase. Bottle-necks in the educational and health system and the insufficient provision of housing must also be counted among them. While per-capita living space of China's urban population still amounted to 6.3 square metres in 1949, it had shrunk to 3.6 square metres by 1978. It is certain that this decline to extremely low standards was also caused by the neglect of 'unproductive' investments for private consumption during the Mao era. Long-term remedies could only include a reduction in population increase, high additional investments and stimulation of private house building. Since the 1980s, large-scale construction and housing reforms have again raised figures for urban housing beyond the pre-revolutionary levels, but inadequate housing as the number one grievance in China's cities has only recently become a little less urgent.[38]

Together with concern for the well-being of mothers with many children, the difficulties of providing universal education for the ever-growing number of school-age children have been advanced as the first reasons for proposing birth control in 1954 and 1955. In later years, projections of school enrolment have not drawn the same amount of attention that has been paid to the problems of feeding, employing and housing China's population. However, a periodically repeated commitment to raising educational standards has extended the period of compulsory education and added pressure to the demographically induced rise in the demand for schooling. Some problems faced by the nation can be glimpsed from a report on the situation in Shanghai's elementary schools. Large groups of children born in the early 1980s entered the city's schools in the second half of the decade, creating bottle-necks in teaching capacity. In February 1986, Shanghai newspapers urged their readers to prepare for instruction by shifts and to make arrangements for the supervision of unattended children. Although the different age structure in other provinces leads to notable differences, a long-term increase of the school population may be discerned. In 1980, enrolment in Chinese elementary and junior high schools reached an all-time high. After a marked drop over the rest of the decade, the numbers of school-age children have again risen slightly in the 1990s.[39]

Finally, demographic growth carries definite implications for China's environment. Although the ecological difficulties of the country are well known to Chinese specialists, and the link between population development and environmental protection has been stressed by a central work conference devoted to that subject in March 1998,[40] ecological questions command a secondary position in public life and economic decision-making. Just as in other developing countries, environmental policies are often regarded as a luxury that the nation has to defer to later stages of development. The only exception to this rule is the chronic lack of water resources in China. It has already produced symptoms of crisis, provoking concern for long-term water supply and demand.[41] But air and soil pollution, deforestation, erosion and desertification seem to progress rapidly too. Demographically conditioned factors like hunger for land, over-exploitation of natural resources and low productivity are the basic factors looming behind them.[42]

In the 1980s and 1990s, China's economic boom has mitigated some of these problems. But the leadership's mental preoccupation with the 'guoqing', China's special conditions, summed up in the words 'many people, little land for cultivation, and a weak basis', continues to prevail. It is a clear break with the traditional belief in the boundless wealth of the country's resources, and it has led the post-Deng leadership to maintain that population development can only be managed by relying on constraints and control.[43]

4.2 Defining population targets

Projections of optimum population totals have been a major step in setting target numbers for birth planning. The Western ancestry of these exercises leads to John Stuart Mill and his neo-Malthusian followers, who theorized on population totals requisite for attaining maximum social product per capita and on the state of overpopulation setting in beyond that stage. In later political discourse, the concept became vulgarized and suspect. It was partly confused with Malthus' earlier predictions of food constraints checking further population growth, or with the theories on *Lebensraum* (living space) for nations, fashionable during the early half of the twentieth century and leading right up to the world wars. Political embarrassment is coupled with a theoretical problem, since all calculations of either maximum or optimum population have to incorporate suppositions as to the long-term carrying capacity of territories. Historical experience has not vindicated such precise calculations. Time and again, it has taught that carrying capacities or population optimums cannot be fixed definitely but rather depend on ethical criteria, welfare standards and political objectives, as well as constantly changing factors such as economic structure, patterns of trade, technological progress and potentials for substitution. The calculations are usually strong on assessing demand but weak as far as the anticipation of future supply factors is concerned.

In view of the nation's population problems, Chinese scientists and politicians nevertheless felt prompted to again take up the notion of optimum population. First attempts at respective calculations began during the Hundred-Flowers campaign in 1957, when Zhong Huinan, the superintendent of China's leading hospital, introduced the idea of striving for a population limit of 700 million by the year 1967 – 100 million less than the internal projections for that time. Shortly after, veteran sociologist Sun Benwen echoed the arguments of many colleagues and presented a calculation of an expected 770 million for 1967, augmented by a recommendation of 800 million as 'the most suitable population number for China' in the future.[44] As an influential intellectual and former official from the Guomindang period, Sun was not deemed worthy to be cited for reference, but it is surely no coincidence that the 700–800 million figure comes up in a number of contemporaneous Party documents, among them internal speeches of Mao Zedong.[45]

Sun based his recommendation on projections for cultivated area and land reclamation potential, grain production and urban job creation, which he singled out as the crucial bottle-necks. Looking back at his ten-year projections from a historical perspective, most have been rather wide off the mark. While grain production and land reclamation potential were grossly overestimated, job creation was underestimated. Only the demographic calculation was right. Although the population has far surpassed the recommended limits since 1967, it shows no signs of imminent perishing – nor has it reached the desired levels of well-being. There is definite progress; however, the time needed to realize it has been longer than projected. The gap between expected and real outcomes betrays the problems of the approach.

The crisis of the Great Leap and the increase of fertility rates in 1962 prompted the Party to reconsider the case for limiting population growth. A draft plan for birth planning introduced by the Ministry of Health during the Second Work Conference on Urban Affairs in September 1963 urged a lowering of natural increase to 2 per cent by 1965, less than 1.5 per cent by 1970, and less than 1 per cent by 1975. This amounted to the recognition that even under extremely favourable conditions the total population would rise to approximately 790 million by 1970 and to 880 million by 1980 – as a matter of fact, it eventually surpassed the latter figure by more than 100 million. In contrast to the 1957 debates, the 1963 draft plan did not contain any discussion of optimum population numbers and final goals, and when it was endorsed by the Central Committee and the State Council one month later, it was declared applicable for urban areas only.[46] The havoc wreaked by the Great Leap seemed to preclude any comprehensive planning. A few years later, all target figures were made obsolete by the Cultural Revolution.

As with the search for optimum economic development, projections of optimum population numbers resumed at the beginning of the reform period. This time, they were taken up in a much more elaborate form than in 1957 and with the express support of the Party. The methods and hypotheses used for constructing the population optimum in the early 1980s led straight back to the moral dimensions of the problem. Faced with the impossibility of making precise projections for the technological and economic conditions of the future, China's demographers calculated with economic coefficients derived from the analysis of present-day industrial societies. They thereby documented the country's aspiration to attain the same living and working conditions existing in industrialized nations today.

China's leading scientist and politician Song Jian has played a major role in these projections of future developments. After studying systems analysis in Moscow and working as a collaborator of China's famed rocket specialist Qian Xuesen following his return to China in 1961, Song was invested with various positions in the science establishment for applied mathematics and space engineering, rising to Minister of Aeronautics and member of the Politburo in the 1980s. Until 1998 he continued to serve at the helm of the government as State Councilor and Minister of the State Commission for Science and Technology.[47] Between 1979 and 1981, he and other Chinese scientists developed projections for launching China's population on a trajectory to eventual re-entry into the optimum sphere. These calculations were a major step in Chinese demographic modelling prior to the availability of new census materials. Even today, they continue to be instructive for the thinking behind the population policies of the Chinese leadership.

On the basis of long-range trends in China's economic development since 1949, Song projected future growth rates for important macro-economic indicators. He calculated the future stock of fixed assets, deriving employment figures for industry and agriculture by the use of production and employment coefficients. In a further step, he projected employment totals for the tertiary sector by making use of macro-relationships existing in Western industrial societies. These numbers were summed up to a total for the workforce. From this workforce total a desirable population total, as produced by the age structure of a stationary population, was derived. Apart from such economic projections, Song also submitted in-depth studies of long-term trends in China's cultivated area and pasture land, agricultural production and water resources. His calculations resulted in a theoretical optimum of 630 to 700 million people for China – lower than the 800 million recommended in 1957. Adopting the upper limit of this range, he developed various scenarios for population development, passing through a stage of approximately 1.13 to 1.20 billion in the year 2000 and reaching a stable level of 700 million by the end of the twenty-first century.[48]

For Song Jian, the optimum scenario has always been a drastic reduction of fertility levels to one child per woman by the year 1985. Ideally, he proposed to maintain strict one-child policies until the year 2000, after which fertility was to be gradually raised to replacement level. Under such circumstances the desirable level of 700 million would be reached by 2070. In an alternative scenario, he worked with a total fertility rate of 1.5 children per woman for the period 1990 to 2025. This fertility level meant that the population would reach 1130 million in 2000, with a stable level of 700 million only attainable by the year 2090. A third trajectory worked with a total fertility rate of 1.7 for the period 1985 to 2045. It led to optimum population by the year 2110.[49]

Another Chinese study of optimum population levels published in May 1981 proceeded along essentially similar lines. Arguing for an optimum population of 700 million to be reached by the application of birth planning, it frankly admitted that this target figure was half the future population number that would result, if childbearing preferences of the population and considerations of old-age support were allowed to have a greater say in population matters. The study proposed to extend the period of strict one-child policies until 2030 and to raise fertility to the replacement level of 2.16 children per woman subsequently. In contrast to Song, an adjustment of the target figure to 1 billion was admitted, if tight population planning proved to be unenforceable and lower standards of living were accepted. Grain, fish and meat production, land use, water resources, energy consumption and per-capita levels of gross domestic product were treated as key constraints for population growth, with water resources and domestic product per capita being identified as the most critical areas. At the same time, it was revealing for the mental reservations and political motives colouring some discussions of population policy that an additional criterion of 'international weight' was introduced under which a number of 1 billion Chinese was thought to be optimal.[50]

In public discourse of the 1980s and 1990s, such considerations of national grandeur have surfaced only rarely. Instead, the vast majority of contributions to the debate on optimum population levels has focused on the wide discrepancy between desirable and real population numbers. It has been viewed even more dramatically by some Chinese scientists, who in 1981 counselled a lowering of China's population to the level of 1949 within the next seventy years. According to them, there would be 'no need to worry' as 'it would not be too late to readjust' policies after the mid-twenty-first century.[51]

Another advocate of extremely low population targets (though one with less radical solutions) has been Guangzhou futurologist He Bochuan, whose unabashed analyses of the country's basic problems also drew attention from abroad. At the end of 1987 he submitted a study on future challenges for the nation. Employing worldwide standards for cultivated land, nutrition and water consumption, he reached a theoretical optimum of 500 million people. This figure amounted to less than half the number of Chinese living at that time. Explaining the reasons for his advice, He furnished a succinct chain of reasoning: China's population growth produces strong pressures on the country's national resources with negative consequences for the environment; pressures on natural resources lead to economic pressures, resulting in low productivity, high unemployment, inflation and distributional problems; economic pressures translate into social strains as documented by a low standard of social security, a depressed educational level, a decline in morals and growing administrative problems; these factors would finally cause political tension, leading to civil unrest and war.[52]

China's Birth-Planning Commission, in contrast, has been thinking more in practical terms than in theoretical optimums. In the newspaper edited under its auspices, the Commission in December 1987 proposed 0.7 to 1.0 billion people as a desirable population total for China. Later calculations have been even more cautious. Discarding all aspirations for high standards of living, employment and resource consumption within the foreseeable future, they have argued in favour of an 'optimum population suitable for low income levels', which implied a total of 1.3 to 1.5 billion people by the mid-twenty-first century, with a reduction to between 1 and 1.4 billion at its end.[53] Recent projections use the argument that population growth has retarded instead of prevented economic growth. They refrain from linking population targets to pre-set standards of living, and rather concentrate on reconciling the 'reduction of the population's huge pressure on environment and resources, as well as the promotion of a balanced economic development', with warnings against the problems of an ageing population.[54] Since the late 1980s, ceilings for population growth have shown a tendency towards constant upward revision. At present, the country's leading politicians operate with a figure of 1.6 billion, said to be 'the maximum supportable by China's natural resources at current technological levels'. This figure hails from a study by the Academy of Sciences on the maximum production capacity of China's natural resources and is based on only modest standards of living.[55]

Such later modifications are largely driven by a growing awareness of the problems of population ageing. While displaying a sober assessment of the country's economic prospects, they also signal a departure from the Malthusian predicament. Finally, they contain a great deal of scepticism generated by the disappointing experiences with strict one-child policies. In the early 1980s, China's population specialists were more forceful. While He Bochuan refrained from suggesting concrete policy measures, Song Jian and his fellow control theorists phrased their advice unequivocally. In an English-language study published in 1984 for the benefit of the Western public, they sketched a gloomy picture of Chinese development prospects should drastic birth-control measures fail to materialize. Among the prospects was a falling standard of living, expressed in quickly rising death rates as a consequence of persistently high birth rates. Their horror scenario included hundreds of millions of peasant migrants, who would cause a 'lifting of sluice-gates washing away Chinese cities'.[56] The authors therefore insisted on the importance of setting an upper limit for population growth, even if the calculations necessary for this exercise remained theoretically unsatisfactory: 'otherwise, the population would turn into a time bomb waiting to detonate.' Their study ended with a call for drastic measures for the prevention of unacceptably high birth numbers. It contains the core belief of Chinese birth planning until this very day:

> This is the hardest part of the whole issue, for it requires a national consensus and total mobilization, and it involves a lot of unpleasantness in the enforcement of the program. However, such unpleasantness, no matter how awful it may be and what causes lay behind it, should not be allowed to shake our faith in the truth so far sought and the reality it reflects. For the single-child family policy is the first punishment for ignorance of the seriousness of population matters in years past, and, if the single-child family policy is a strong dose that would cure the illness, China had better be prepared again for the unfavorable feedback of the drastic practice in its effect on aging – the second punishment of the dogmatic stubbornness in the 1950s. Then, and only then, can China be rid of the burden of an overtaxing population and channel its people into circumstances that should be much more pleasant.[57]

These passages are outspoken enough. Their authors had crossed the borderline between demographic analysis and political advice.

5 Phases of the one-child policy and its forerunners

5.1 Stir and hush: the muddle 1949 to 1978

Condemnation of birth control as a reactionary policy and an anti-Chinese, imperialist plot characterized the first years of the People's Republic. After tumultuous decades of war and revolution, the nation celebrated large birth numbers as a sign of recovery. China's first modern census of July 1953 seems to have lent renewed legitimacy to the anti-natalist position and triggered Chinese birth-control efforts. In fact, census work continued well into 1954, and official results were delayed until November of that year. The final result of more than 580 million people surpassed the number that had been expected on the basis of estimates from the 1930s and 1940s by approximately 70 million.[1] Provisional numbers from five provinces and sobering internal projections of a population total of 800 million for 1967 were already available in autumn 1953.

The first political leader on record to urge a relaxation of the strict rules pertaining to birth control is the then Vice-Premier Deng Xiaoping. A pertinent internal directive from him to the Ministry of Health dates from August 1953. Nine months later he once again endorsed birth control in a note to a functionary responsible for coordinating government work within the State Council. The note was written in reaction to a letter from the Vice-Chairwoman of the Women's Federation, Zhou Enlai's wife Deng Yingchao, written in May 1954. One month before, she had presided over the meetings of the Second National Congress of the Women's Federation, which saw debates on how to reconcile childbearing, work and household chores for women. This topic had become increasingly significant once new initiatives for the emancipation and employment of women were taken after the founding of the People's Republic and when complaints about firing pregnant women from their jobs appeared in the press. Now, Deng Yingchao took up the pen to complain about a growing but unmet demand for contraceptive devices among women cadres. In order to back up her demands, she attached an invoice from the Soviet Union to her letter, proving that contraceptives were sold in the model country of socialism and did not violate ideological principles there.[2]

In present-day China, Deng Xiaoping is celebrated as the originator of Chinese birth control, and a special booklet has been published for studying his 'thought on population'.[3] This does not necessarily reflect reality however, and may have to do with current political conventions. In spite of his public demurring later on, Zhou Enlai seems to be an equally likely candidate for the role of political instigator of birth control. Whatever the case may be, there are unmistakable signs that thinking on population issues differed among the leadership at a rather early date and low-key initiatives against the views of Mao Zedong were taken. However, precisely because of these differences, open debate of the issue was muted and conducted by proxy figures.

In public discourse of the 1950s, the person accredited as the first to warn against unrestrained population growth was Shao Lizi, a veteran politician from the Guomindang period, who stayed on the Chinese mainland and continued to occupy honorary positions. In September 1954, he used the inauguration session of the newly convened National People's Congress to deliver a speech that included passages on the desirability of some form of birth control. In keeping with the times, he justified his politically sensitive remarks by quoting Lenin on the need to abolish anti-abortion laws and to spread contraceptive knowledge. This was a shrewd argument, side-stepping both Stalin and Mao. Another article by Shao in December 1954 further outlined his views.[4]

Shao was soon joined by Party Vice-Chairman Liu Shaoqi. Speaking before an internal government meeting, summoned in December of that year for the discussion of census results and population problems, Liu registered his advocacy of birth control and his concern for a lack of sufficient food and clothing, medical and educational provisions for the growing population. He expressly rejected Stalin's campaigns for furthering motherhood as unsuitable for China, but in recognition of the widespread opposition to birth control within the country, he pleaded for cautious moves. He proposed that a debate on the issue be waged strictly inside the Party, the press should refrain from starting birth-control propaganda, relevant medical information should be published without advertising, and women cadres should pass on oral advice only. In January and February 1955 a newly instated *ad-hoc* commission, comprising representatives of the ministries of health, light industry, commerce and foreign trade, as well as the Women's Federation, took up the study of concrete measures for birth control. Its recommendations were endorsed by the Party's Central Committee in an internal directive of March 1955. The Central Committee acknowledged a growing demand for contraceptives among urban cadres and workers, and linked birth control to the economic well-being of the country. At the same time, it supported the import, production and sale of contraceptives to married couples of reproductive age in the cities. However, despite a few press articles in support of birth control, debate on the topic was again stifled at the 1955 session of the National People's Congress. For many cadres a reference to the pro-natalist policies of the Soviet Union sufficed to turn birth control in China into a non-issue. The Party press continued to bemoan the lot of childbearing women in capitalist countries, while it praised their happy life in socialist societies. Both Liu's speech and the directive were treated as internal documents unsuitable for public consumption. They have since come to light after a delay of more than three decades.[5]

The directive of March 1955 was based on a report of the Party cell in the Ministry of Health containing a self-criticism and a number of interesting points. It revealed that back in January 1953 the Ministry had prohibited the import of contraceptives as not being in accord with the country's policy. It had also stalled the efforts of Vice-Premier Deng Xiaoping to relax the almost complete ban on contraceptives, sterilizations and abortions. This ban was contained in provisional rules of the Ministry from December 1952, superseding internal regulations from April 1950 that allowed sterilizations and abortions in cases of medical complications only and threatened prosecution of women who underwent illegal surgery.

When revised rules were finally promulgated in July and November 1954, they ordered the introduction of selling and producing contraceptives, but specifically excluded the rural areas from selling them. Moreover, the rules still limited sterilization to medical conditions, the sole exception being mothers of six children or more who had obtained the prior consent of their husband, superior and doctor. The conditions for abortions were similarly tight, with social indications restricted to a few exceptional cases. Although in 1955 the Central Committee also indicated tolerance of contraceptive surgery in case of conflicts between childbearing, economic considerations and work demands, the Ministry of Health acted on this recommendation only after a delay of one year and relaxed the requirements in a circular of March 1956. A new minimum number of four children was set for having an abortion. A further ministerial directive of August 1956 spoke of 'a democratic right of contraception' and advocated birth-control propaganda in the rural areas too. No precise information on the reasons for the Ministry's stalling is available, but in view of Mao Zedong's repeated interventions in the Ministry's work and his attacks on its supposed lack of ideological commitment, it may be speculated that perceived pressures from the Chairman and his followers were the ultimate cause of the delay.

It took a further year and another circular of May 1957 to abolish various medical and social indications, or the minimum of four children, as strict preconditions for having an abortion. The new rule required merely proof of health problems or of an unspecified excessive number of children. At the same time the manifold consent requirements were lifted, and the principle of paid leave from work for abortions and sterilizations due to medical indications was laid down. Only Shanghai and Zhejiang acted noticeably faster by introducing such changes in 1955. However, despite a plea from the Trade Union, women who desired sterilization because of a large number of earlier births still had to foot the expenses.[6]

Support for birth control was anything but unequivocal. Despite brief positive references to the subject in the January 1956 draft of a Twelve-Year Programme for Agricultural Development and in a report by Premier Zhou Enlai before the 8th Party Congress in September 1956, Party circles continued to oppose all measures reminiscent of Malthusianism and smacking of immorality. Many audiences reacted angrily to internal presentations of birth-control advocates. For years, leading politicians, including Mao Zedong himself, continued to bemoan the stubborn resistance caused by traditional familism among the peasantry. Essentially, the first birth-planning campaign of 1954 to 1958 was restricted to educational work of the Women's Federation and the health clinics, which started to propagate late marriage, to offer contraceptive counselling, or to render abortions and sterilizations in a few special cases. Media coverage was largely confined to public debate in 1957 and early 1958, and only a few cities advertised new preventive techniques by holding large exhibitions. Although the sale of contraceptives and the establishment of their production were major breakthroughs, supply trailed behind potential demand for a long time. Basically, the activities were confined to the population of the big coastal cities and a few places in the hinterland. Only Hebei province started experimenting with rural birth control in 1954, subsequently expanding such efforts to the whole province. Some areas of Shandong province followed suit in March 1956, with Hunan joining a year later.[7] The pace in different areas of the country is shown in Table 1, which provides an overview of birth-control development by province. This gives rough indications only, as both urban and rural initiatives are lumped together, and the impact of the various initiatives is hard to evaluate.

The contradictions surfaced in the Hundred-Flowers campaign. On 5 March 1957, one week after Mao had personally championed birth control in internal speeches for the first time before the Supreme State Conference, an editorial in the *People's Daily* came out publicly in support of birth control. Leading intellectuals from the pre-revolutionary period suddenly emerged after years in the shadows, and used various forums convened by academic bodies or united-front organizations in order to speak out, restate their anti-natalist views, and criticize the delays. The roster of participants in the debates of spring 1957 reads like a Who's Who of social science in pre-communist China: it included the founding fathers of Chinese demography Chen Changheng and Chen Da, the influential sociologists and reformers Sun Benwen, Fei Xiaotong, Li Jinghan, Zhao Chengxin, Pan Guangdan, Wu Jingchao and Wu Wenzao, or Ma Yinchu,

Table 1 Beginning of provincial birth-planning activities: year of earliest reference

1954	Beijing, Tianjin, Hebei, Shanghai, Zhejiang
1955	Jiangsu, Fujian, Hunan
1956	Shanxi, Liaoning, Jilin, Heilongjiang, Shandong, Henan, Guangdong, Sichuan, Yunnan, Qinghai, Xinjiang
1957	Jiangxi, Shaanxi
1962	Hubei
1963	Anhui, Hainan, Guizhou
1964	Guangxi, Gansu
1971	Inner Mongolia
1972	Ningxia
1975	Tibet

Source: provincial information in ZJSQ 1997, 1259–1386 and Zhongguo renkou congshu 1987–93, 32 vol.

the famous educator, economist and Chiang Kaishek-critic, who served as president of Beijing University in the 1950s. Once again, they based their arguments on China's lack of sufficient cultivated or reclaimable land, the shortage of capital for economic construction and the threat of future mass unemployment. However, interestingly enough, the majority of them favoured methods of birth control such as late marriage, birth spacing, contraception and voluntary sterilization, taking quite explicit stands against abortion. It was conspicuous that an influential group of Marxist scholars around Wang Ya'nan and Sun Jingzhi continued to oppose the whole idea of birth control throughout the discussion.[8]

The great debate on birth control became entangled in the sharp volte-face of the Hundred-Flowers campaign in June 1957, the beginning of an anti-rightist rectification campaign, the intense inner Party wrestling over past culpabilities and the future policy line, and Mao Zedong's own contradictions. While first clarion calls for 'settling accounts' with the 'rightist conspiracy to reinstate bourgeois sociology and accomplish the restoration of capitalism' appeared in the Party organ in October 1957, the Chairman endorsed birth control once again at the 3rd plenary session of the 8th Central Committee that met at the same time. His support was not conclusive however, and contained the advise to continue the debate for some years. When a revised version of the Twelve-Year Programme for Agricultural Development in 1956–67 was promulgated in the same month, the suggestion to extend birth control to all densely populated areas of the countryside was taken up. Point 29 of the Programme mentioned it briefly, stimulating the propaganda to quote excited peasant women with the remark: 'Chairman Mao is caring so much for us that he even gives thought to our childbearing!' This prompted some provinces to begin drafting provincial twelve-year plans for birth control.[9]

One of the last major events of the first campaign was a national birth-control conference, which met in March 1958 and passed a resolution on spreading the movement to the whole country. At the same time, a number of provinces proclaimed fixed goals for lowering population increase, and the Ministry of Health urged integrating birth control into the set of target figures for the Great Leap. In May 1958, a national conference convened in Fushan county of Shandong province once again endorsed rural birth planning. One month later, the *People's Daily* still printed two controversial articles on the matter.[10]

However, these were victories on paper only, and soon gave way to a policy reversal. At the peak of the Great Leap Forward between 1958 and 1961 birth-control propaganda ceased altogether. Both Mao Zedong and Liu Shaoqi started to criticize anti-natalist views. The great majority of dispensaries offering contraceptive counselling closed down, and the Party press began to hammer the idea into everybody's head that 'the more people there are, the more, faster, better, and thriftier can we build socialism'. At the Beidaihe Conference of August 1958, which ushered in the people's communes, Mao Zedong raised his personal ceiling for future population numbers from 800 million to '1 billion and some hundred millions more'. And the Central Committee resolved in December

1958 that the future problem would be lack of manpower rather than overpopulation. A lone voice continuing the warnings against further unlimited population growth was economist Ma Yinchu, the famed President of Beijing University and one of the most vocal proponents of birth control. Even in November 1959 and January 1960, he still managed to publish rebuttals of the more than 200 attacks on his views that had appeared since October 1957, but in March 1960 he was accused of propagating Malthusianism and finally deposed.[11] The power behind this dismissal was none other than Mao Zedong himself.

China's second birth-planning campaign of 1962 to 1966 was conducted under similarly difficult circumstances. Begun as a reaction to the national crisis after the Great Leap Forward, it continued to struggle against the resistance of the Party's left-wing ideologues. Its point of departure were the difficulties of feeding, housing and employing the urban population, which after the in-migration of approximately 10 million peasants during 1958 had swollen to unprecedented numbers. Reducing the city population by limiting its natural increase and by returning the migrants to the countryside became one of the most urgent tasks. Initial suggestions to this effect were presented by Politburo member Chen Yun in June 1960 but it was another two years before action was taken. In 1962 and 1963 Premier Zhou Enlai used a series of conferences to initiate a large-scale resettlement programme and to propagate the idea of birth control, which in his opinion had to extend to the countryside. His suggestions came in the wake of a devastating famine that reduced many peasants to eating tree bark and cost the lives of up to 30 million people.[12]

The first signs of change were seen in Shanghai in March 1962, when the municipal Party Committee and the urban mass organizations started to revive birth-control activities. One month later, an internal circular of the Ministry of Health bemoaned the nationwide cessation of birth-control propaganda, the closure of most offices for contraceptive counselling, and the shortage of contraceptive supplies and abortion facilities in view of rising demand. In some rural areas, oral propaganda and personal persuasion to respect a limit of two children were introduced in autumn 1962.

The Central Committee and the State Council finally acted in December 1962. In a new directive they called for the resumption of birth control, wider access to contraceptives, and the spread of the campaign to densely populated rural regions. Yet typically they legitimized the campaign again with the usual innocuous health arguments and did not spell out the economic reasons behind the renewed drive to limit population numbers. An internal report of the Ministry of Health from July 1963 followed up with concrete suggestions for the establishment of a birth-planning organization, and the Second Work Conference on Urban Affairs, convened by the Party's Central Committee and the State Council in September and October that year, resolved to cut the population's natural increase by more than half within the next decade. However, contrary to proposals of the Ministry, this plan was confined to urban areas.[13]

Local guidelines advised having only two or three children per family. However, there were no clear rules on the subject, and the big national dailies kept silent on the matter. Steps such as the propagation of late marriage, the reopening of health offices for contraceptive counselling, and the complete liberalization and free performance of abortions were taken in 1963. The establishment of a State Birth-Planning Commission and the enactment of budgetary provisions followed a year later, but, with a few notable exceptions, such as rural areas in Hebei, Shandong and Hunan provinces, the campaign continued to be largely confined to the big cities. A central work conference in October 1965 finally called for shifting the focus of birth control to the villages. This drew other provinces such as Jiangsu, Liaoning and Sichuan into the orbit of birth planning, and succeeded in mobilizing around 20 per cent of all counties with 40 to 50 per cent of the rural population.[14]

Since the very start of the campaign, all activities had been overshadowed by the intensifying ideological struggle within the Party. In 1966 and 1967 most efforts collapsed in the turmoil of the Cultural Revolution. In some instances, they were branded as 'revisionist'. When in November 1968 the *People's Daily* attacked Liu Shaoqi for the 'nonsense' of linking birth control to population problems, it became clear that the rationale of birth planning was as contested as ever.[15] Only in Shanghai did birth-control measures continue more or less unabated. In some areas, such as Jiangsu, Shandong or Guangdong, they were taken up again in 1969; in most others the paralysis continued until 1971/72. Birth control suffered from the attacks on bourgeois academic thinking and bureaucratic regulations. Administrative functions, budget appropriations, as well as the production and distribution of contraceptives, were heavily affected.

The Ministry of Health as the central state organ in charge resumed some activities in 1968 under army tutelage. In a major initiative of May 1970, its Military Control Commission decreed that henceforth all contraceptives were to be distributed free of charge. On the instigation of Premier Zhou Enlai, the Commission also authored a joint report with the Ministry of Commerce and the Ministry of Fuels and Chemical Industry, dated February 1971, that announced the intention to revive birth-planning work and all related activities for the production and distribution of contraceptives. In the same year population targets (natural increase down to 1.5 per cent in the countryside and 1 per cent in the cities) were integrated into the new five-year plan for 1971–75. They signalled that the original target figure from 1963 for the end of the plan period (natural increase of 1 per cent for the whole country) had been abandoned as unrealistic. At the same time a propaganda drive focusing on the theme 'One child isn't too few, two are just fine, three are too much' commenced. Once again it relied on the efforts of Zhou Enlai, who used ingeniously edited Mao remarks of 1957 to circulate an internal government endorsement for the third birth-planning campaign in July 1971. Further crucial elements of policy such as late-marriage requirements of 23–25 years for women and 25–28 years for men, plus a birth-spacing rule of four to five years between the first and the second child, were introduced in 1972 and 1973.[16]

The campaign intensified when in 1973 the national dailies finally started a press campaign in favour of birth planning. In July of that year, a new Leading Group for Birth Planning under the State Council was installed. This organ was responsible for convening a national birth-planning conference in December that year, which endorsed the newly coined slogan 'Later (births), Longer (intervals), Fewer (children)'. It also served as the model for parallel organizations on the lower levels that soon extended to the counties or even beyond them. The five-year plan for 1976–80 lowered targets for natural population increase further to 1 per cent for the countryside and 0.6 per cent for the cities. Birth-control recommendations became increasingly tighter and were extended to all rural areas, where the collective institutions of the people's communes, the newly resurrected Women's Federation, and a drive to install barefoot doctors and medical institutions in the countryside served as important transmission belts. But the greatest successes continued to be achieved in the major cities. Shanghai in particular served as the model for the whole country. In 1973 and 1974, the municipality spearheaded a system of monthly inspections and half-yearly adjustments in order to check implementation of plan targets for late marriage and fertility reduction. Some regions seem to have introduced formal birth permits for third children of workers and staff in spring 1973.[17]

In contrast to the muted and largely futile efforts of the two earlier birth-planning campaigns, the third campaign achieved the halving of the total fertility rate between 1971 and 1978. This remarkable feat could not make up for the economic dislocation in the last years of Mao's rule, however, and it proved to be a source for bitter quarrelling in the subsequent decade.

5.2 Drums and gongs: the campaign 1979 to 1983

The search for the origins of the one-child policy leads back to the great stock-taking of economic and social conditions in China, initiated after the death of the Great Helmsman. Moves for a further tightening of the policy seem to have begun in December 1977, when the State Planning Commission decided on demographic targets for the following two one-year plans as well as for the mid-term perspective until 1985. In February 1978, these targets were deliberated by a national birth-planning conference and announced during a session of the National People's Congress convened by Mao's successor Hua Guofeng. According to the documents passed by the session in March, China's natural population increase was to decline to an annual average of 1 per cent by 1980. This equalled the old target figure for 1975 and indicated that some upward revision of the figures had already taken place. Birth planning was included among the catalogue of state objectives in the newly revised constitution.[18] In line with the new policy, the State Council's Leading Group for Birth Planning was reorganized and broadened to include a wider range of members from other bureaucracies. Directives endorsed by the State Council and the Central Committee urged coordination between birth planning and all social welfare policies.[19]

It took almost another twenty years to attain natural increase by a rate of 1 per cent. Even more unrealistic have been the long-term plans envisaging the decline of natural increase to 0.5 per cent by the year 1985 with a further decline to zero growth by the turn of the century. Such long-term plans were debated during a number of Politburo meetings and work conferences between March and May 1979. Senior leaders Deng Xiaoping, Chen Yun and Li Xiannian dominated the discussion of birth-control policies with warnings against excessive demographic growth and calls for the scrapping of taboos in population policy. The earliest mention of a lowering of natural increase to 0.5 per cent by 1985 may be found in an internally disseminated speech by Deng Xiaoping dated 23 March 1979. In May that year, Deng reiterated his commitment by stating before a work conference of the Central Committee: 'We must lower population increase to 0.5 per cent by all means. For this goal both administrative and economic methods can be used. Everything which effects a decline of growth rates must be seen as a great victory.'[20]

One month later, the extremely low new target figure was publicly announced in a government report by Hua Guofeng. Zero population growth by the year 2000 in turn is mentioned first in internal explanations by Chen Muhua, the newly appointed director of the Leading Group for Birth Planning, who alluded to it on 26 June 1979 after a meeting of the Central Committee Secretariat. The new target was made public by the Party organ in August that year.[21]

A number of factors contributed to the inability of the Party to realize these plans, foremost among which was policy formulation in Maoist campaign style. Desirable population targets were set and combined with other desirable economic indicators into a grand plan. Yet neither were concrete steps for implementation specified, nor were complicated interrelationships taken into account. In particular, this applied to internal demographic processes conditioned by the age and sex structure of the population. These were completely underestimated in 1978/79. Also neglected were the many-faceted side-effects of modernization policies, which in later years were to act as powerful constraints on birth planning.

However, even if the Party leadership had shown an interest in more precise analyses, it would have lacked the necessary data. China's last population count had been staged fifteen years before and had provided only rather crude numbers. Demographic research in China recovered only slowly from decades of proscription during the Mao era. In September 1979 the 97-year-old Ma Yinchu was rehabilitated after suffering almost twenty years of continuous criticism. In April 1980 demographic study courses at a number of universities were restored, with a Chinese Association for Population Studies founded at long last in February 1981.[22]

It was therefore more than unclear how to realize the ambitious population plans. As a first step, in October 1978 the State Council decided to act on recommendations of the birth-planning conference and to establish birth-planning bureaus in all counties as well as cadre posts for birth planning in people's communes and large factories all over the nation. These were given the duty to propagate the one-child family, to tolerate families with two children but to forestall any additional births. More stringent policies for the cities had apparently already been devised in 1978: while in the future 50 per cent of all rural deliveries were to be first births, this was set at 80 per cent for urban areas.[23] The one-child policy started to loom on the horizon.

Implementation of these guidelines was to be realized by a new system of incentives for one-child families and sanctions after the third child. In January 1979, these measures were discussed for the first time at a Beijing conference of directors from regional birth-planning bureaux, who studied relevant model regulations from Tianjin and Guangdong. These provisional regulations also served as the basis of a national birth-planning law, a draft of which was discussed by the conference without being ratified at that time. On the regional level, the process of drafting birth-planning rules proceeded at a faster pace. Until November 1979, twenty-seven provinces, autonomous regions and centrally administered cities had passed provisional birth-planning rules.[24]

In the early years, the population policy directives of the leadership met with differing responses at the grass-roots level. Steven Mosher, who pursued field research in a village of the Guangdong Pearl River delta in 1979 and 1980, reported tough coercive measures for implementing the birth-control directives from the provincial capital and from Beijing. The arsenal of severe sanctions included compulsory attendance at mass meetings and incessant group discussions for pregnant women, who were threatened with high fines for non-attendance, threats of dismissal from work, as well as forced sterilizations and abortions even after the sixth month of pregnancy. In addition to the fourteen years of 10 per cent income deductions stipulated by the Provincial Revolutionary Committee of Guangdong, the local people's commune ordered still further income deductions, a one-off fine of 300 yuan, as well as a doubling of health insurance fees. Whoever ignored the official two-child limit was driven to financial ruin.[25]

During repeated visits to a Guangdong county at around the same time, the American anthropologists Potter and Potter recorded quite different experiences with the one-child campaign. In 1979, this county did not impose any fines even after the fourth child. In particular, it did not enforce any punishment for couples without male offspring. In the people's commune studied by Potter and Potter, the one-child campaign only began in June 1980. It was practised in a mild form, working with quite affordable fines for children born outside the birth plan. Coercion and mass abortions were first recorded by Potter and Potter in 1981.[26]

The reports quoted above hail from the very same region and give reason to reflect on the execution of the government's directives in 1979. These directives were seemingly implemented in a highly diverse manner. The leadership must have been somewhat dissatisfied with the results of the campaign, prompting Chen Muhua to urge a further strengthening of guidelines at a new conference of directors of regional birth-planning bureaux held in December 1979. She demanded to 'shift the emphasis of birth planning to propagating the one-child family', and she praised a model commune in Gansu which demanded written commitments from all married couples to respect the birth plan. In a circular to all Party members dated January 1980, the Secretariat of the Central Committee sanctioned such calls by calling for legal, economic and administrative measures in favour of one-child families. These formulations were explicit borrowings from the directives of Deng Xiaoping.[27]

The support of China's demographic circles for the new policies was less than unanimous. A December 1979 conference, convened in Chengdu to prepare for setting up the Association for Population Studies, witnessed vehement debates on the consequences of one-child policies for old-age support. Among the most explicit opponents of the policy was a leading scholar from the Shanxi Academy of Social Sciences, who continues to be a prominent critic of the one-child policy today and who coined the notion of a future 4–2–1 constellation: one grandchild would have to shoulder support for two parents and four grandparents.[28] Other demographers from Beijing spoke out in favour of comprehensive state support for the elderly, urging a struggle against the discrimination of women and more consideration for population growth in economic planning. However, although they supported one-child propaganda and incentives, they carefully refrained from endorsing a complete ban on second births.[29]

One month later, however, the tide finally turned and the recommendation of one-child families became a one-child limit. Chen Muhua demanded that in the future 95 per cent of urban and 90 per cent of rural women should give birth to one child only. Shortly afterwards, the Party paper pointed out that only in this way could population targets for the years 1985 and 2000 be met. For the first time, the magic number of 1.2 billion people by 2000 acquired the quality of a fixed upper limit. It was based on remarks by Party elder Li Xiannian at the April 1979 work conference of the Central Committee and ultimately resulted from the calculations of Song Jian.[30]

This was a time of continued discussion on China's economic backwardness, population problems and strategies for modernization in the highest leadership circles of the Party. Projections undertaken in 1979 and published in February 1980 by control theorists and demographers Song Jian, Tian Xueyuan, Li Guangyuan and Yu Jingyuan exerted a strong influence on the leadership's thinking. Working with different fertility levels of 3.0, 2.3, 2.0, 1.5 and 1.0 children per woman, the scientists submitted different scenarios for China's future population growth. They demonstrated that by retaining a two-child policy, the upper limit of 1.2 billion in the year 2000 would be breached. Shortly after, this led the birth-planning authorities to adopt average fertility levels of 1.5 to 1.7 children per woman for their internal calculations.[31] New guidelines were proposed in a letter addressed by the Party's Vice-Chairman and Minister of the powerful State Commission for Finance and Economics, Chen Yun, to Chen Muhua, the minister responsible for birth planning. Chen Yun demanded:

> First, we have to whip up public opinion in a big way; second, we have to pass laws urging one child per couple; third, we have to provide incentives for single children as for instance in work allocation; fourth, we have to promote eugenics and better birth-planning techniques; fifth, we have to further develop social security – peasants who have lost their work ability have to get a monthly allowance of five yuan.[32]

In early September 1980, Deng Xiaoping proclaimed his support for a one-child campaign during an inspection trip to Sichuan:

> In birth planning, we must definitely keep propagating that every couple has only one child. We cannot make concessions here. There is no hope for the Four Modernizations, should this lever be broken. It is of major importance for the national economy.[33]

The Party Central Committee heeded the calls and addressed an Open Letter to all members of the Party and the Communist Youth League on 25 September 1980. This letter reaffirmed the one-child policy, which meanwhile had been also sanctioned as a binding target for the government. It reconfirmed the limit of 1.2 billion Chinese for the year 2000, without setting precise targets for the ensuing period. While this sealed the change from two-child to one-child policies, the Party still made a number of concessions, among them the offer that 'persons in real difficulties defined by pertinent rules' could obtain special permission for second births. China's national minorities were to be subject to a loose form of birth planning only. Finally, the Party pleaded for a free choice of contraceptive methods and emphasized the use of incentives rather than sanctions.[34] It remains unclear, however, to what degree such concessions were put into practice. There are numerous indications that many cadres perceived the one-child propaganda as a one-child command, that special permits for second births were refused, and that the free choice of contraceptive methods remained on paper only.

Indeed, uneasiness about the course to be followed seems to have continued throughout the year 1980. There are a number of statements from high-level politicians opposing forced abortions and excessively hard measures such as a complete freeze of wage payments, the withdrawal of grain rations and the expulsion of Party members violating the one-child rule.[35] Opinions on these points seem to have been divided, since the Central Disciplinary Commission of the Party revised its former stand against disciplinary punishments of cadres opposing birth planning in July 1980.[36] The high number of abortions and sterilizations in the years 1979 and 1980 also point to a successive tightening of the campaign.

Instability characterized the situation in 1981. The Party continued to press for a more thorough implementation and legal safeguards in support of the one-child policy. In January 1981, it used a conference of the Association for Population Studies to form a research group for the study of the long-term carrying capacity of China's territory and her economy. The national organization of China's demographers also submitted proposals for differentiated birth planning among the national minorities that aimed to restrict their freedom to refuse birth control.[37] At the same time, China's courts began to pass sentences in rural areas against the widespread removal of IUDs. The Party press renewed its propaganda for written commitments obliging both peasants and cadres to respect the one-child rule. It urged the establishment of a system of economic incentives and sanctions for both agricultural production and birth planning.[38]

Of major importance was the decision in March 1981 to transform the State Council's Leading Group for Birth Planning into a state commission with its own vertical organization and subordinate offices in all parts of the country.[39] For the first time, organizational arrangements were established to help turn the one-child campaign into professionalized birth planning, yet reports on new coercive measures continued to leak through in 1981. A report gained notoriety on the 'mobilization' of the population in Huiyang district, Guangdong province. It documented the fact that pregnant women without birth permits were marched off in handcuffs to undergo forced abortions. While peasant families who violated the birth-planning rules were refused water and electricity supplies, activists unroofed their houses. The Party Secretary responsible for these actions was later awarded a special commendation for 'patient and careful ideological work among the masses'.[40]

It is hard to pass judgement on the representativeness of these and similar reports. For while the account cited above documents a brutal attack on the peasant front of widespread passive resistance, other reports on the situation of birth planning in 1981 point in exactly the opposite direction. For the first time, the consequences of China's new marriage law were felt. After prolonged controversy, this new law was passed in September 1980 by the National People's Congress. It effectively lowered the age limit for marriage to 20 years for women and 22 years for men. This liberalization of former rules documented the willingness of the Party to meet the prevalent wishes of the population. Moreover, many experts had urged more chances for self-realization in private life in order to combat an increasing number of illegal marriages and sex crimes, growing juvenile delinquency, as well as the lack of sufficient entertainment opportunities in public life. The consequent run on marriage-registration offices raised the number of marriages in 1981 by nearly 50 per cent in comparison to the previous year. In subsequent years it effectively lowered the average marriage age and neutralized the effects of the one-child policy to a large degree.[41]

Initial signs of yet another important change in the overall framework of birth control began to appear in 1981. Above all, this concerned the negative consequences of agricultural decollectivization for birth planning. With the resurrection of the petty peasant economy, incentives and sanctions devised under the old system of people's communes became ineffective, robbing the Party of its control over peasant income, land use, collective welfare funds and cadre recruitment at the grass roots. In the villages large numbers of one-child certificates were handed back, and reports on the decreasing effectiveness of birth control multiplied. This was first documented in the minutes of a telephone call in April 1981 between Hu Qiaomu, the then Deputy General-Secretary of the Party, and the Minister of the Birth-Planning Commission, Chen Muhua. Hu demanded from Chen new proposals for birth planning, arguing that in the course of decollectivization the old methods no longer worked.[42] Premier Zhao Ziyang confirmed this state of affairs in his government report of November that year. The session of the National People's Congress at which his report was delivered also witnessed complaints about lagging efforts of birth-planning cadres, glaring gaps in the financing of birth control, insufficient supplies of contraceptives and opposition to the sanctions stipulated by birth-planning rules.[43] Chen Muhua was forced to declare unequivocally: 'Recently, we have seen quite a number of debates on birth planning. It is claimed that the one-child propaganda will be terminated, and two children will be permitted. Such declarations are groundless.'[44]

In fact, they were not groundless at all, for in summer 1981 the Secretariat of the Central Committee conducted a large-scale enquiry among provincial Party committees, birth-planning cadres and population experts that produced two proposals for a change of policy: the return to the former two-child rule or second-child permission for peasants with only one daughter. It was the general consensus that most peasants with one son could eventually be persuaded to renounce a second birth, but rural families with only one daughter stubbornly insisted on the right to have another child.[45]

When the Central Committee finally took a stand in February 1982, it opted for rather mute concessions. In a joint directive with the State Council, it re-emphasized that only those in real difficulties would be granted second-child permits. Although the right of national minorities to special treatment was conceded once again, for the first time these minorities were obliged to acknowledge at least the principle of birth planning. Through this directive the Central Committee attempted to systematize the different local formulas for incentives and sanctions. It advocated linking new rural responsibility systems for agricultural production and peasant income with birth planning by introducing relevant passages into all contracts.[46]

The Central Committee's intervention provoked a new wave of regional birth-planning regulations, which laid down more specific rules for second-child permits. In early 1982 such permits were only granted under three rather restricted conditions, but an August 1982 work conference decided to extend second-child permits to seven further types of cases. The conference underlined that henceforth regular work would replace the former campaign-style efforts for birth control. Propaganda and educational work would be given priority over economic sanctions, and effective contraceptive measures would be preferred over later abortions.[47] However, the belief of the Party in the efficacy of the new birth-planning bureaucracy seems to have been limited, since while the thrust of such guidelines was directed against acts that Politburo member Wan Li in November termed 'coercion, commands, and methods far removed from the masses',[48] the Central Committee decreed at the same time:

> Propagating one-child policies comes first, problems arising from this come second. Birth planning implies heavy responsibilities and great difficulties. It is understandable that certain problems develop in the course of this work. They should not be exploited for excessive criticism.[49]

When the country's constitution was revised once more in December 1982, it strengthened the commitment for birth planning by including it among citizens' duties and the tasks of lower level administrations – steps without precedent in world history.[50] This is the basis on which the Birth-Planning Commission began to prepare a special month of one-child propaganda activities that showed all the signs of a new shock campaign. On 22 November 1982, Qian Xinzhong – a Party veteran in health work since the 1930s, who acted as China's last Minister of Health before the Cultural Revolution and became her new Minister of the State Birth-Planning Commission in May 1982 – had already written to the Party secretaries of China's fifteen most populous provinces:

> We suggest that you combine the propaganda month with the implementation of contraceptive measures for married couples. In particular, one spouse of rural couples of reproductive age with already two children should be mobilized for sterilization. The only exception are persons successfully using IUDs for more than five years, those who will be beyond reproductive age shortly, who are sterile, or belong to national minorities. We have to struggle for a complete sterilization of all target persons during this winter or in the next year. At the same time, we have to go all out to struggle for early abortions among women with pregnancies outside plan.[51]

The propaganda month of January 1983, which was emphatically endorsed by the Central Committee,[52] produced the intended results: 1.37 million propagandists, 138,000 doctors, medical assistants and nurses, as well as innumerable cadres, moved to combat the prevalent disinterest in the one-child policy. Their efforts resulted in 2.68 million new sterilizations as well as 0.21 million other contraceptive measures taken in January 1983 alone – the highest monthly record ever since the beginning of the one-child policy.[53] All statements against coercive measures and commandeering ceased, while record numbers of sterilizations and abortions continued for the rest of the year. Party leaders pronounced their express support for the new campaign. The most unreserved encouragement came from State President Li Xiannian, who in July 1983 registered his concern about the continuing high number of second births, and assured Qian Xinzhong: 'The Standing Committee of the Politburo supports you. It does not matter if problems come up in your work. Stiffen your back for a couple of years, things will get better later on.'[54]

Nevertheless, even during the mobilization campaign of 1983, Chinese policies have not been without ambiguity. While propagandists in the villages of the country beat drums and gongs, planners started fine-tuning the new five-year plan passed in December 1982 for the period 1981 to 1985. Without much ado, this plan had quietly set a new course for birth planning that could only be termed sensational: a natural population increase of 1.3 per cent by the year 1985 rather than an increase of 0.5 per cent was striven for.[55] The change could not have been more dramatic, but in common with Chinese propaganda usage, it was presented as a self-evident small 'adjustment'. When a Kunming conference of the State Birth-Planning Commission in March 1983 discussed the adoption of regionally differentiated policies and the departure from the hitherto almost uniform one-child rule, the outlines of the new course became clearer. The conference recommended that in drafting future long-term plans, more attention should be paid to regional differences and natural resources, environmental conditions, economic structures and social affairs.[56]

Renouncing the radical lowering of fertility levels envisaged in 1978 signalled that, despite all the propaganda, education, regulations, incentives and sanctions, the one-child campaign encountered serious problems in gaining acceptance. It is therefore indicative that in August 1983 the Association for Population Studies turned the tables on prevailing birth-control thinking, and for the first time deemed the family size preferences of peasants worthy of a discussion.[57]

But other factors also played a role. At the end of 1982 the provisional results of the new population census of July 1982 and of the national fertility survey of September that year became available. For the first time in Chinese history, population numbers came into being that were sufficiently reliable and structured to permit more detailed planning. More than ever before, the problems of population ageing induced by a radical one-child policy aroused general interest, and individual Chinese demographers began to doubt the population target of 1.2 billion for 2000. One among them was Tian Xueyuan, Director of the Institute of Demography of the Academy for Social Sciences. He presented new projections, the medium and high variant of which reached population totals beyond the 1.2 billion limit for 2000. Moreover, they assumed a general resurgence in fertility levels after the turn of the century.[58] When the Minister of the State Birth-Planning Commission was dismissed after compromising himself in the controversial campaign against spiritual pollution, everything was ready for a general change of course.

5.3 Small holes and big gaps: the relaxation 1984 to 1985

The relaxation of rigid one-child policies in early 1984 and the temporary renunciation of further campaigns and coercive measures are intimately related to changes in Chinese domestic policy at that time. The campaign against spiritual pollution, abandoned by intervention of the then General-Secretary of the Party Hu Yaobang, gave way to a fresh wave of liberalization. Above all, the new course was directed against leftist forces who opposed the continuation of economic reforms and the cooptation of intellectuals to leading positions. The impact of this new trend was soon felt in population policy, too. At its meeting in January 1984, the Secretariat of the Central Committee, chaired by Hu Yaobang, spoke out against any 'commandeering' in family planning. It called for a defeat of the lack of acceptance of birth control among the population by using new initiatives. However, all new policies were conditional on the demand that the successes of population policy secured so far should not be called into question.[59] One month later, the Secretariat received an internal report with a far-reaching proposal. Pointing to the widespread opposition to the one-child policy and the problems of implementation, it urged a return to a conditional two-child policy. All peasants who consented to a late birth of their first child and to an extended birth interval of eight to ten years should be allowed to have a second child. While the one-child propaganda in rural areas should be continued, there should be no fixed requirement, and policies should only aim at a realistic proportion of 30 per cent of one-child families.[60]

Two new conferences of directors of regional birth-planning bureaux discussed these initiatives, before another meeting of the Secretariat of the Central Committee finally adopted a decision on 19 March 1984. The new decision emphasized that, small exceptions apart, the one-child policy should continue in the urban areas of China. Different rules were to apply for the countryside, however. While propaganda for the one-child family was to continue in the villages, special permits for second children should be granted to a greater degree than hitherto. Again, it was stressed that only 'persons in real difficulties' should benefit from these new regulations. However, this time, the formulation also included rural households suffering from a lack of manpower and experiencing economic hardships due to the birth of only one daughter.[61] The reformulation of population policy culminated in the decision of the Central Committee Secretariat of 12 April 1984 to endorse a report of the State Birth-Planning Commission with suggestions for new birth-planning approaches. This report was circulated as Document No. 7/1984 in the internal bulletin series of the Central Committee. Constituting one of the most important documents of Chinese birth-control policies, it has been quoted incessantly by politicians, academics and press commentators in the country. Although the full text was publicized only with a delay of thirteen years, its main message was spread by way of internal Party channels and a host of references in contemporary pronouncements.[62]

The most important provision of the document was the extension of rural second-child permits, which were allowed to increase from 5 per cent to a future 10 per cent of all current births. New types of exemptions from the one-child limit were allowed, among them the rule that spouses who themselves were single children could have two births. This rule was seen as a gateway to a future transformation of policy, since such families would become increasingly prevalent after 2000. On the other hand, the document also urged the strict prevention of all non-authorized second and higher order births. The new margins for second births were only to be realized after applicants obtained proper permission within the population plan. Just as carefully balanced were the special rules for national minorities, who were now unequivocally included among Chinese citizens with a duty to practise birth control. While smaller minorities with fewer than 10 million members were granted a general second-child permit, third births were subject to special conditions, and higher order births were strictly forbidden. The slogan coined by the circular for the new policy guidelines was borrowed from local experiments that had begun in Shandong province two years earlier. It was typical of the combination of flexibility and strictness in Chinese pronouncements: 'Open a small hole to close a big gap (*kai xiao kou, du da kou*)!'

Similar dialectics also characterized the attitude of the Party Secretariat in regard to the use of coercion. On the one hand, it pleaded for 'putting birth planning on an acceptable, reasonable basis that will be supported by the masses and can be implemented by the cadres'. In the same context, the Central Committee criticized the widespread attitude among cadres that 'coercion and commands are unavoidable'. Emphasis was put on the voluntariness of sterilizations, regard for special circumstances and abortions only according to strict medical rules. However, the Party Secretariat also tried to forestall 'excessive criticism' of cadres, 'in order not to dampen their enthusiasm'. Leaving no doubt that relaxation was not to mean an abandonment of family planning, the circular finally ordered a large-scale extension of birth-control organization and personnel at the grass-roots level.

Document No. 7/1984 of the Central Committee ushered in a new round of birth-control measures at the provincial level. Following its dissemination within the Party, a large number of new rules and interpretations clarified its main lines of departure. A new list of fourteen types of cases eligible for special second-child permits was drawn up, more than in all former documents. In addition, trial policies for even more far-reaching exemptions from the one-child policy at the regional level were sanctioned. Between December 1984 and the end of the following year, a list of experimental areas was drawn up. Forty-four counties were empowered to try out different forms of second-child permission, among them differentiated policies for divergent types of areas within a county and exemptions from the one-child rule for all peasants with only one daughter. The most wide-ranging trial policies were adopted in counties experimenting with a global second-child permit for peasants who practised prolonged birth spacing.[63] Other localities ventured to grant additional second-child permits only if a whole village community was able to demonstrate full compliance with the population plan. Finally, birth-planning bureaux became established in all rural towns, as well as at the level of street committees of medium-sized and large cities. Large enterprises and state organizations were also ordered to establish birth-control bureaux with their own personnel.

Interpretations of the document have been diverse, demonstrating that its carefully balanced clauses could be cited for quite different purposes.[64] Two interpretations may be cited as representative examples of such different lines of argument.

Six weeks after the issuing of the circular, two leading cadres of the State Birth-Planning Commission disavowed a simplified understanding of the one-child policy. They pointed out that under specific conditions this policy covered second-child permits for people in difficulties. In an extensive discussion of experiments in Mian county, Shaanxi province, begun in 1982, they discriminated between three areas with different economic, social and environmental conditions practising three different sets of two-child policies. Overall, this amounted to an extension of second-child permits. On the other hand, the birth-planning cadres also argued in favour of strict adherence to all relevant guidelines. In particular, they called for a reduction of higher order births beyond the second child, which still amounted to more than 24 per cent of all current deliveries. In regard to contraceptive methods, they declared: 'As far as contraceptive methods are concerned, we should not demand the use of one and the same method from the masses.'[65]

The Party Committee of Guizhou province obviously faced different problems. Debating the question of how the authority of birth-planning cadres could be upheld in a criticism of coercive measures, it proclaimed in a circular dated 27 July 1984:

> The province accepts main responsibility for some mistakes that have been committed in individual places and units. Under no circumstances is the perfection of the Party's concrete measures and regulations allowed to dampen the zeal in implementing birth-planning policy or to shake our resolution to keep the population within 1.2 billion at the turn of the century.[66]

While such reactions betrayed the fear that the relaxation of policies would discredit birth planning *per se*, other actors understood the circular of April 1984 as a signal for even more flexibility. This is demonstrated in a letter of July 1984 which two cadres of the Birth-Planning Commission addressed to the then Premier Zhao Ziyang. In their letter, they submitted the question whether the population target of 1.2 billion by 2000 should be taken as a fixed plan target or whether it should be interpreted as a rough indicative guideline only. Annotating the letter, Zhao Ziyang spoke out in favour of flexibility – a position that provoked the irreconcilable hostility of the advocates of a hard-line one-child policy. The hard-liners interpreted the 1.2 billion target for 2000 as an upper limit, the lifting of which would gravely endanger the realization of China's economic objectives and long-term development perspectives.[67]

Four weeks later, participants at a population conference in Chengdu did not beat about the bush. Demographers and birth-planning cadres discussed the consequences of agricultural decollectivization for birth planning. They reported strong pressures from the peasantry for permitting second children, and they generally deemed a two-child policy to be much easier to implement. Long debates centred on the implications of the abolishment of people's communes: agrarian reforms would restrengthen the economic position of the family, which in the face of low individual incomes kept functioning as an indispensable unit for production and consumption. Because of the low degree of mechanization, human labour and craftsmanship remained of major importance, with an accordingly strong reliance on male manpower for carrying out basic family functions. The following alternative proposals to the current one-child policy were submitted at the conference: 'Each couple should be allowed two children, but the second child should only be borne by women between 30–34 years of age.' 'If peasants in the countryside agree to later sterilization, they should all be permitted a second child.' Another suggestion debated at the conference was the progressive taxation of higher order births.[68]

As the political constraints continued to be sensitive, no clear reactions to these proposals ensued. At a conference of the Tianjin Birth-Planning Commission in October 1984, Deng Xiaoping reconfirmed the validity of the

1.2 billion limit. His remarks were made during a discussion of planning targets for 2000, which also covered initial experiences with the new experiments for second-child permits. These remarks should be read as a restrictive attitude *vis-à-vis* new proposals for relaxing birth control.[69]

The concrete consequences of such demands for strict adherence to the 1.2 billion population goal remained unclear, however. For while in 1985 the per centage of authorized second and higher order births was raised to 20 per cent of all current deliveries, a lengthy investigation of 'China in the Year 2000', submitted to the State Council in May of that year, warned that the 1.2-billion limit could not be met.[70] For the first time, a number of new regional birth-planning regulations for the migrant population documented the growing concern of the authorities about their loss of control.[71] Premier Zhao Ziyang, however, continued to hold on to his views about flexible birth planning. In an interview with a journal published by the Food and Agriculture Organization (FAO), he formulated that China's population should be limited to about 1.2 billion by 2000.[72]

In accord with this position, the Birth-Planning Commission and academic advisory bodies adopted similar stands. In November 1985, the first outline results of the national research project on 'China in the Year 2000' were presented to the public. The authors of the chapter on population and employment, who worked in a research centre of the State Council, submitted a medium projection of 1.248 billion people by the turn of the century. This number was based on total fertility rates of 2.1 by 1985, 1.9 by 1990, 1.75 by 1994, and 1.6 by 2000 – a long way from a categorical one-child limit. Introducing alternative calculations with a continuing high fertility level of 2.2 to 2.4 children per woman, they reached numbers of 1.30 to 1.36 billion people by 2000. The scientists pleaded for lowering the total fertility rate to 1.5 by 1990 in order to comply with the 1.2 billion limit for 2000 and to keep within a maximum of 1.3 billion by 2020, but the text of their analysis does not display much credence in the attainment of these goals.[73]

Quite the opposite: the different scenarios betrayed much uneasiness about current fertility levels. During a population conference in November 1985, many scientists argued for stalling recommendations until new survey data became available.[74] The advocates of two-child policies felt encouraged by a new study on alternatives to the one-child policy published by the New York-based Population Council at the end of 1985. This study, which became widely known within China, recommended a socially more acceptable two-child policy with a late-marriage age of at least 25 years and four to six years of birth spacing. The authors estimated that by the mid-twenty-first century such a policy would result in a population total only 5 to 7 per cent higher than the one projected under a strict one-child limit.[75] However, the proposal shifts the problem to adherence to late-marriage, late-birth and birth-spacing rules. In the 1980s, these norms proved to be extremely hard to enforce. Furthermore, it requires that third and higher order births be effectively prevented – a premise that, in view of the strong cultural son preference, is anything but a matter of course.

In this complicated situation, the State Birth-Planning Commission held to its line of flexibility coupled with policy experiments. In a speech before the Central Party School, the Minister of the Commission, Wang Wei, explicitly opposed a 'conquering mentality', 'commandeering' and all cruder forms of one-child policies. In October and November of that year, he and his deputy Chang Chongxuan sketched diverse forms of differentiated birth planning. They discriminated between five to seven different types of areas with divergent rules for second-child births: (1) areas permitting a second child only for special hardship cases; (2) areas permitting a second child for peasants with only one daughter (this applied to two-thirds of Shandong, the South of Zhejiang, as well as to Guangdong and Guangxi); (3) areas with general second-child permit for those with sufficient birth spacing (Ningxia, mountainous areas in other provinces, minority and border areas, experimental counties); (4) areas with graded second-child permits conforming to different economic levels within the region (Shaanxi plus parts of Gansu and Sichuan provinces); (5) areas that linked an extension of second-child permits to a lowering of higher order births (Gansu); (6) areas with a global second-child permit for those practising late marriage with late birth; (7) national minority areas with special rules.[76]

This classification marked the zenith of the liberalization in birth planning. Later accusations against the promulgators of these policies claimed that 'the former leading cadre of the department in charge' had pleaded for 'slow, moderate changes' in the direction of a two-child policy. He is rumoured to have stated that 'the small hole could be enlarged even more and need not be fixed'.[77] It is not far-fetched to speculate that the objects of these veiled accusations could only have been the then Minister of the Birth-Planning Commission, General-Secretary Hu Yaobang's long-time associate Wang Wei, and Premier Zhao Ziyang as his direct superior. Even after indications for a new wave of births multiplied in late 1985, these politicians continued to uphold the relaxation of policy.

5.4 Tit for tat: the controversy 1986 to 1989

The comparison of China's population total and vitality rates at the end of 1985 with the targets of the sixth five-year plan for the period 1981 to 1985 substantiates a remarkable degree of plan adherence. Natural increase was only minimally above target, and the population total for the end of 1985 conformed exactly to the target number fixed at the time of plan promulgation in 1982: 1.06 billion. This is the state of plan fulfilment if plan targets are compared with later data based on the 1990 population count.[78] In late 1985, China's politicians believed in an even better situation, for incomplete numbers of various sample surveys since 1982 seemed to document a birth rate and a natural increase slightly below target.[79]

These positive experiences encouraged the planners to project similar developments for the seventh five-year plan for the period 1986 to 1990. Basing themselves on the vitality rates of 1985, they extrapolated a slightly lower average figure for the succeeding plan period. The target number for total population in 1990 was set at 1.113 billion.[80] In reality, however, population growth during the seventh five-year plan exceeded this number by 20 million. There are a number of reasons are for this deviation, among them the under-reporting of birth numbers which had already begun earlier, the lowering of the marriage age and the age at first childbearing, the contraction of birth intervals, as well as fertility rates distinctly above the projected level. Already in 1987, many of these problems became apparent. It is remarkable, however, that even in 1989 the State Birth-Planning Commission continued to project 16 million people fewer than enumerated in the new census of 1990.[81] Shortcomings of the statistical system evidently played a role, too.

However, political factors also figured in the emerging dispute on the causes of the considerable breach of plan targets. Starting in 1986, a major controversy erupted on the future handling of second-child permits. Two positions may be observed in this internal debate, which only partially surfaced in public. On one side, there were those Chinese demographers, statisticians and birth planners who maintained that birth control hitherto had been unrealistic and incommensurate with China's new situation after the decollectivization of agriculture. They called for a gradual extension of second-child permits in the countryside. The opposition consisted of hard-line advocates of the one-child policy who warned time and again against the negative consequences for the economic and ecological future of China, brought about by a relaxation of population policies. They urged a restriction of second-child permits to a small number of strictly defined special cases only. As both camps started to realize the full impact of China's demographic structure in 1986, the controversy became acrimonious. Foremost among the newly realized circumstances was the fact that those born between 1962 and 1973 were now of marriageable and reproductive age, creating additional hardships for birth planning in the mid-1980s.

Such basic differences of opinion and perception governed the drafting of a new circular of the Central Committee, which, according to varying interpretations of the opposing camps, was to either augment or replace the preceding Document No. 7 of 1984.[82] While it reconfirmed the broadening of second-child permits and emphasized the stand against coercion, commandeering, and other 'uncivilized practices, which are quite serious in some places', the new CC Document No. 13 of May 1986 noted laxness and a 'loss of control' in other areas. It called for strict adherence to population targets formulated two months earlier in the seventh five-year plan. Birth-planning regulations were to be scrupulously obeyed in the future. Particular emphasis was put on future work in rural areas lagging behind in birth control. Furthermore, the Central Committee decreed a recruitment drive for birth-planning personnel at the grass-roots level, and it called for improved coordination between all authorities concerned.

After the issuing of Document No. 13, another internal circular urged investigations to discover the reasons for the resurgence of birth numbers. In line with the two documents, new directives recommended the introduction of written commitments compelling all peasants with second-child permits to renounce further births. In order to reinforce the message, the authorities again pressed for experiments with collective liability. Many regions were urged to issue second-child permits only in villages that had fulfilled all birth-planning targets concerning maximum birth numbers, propaganda work, medical and technical services, cadre recruitment and other regular duties. In future, all administrative units of the People's Republic were to make their First Party Secretary take personal responsibility for birth planning.[83]

New projections, published four weeks after the circular, revealed the alternatives faced by the Central Committee. A research organ close to Song Jian, Institute No. 710 of the Ministry of Aeronautics, presented alternative calculations for population totals resulting from either a tight one-child policy, a restriction of fertility rates to an average 1.5 children per woman, second-child permits for all couples with only one daughter, third-child permits for all couples with two daughters, or a general second-child permit for those practising extended birth spacing. Projections for 2000 varied between a minimum of 1.19 billion under a tight one-child policy and a maximum of 1.25 billion in the case of a general second-child permit. They diverged to a larger degree for 2100, ranging between a strict one-child variant of 1.10 billion and a two-child alternative of 1.6 billion.[84]

Pressures to respect the 1.2 billion limit in 2000 must have been strong, for in July 1986 the State Council's Centre for Development Research had to submit an internal self-criticism for its projection of 1.25 billion by 2000.[85] Birth-planning conferences held in the second half of 1986 underlined the leadership's intention to strengthen birth planning. This was testified by a joint work conference of the Birth-Planning Commission and the Ministry of Finance to discuss financial aspects of birth planning.[86] In December 1986, Premier Zhao Ziyang used a new national work conference on birth planning to assume the role of warner, admonishing strict adherence to the one-child policy.[87]

Yet once again Zhao Ziyang supported all current experiments with additional second-child permits, a position that was also endorsed by Wang Wei in his capacity as Minister of the State Birth-Planning Commission. Nevertheless, his remarks before the work conference clearly mirrored the defensive posture which liberals had to adopt in view of the resurgence of birth numbers. Wang Wei made his future support for new experiments dependent on prior approval, organization and evaluation by the centre. According to him, the resurgence of birth numbers was primarily due to the age structure of the population and to the rise of marriage numbers after promulgation of the new marriage law in 1980. In contrast, births outside plan would contribute to the resurgence by an estimated 30 per cent only.[88] Other leaders of the Birth-Planning Commission pointed out that growing migration and special permits for second births were additional reasons for the rise in birth numbers. They too insisted that lax birth control contributed only one third to the unexpected growth of birth numbers.[89]

Fifteen months later, the opponents of liberalization were viewing things quite differently. In their opinion, the age structure of the population contributed to the resurgence of births by only 17 per cent, while political mistakes were responsible for the rest.[90] Such global accusations in turn were not accepted by the advocates of extended second-child permits. In their analyses, they cited a multitude of other causes for the rise of the birth rate. Foremost among them were special liberties for the national minorities enjoying much greater concessions than Chinese peasants at large, the lowering of the average marriage age, the decrease in birth intervals, and lax control of medical certificates and documents required for second-child applications. The growing intricacies of birth planning as well as the widespread falsification of statistical reports were cited as further reasons.

For one, the numerous additions to the list of causes for the breach of population targets demonstrate the complexity of Chinese birth planning, but of course, they also serve a political function. For while it was mainly the Birth-Planning Commission that had to take responsibility for raising the share of second-child births, marriage registration and medical certificates, minority policy and statistics were within the jurisdiction of other departments. More recent analyses have vindicated the liberal position. A study of birth rate changes between 1984 and 1987 attributes 47 per cent of the increase to unfavourable changes in age structure, while it appropriates 27 per cent of the blame to the decrease in marriage age, and only 18 per cent to a rise in marital fertility; another calculation for the continued increase between 1986 and 1989 attributes 49 per cent to the influence of age structure, 13 per cent to the renewed decline of the marriage age and 35 per cent to a drop in marital fertility.[91] It should be mentioned, however, that these computations employ base figures that have been revised ever since due to the resurfacing of non-registered births.

However, in late 1986 the Birth-Planning Commission had to face increasing pressures. At its work conference of December that year it passed a resolution according to which new regional birth-planning regulations were not to contravene national policies in the future. In January 1989 a circular repeated this admonition, urging all lower units to submit a copy of local regulations to the State Birth-Planning Commission before final promulgation.[92] Seemingly a matter of course, these resolutions once again disclose the degree to which everyday political life in China diverges from the image of a centralist, totalitarian state. Annual sample surveys on population dynamics have revealed continuous breaches of the population plan and a general loss of control since 1986, with the micro-census of July 1987 resulting in the same conclusion.[93] As of today, we know that this was a false alarm, for the shares of second and higher order births had exceeded the projected levels already at an earlier date. Higher parity births in particular did not register the decline envisaged by the promoters of second-child permits, leading to the accusation that in allowing second births the liberals had obtained third ones.[94]

When these developments caught the attention of the government, it reacted with a series of new regulations and decrees. In 1987 new birth-planning rules were issued for all problem groups of the population: the fast-rising numbers of the self-employed in trade and small industries, the allegedly rapidly increasing number of migrants with births outside plan and peasants in backward areas not respecting the legal age limit for marriages.[95] Moreover, high-ranking politicians began to concern themselves with the organizational problems of birth planning. An example is the wife of former State President Li Xiannian, who, at the April 1987 session of the National People's Congress, put on record her demands for budgetary increases, more cadre recruitment and wage raises for the Birth-Planning Commissions.[96]

However, the controversy continued as to how to treat second-child applications in the future. In his speech before the first conference of directors of regional birth-planning bureaux convened in May 1987 after the fall of former Party General-Secretary Hu Yaobang, Wang Wei repeated his view that the resurgence of birth numbers was quite normal, caused primarily by the age structure of the population, namely the large numbers of young people entering marriageable and reproductive age. The high number of births outside plan was commented by him with the remark that 'this is not a problem of policy but rather a problem of implementation'. Against this background, the conference resolved to uphold strict one-child rules for the urban areas and to enforce more strongly the prohibition of early marriages. On the other hand, it also legitimized preparations for introducing a global second-child permit for peasant families with only one daughter that had been initiated in three provinces of the country since 1986.[97]

But these decisions did not result in a resolution of the controversy. It took only two months to demonstrate that differences of opinion endured among the leadership. Zhao Ziyang, who rose to Party General-Secretary after the demise of Hu Yaobang, issued a new directive on the continuing debate concerning the question of, whether the resurgence of birth numbers was caused by the relaxation of the 1.2 billion population target for 2000, or whether it was due to the policy of 'the small hole'. In his directive of 22 July 1987 he stated:

> Neither the 'circa 1.2 billion' nor the 'small hole' are the crux of the problem. However, the current reincrease of the birth rate must be taken seriously, and present policies must be applied thoroughly. Higher-order births, early marriages, and early pregnancies must be solved. Indeed, there now are some places where policies are lax, and things drift without direction. This must be corrected.[98]

While this directive supported the course charted by Wang Wei in May 1987, Chang Chongxuan, the Deputy Minister of the State Birth-Planning Commission, clearly deviated from the position of his superior. In July 1987 he declared:

> While upper levels discuss whether second-child permits for one-daughter families are suitable or not, second births have become prevalent at the grass roots, and higher-order births are increasing everywhere. ... Not relaxation but rather restriction is the order of the day.[99]

A conference chaired by Chang urged that the 1.2 billion population limit for 2000 should be respected by all means. Special permits for second births should not be widely issued for a whole township but rather restricted to individual villages only.[100] A joint circular of the Birth-Planning Commission, the Ministry of Civil Administration, the Ministry of Justice and the Women's Federation issued in December 1987 urged a large-scale campaign against early marriages, which were said to have reached an average level of 15 to 20 per cent in rural areas.[101]

But even this did not end the controversy. Opinions on the question whether it would be both possible and advisable to comply with the 1.2 billion population target for 2000 must have raged back and forth, as in December 1987 Wang Wei requested new instructions from Party General-Secretary Zhao Ziyang. He again posed the question of, whether target numbers in the population plan should be interpreted as recommendations or as fixed upper limits. Zhao Ziyang replied: 'Isn't the formulation circa 1.2 billion? In general, "circa" means approximately 5 per cent.' Wang Wei used this instruction to stipulate that in future no maximum numbers for second-child permits need be laid down. In public and non-public pronouncements, his commission began to calculate with alternative target numbers, ranging from 1.23 billion to more than 1.30 billion in 2000.[102] Many provinces followed suit and in 1987 raised their population targets for the year 2000.[103] The need to comply with the population targets of the seventh five-year plan was thereby whittled down more and more. In their internal statements, many participants in the debate welcomed this state of affairs, since they felt frustrated by 'unreliable statistics', 'insufficient estimates' and 'too restrictive plan targets'.[104]

In January 1988 the long simmering conflict finally came out into the open. In an article published in the Party newspaper, the advocates of hard-line one-child policies berated an irresponsible increase of both authorized and non-authorized second births, the counter-productive consequences of decollectivization, and the decreasing effect of penalty payments that were voluntarily paid by peasants in line with the motto 'Let's spend some money to buy a son'. The hard-liners' vehemently proclaimed appeal in favour of keeping the original targets provoked the dismissal of Wang Wei a week later. He was replaced by the new minister Peng Peiyun, the daughter of conservative Party elder Peng Zhen, as head of the State Birth-Planning Commission. This was the third change of personnel in this position within a few years. Because of its direct political impact and its extraordinarily frank line of reasoning, the article deserves to be quoted at length. The following passages summed up the paradigmatic approach of the hard-liners:

> If natural increase will not be reduced, China's population will grow to 1.285 billion or even more by the turn of the century. One wrong move, and the game is lost. ... Frankly, the one-child rule is no absolute truth. But we have to hold fast to it in view of the critical situation in population growth. It is a policy in accord with the overall interest of the state. We have no other choice.
>   It is both sensible and reasonable to concede a favorable treatment to families in difficulties and to grant them permission for two children. This

is a special measure, documenting our desire to gradually improve birth planning. But the crux of the problem is, when and how to grant this favorable treatment. If it is conferred on the peak of a birth wave, and if no measures for effective birth control are adopted at the grass roots, many problems will ensue.[105]

Six weeks later, China's second important national daily followed in step. In an article on 'The crisis of birth planning' it declared:

> It is surprising that the one-child policy, which is of far-reaching importance for the national economy and the living standard of the population, has been breached on upper levels. And this has happened even against the remonstrations of some demographers. What an important role the interference of cadres can play! In the majority of rural areas, this breach of policy has not only fostered many second births but also higher-order births. ... Population growth outside plan amounted to 3.35 million in 1986. Among this number, only 0.6 million were attributable to changes of the population age structure, while the breach of birth-planning policy must be blamed for the rest, more than two million.[106]

Many readers must have realized that the power behind the dismissed minister Wang Wei was no less than Party General-Secretary Zhao Ziyang, who had endorsed the relaxation of birth planning. During a meeting of the Standing Committee of the Politburo convened at the end of March 1988 for a resolution of the dispute, Zhao successfully resisted new qualifications for second-child permits. He is said to have expressly supported the eligibility of peasants with only one daughter for such permits. The minutes of this meeting were later circulated as a guideline document within the birth-planning bureaucracy. The carefully thought-out phrases display some of the difficulties of reaching a consensus between the opposing arguments. The minutes stated:

> With the exception of specially exempted cases, cadres, workers and staff in the state sector, as well as other urban inhabitants, are allowed one child only; in the countryside, persons in real difficulties, including households having only one daughter and desiring a second child, may give birth to a second child, provided proper permission is obtained and an interval of some years is respected; third births are allowed under no circumstances.[107]

But even the many legal provisos of these carefully crafted clauses could not reconcile the opposing views. Peng Peiyun thought herself in line with the Politburo when she declared at an international population conference in Beijing: 'Rural couples with only one daughter are allowed a second child, provided they respect a planned birth interval.' Although the government's English-language *China Daily* printed a verbatim record of this statement, the legitimization of families' preference for sons was censored by the Party organ. In the report in the *People's Daily* on Peng Peiyun's speech, the relevant passage read: 'Rural couples who are in difficulties and desire a second birth are allowed a second child, provided they respect an interval of some years and the plan.'[108] The censors could refer to the government report of Premier Li Peng, presented to the National People's Congress one week before the meeting of the Standing Committee of the Politburo. Although Li Peng had used Zhao Ziyang's controversial formula of 'circa 1.2 billion at the turn of the century' in his report, he also added: 'Preferential conditions for rural families in real difficulties must be handled in a strict way.'[109]

A few days later, Peng Peiyun alluded once again to the continuing controversies. Speaking to the directors of regional birth-planning bureaux, she referred to the various alternative policies discussed in the small circle of the five senior Party leaders:

> Some people feel that it has been wrong to 'open a small hole'. They think this was just 'the will of some high cadres' not in accord with realities . . . . Other comrades feel that it would be best to generally permit second births in accord with the wishes of the masses. This would be also much easier to implement than just opening a hole for families with only one daughter. Although such arguments have their merits, we cannot yet put them into practice. I reported to the meeting [of the Standing Committee of the Politburo] on 31 March. Judging from the experiences with some local trial procedures, the results of a policy of late marriages with extended birth spacing were good – no matter if they involved advanced localities like Yicheng County in Shanxi or lagging places like Xinrong district in Datong City. Work should only be carried out in a strict and careful way. Some comrades therefore had proposed to implement such experiments on a larger scale. I asked the Central Committee for their consent. But the clear answer of the leading comrades of the Central Committee was that an extension of second-child experiments would not be advantageous right now, as we presently do not yet grasp whether population development can be controlled by permitting second births . . . .
>
> If the majority of peasants does not accept it, it is hard to realize our policy, or it cannot be realized at all. Peasants, including lower-level village cadres, can devise many countermeasures against us. This would not only lead to a deterioration of relations between the Party and the masses – it would also frustrate the goal of constraining population growth. On the meeting of 31 March, some leading comrades of the Central Committee have repeatedly raised this point.[110]

These comments of the highest Party organ touched on many sensitive areas of the one-child policy. It revealed the general unpopularity of birth control among both the peasants and the cadres responsible for implementation. Furthermore, the comments testified to the far-reaching influence of the alternatives to the one-child policy formulated by Chinese experts since the early 1980s and supported by the New York-based Population Council in late 1985. As it turned out, the experiments with a policy of late marriage and extended birth spacing that inspired Peng Peiyun's positive comments conformed precisely to the suggestions of some Chinese population experts who continue to maintain their long-held criticism of the one-child policy to this day. The Yicheng experiment was begun in July 1985 during the Hu Yaobang era and has been extremely contentious. Its advocates have commended it for reducing fertility, avoiding the negative side-effects of the one-child policy, and diminishing antagonism between the Party and the peasantry. But it has also evoked strong opposition. Hard-liners have doubted its transferability, denounced it for promoting laxness in birth control and associated it with the resurgence of fertility during the mid-1980s.[111]

In view of the clashing arguments and the daunting complexities of population development, even the highest Party organ preferred to temporize and to refrain from taking an unambiguous stand. While it refused to grant a global second-child permit to peasants, it still legitimized the continuation of the new experiments initiated by Wang Wei in 1984. Just as telling for the style of political controversies in China are the great liberties of interpretation taken by the provinces in defining the extent of local experiments with expanded second-child permits. In 1986, nine provinces authorized such permits for peasant families with only one daughter. One year later, the list had grown to include fourteen provinces; six provinces went even further and granted permission to any peasant respecting the required birth interval. In many cases, the 'local limitation' of experiments had grown to involve a whole province. The Birth-Planning Commission adopted a contradictory course. While principally supporting the continuation of trial policies in a circular of May 1988, it cut down the number of centrally endorsed experimental counties to thirteen, leaving the provinces with the choice to prolong the other experiments on their own.[112]

Such conflicting signals produced confusion at grass-roots level. A circular of high-level army authorities dated August 1988 is revealing in this regard. Referring to the minutes of the meeting of the Standing Committee of the Politburo, it contained the following statement:

> We have to put up some action against the widespread feeling of the cadres and masses that 'policies have become relaxed' and 'control measures have softened'. All have to clearly recognize that the resurgence of the birth rate during the last two years has not been caused by present policies.[113]

Equally revealing are the minutes from the meeting of the Shandong Birth-Planning Commission in July 1988:

> Some committee members proposed to revoke the former rules on second-child permits for all rural couples with only one daughter, since this would constitute a big gap. But in view of the fact that this policy has been enacted for years and has been confirmed by the center, it was not changed during the revision of rules. However, in the process of implementation all loopholes must be closed.[114]

However, the worst was yet to come. In addition to permanent controversies among the top leadership and motivational problems at grass-roots level, Chinese birth planners were also plagued by growing corruption and falsification of statistical reports. Even more devastating were the results of a new sample survey on population fertility, organized by the Birth-Planning Commission in mid-1988. It confirmed the extraordinarily large extent of under-registration in the records of the birth-planning authorities. According to the first summary conclusions of Peng Peiyun in November 1988, in five provinces this under-registration amounted to up to 5 per cent of all births, in three provinces it increased from 10 to 20 per cent, in six provinces from 20 to 30 per cent, in thirteen provinces from 30 to 40 per cent, and in two provinces it surpassed even that level.[115]

It therefore came as no surprise that a new joint circular of the State Birth-Planning Commission and the Central Committee's Propaganda Department in late 1988 once again spoke of a 'crisis of birth planning'. The leading cadre responsible for birth-planning legislation in the National People's Congress illustrated the extent of this crisis by outlining eight major problem areas: rural births outside plan; lagging birth planning among the urban self-employed; illegitimate children of unmarried partners and couples under the legal marriage age; lack of birth control among the migrant population; erosion of economic sanctions; increasing attacks on birth-planning personnel from among the population; lack of personnel, low wages and an overload of work for the Birth-Planning Commissions; and glaring gaps in financing.[116]

This was the situation faced by seven research institutes in 1989, when they were assigned the duty of new population projections for the eighth five-year plan for the period 1991 to 1995. The projections presented by the institutes confirmed the pessimistic views on the future for birth planning in the 1990s. Most were based on the expectation that the total fertility rate would clearly surpass a level of two children per woman during the last decade of the century. Medium projections for 2000 ranged from 1.270 billion to 1.299 billion; the lowest projection amounted to 1.248 billion for that year; the worst-case scenario reached 1.323 billion.[117]

On the basis of such developments, the margins for second-child permits continued to shrink. Some areas began to backtrack on earlier promises to peasants by revoking second-child quotas and doubling fines for unauthorized births. A further meeting of the Standing Committee of the Politburo, convened on 23 February 1989 for a new discussion about birth planning, resolved to prevent unilateral action by individual provinces. On the other hand, it once again heeded a new intervention by Zhao Ziyang in favour of second-child permits for rural families with only one daughter. Advocating 'an unwavering policy ... without loosening or tightening', the Standing Committee urged 'the earnest implementation of present policies instead of policy changes'.[118] Speaking to the annual conference of directors of regional birth-planning bureaux in February 1989, Premier Li Peng called for a reconfirmation of the 1.2 billion population target for 2000.[119] Nevertheless, no answers were given to the crucial question: How to reach the old targets in view of the new birth wave and the pessimistic projections?

At least in the organizational sphere, new efforts by the Party could be demonstrated: 8,000 new cadre positions for county Birth-Planning Commissions were budgeted for in 1989. This was a major feat in a time of economic crisis that witnessed general budget cuts and a streamlining of the bureaucracy. Furthermore, the State Council decided to link future subsidies for poverty regions and relief for needy persons to birth-plan adherence of the areas or the individuals concerned.[120] At the end of March 1989, General-Secretary Zhao Ziyang finally decreed a preliminary freeze of further experiments with second-child permits. Current experiments were allowed to continue, however. If they produced good results, they could be generalized later on and serve as the basis for new legislation.[121]

These new guidelines could not alter the fact that keeping the population within a limit of 1.2 billion by 2000 would be outright impossible. At the end of 1988, twenty-five provinces had already breached their population targets of the seventh five-year plan. This was a cruel blow for the Party, which for many years had gone all out to stage propaganda campaigns for adherence to these population limits. During a new plenary session of the National People's Congress in March 1989, Premier Li Peng wriggled out of the dilemma in time-honoured fashion. He simply did not mention population targets in his government report. At a forum of regional Party leaders held a week later, he explained his new understanding of the situation as follows: although the 1.20 billion limit for 2000 should be reconfirmed, it could be interpreted as 1.25 billion. Li Peng was certainly not unhappy with the attitude of the majority of delegates to the People's Congress who deleted a reference to second-child permits for peasant families with only one daughter from his government report. He emphasized that such permits would not be granted automatically but rather had to be based on written applications and well-founded reasons.[122] Shortly after, this did not prevent Politburo member Tian Jiyun, a politician close to Zhao Ziyang, from publicly reiterating second-child permits for rural families with only one daughter.[123]

It would have been logical to expect that the Tian'anmen crisis of June 1989 and the consequent fall of Zhao Ziyang would put an end to the controversy. However, instead of a return to the hard-line one-child policies of the early 1980s, the stalemate continued. Minister for Birth Planning Peng Peiyun used the annual summer meetings of China's leaders in the sea resort of Beidaihe for opposing any attempts to use the demise of Zhao Ziyang in attacks on rural second-child permits. Her pertinent remarks are recorded for 25 July 1989. At the 5th Plenary Session of the 13th Central Committee of the Party in October 1989, however, the Minister at least verbally gave ground to the hard-liners. She reported that henceforth the term 'second-child permits for families in real difficulties' should replace the formula of permits for 'rural families with only one daughter'.[124]

5.5 Law and order: the administration 1990 to 1999

Peng Peiyun's wish to insulate birth planning from the policy changes provoked by the Tian'anmen events was not fulfilled. Instead, the advocates of tough one-child policies used the 5th National Conference of the Association for Population Studies in January 1990 to stage violent attacks on the extended second-child permits authorized by Zhao Ziyang and Wang Wei. The camp of hard-liners comprised control theorists, cadres of the planning authorities, and representatives of the legislative and juridical system who complained about the high number of excess births during the seventh five-year plan. The measures advocated by them for coping with the alleged population crisis have been carried out to a remarkable degree. They constitute the core of the administrative strategy that characterizes Chinese birth planning since 1990.[125]

The following proposals were presented by the hard-line critics: (1) introduction of new laws and guidelines for planning procedures, eugenics, marriage registration and migration; (2) regular cadre evaluations for monitoring the enforcement of regulations and the correctness of statistics; (3) more birth-control propaganda in the media, and in literature and art; (4) a population tax with high social fees for above-quota births, a light taxation of authorized second births, and tax holidays for one-child families; (5) the extension of rural old-age support, preferential production credits and allocations for peasant one-child families; (6) a definite break with the widespread rural practice of increased land allotments and housing plots for all new-born children, no matter whether they were born with or without permission; (7) more recruitment of birth-planning personnel, budgetary increases, wage raises and bonuses for the birth-planning authorities; (8) a large-scale development of citizens' birth-planning associations; (9) clear-cut rules for IUD insertions and sterilizations, as well as additional research efforts for long-term contraceptives. Finally, the critics called for a new Open Letter of the Central Committee in order to counter the symptoms of disintegration in birth planning.[126]

Even more far-reaching proposals had been made a year before, when some Chinese authors openly professed to 'the necessity of coercion and control' in birth planning, urging the establishment of a 'population police', 'population courts' and severe punishment for determined violators of policy. The instigators of these proposals could not hide their despair, however, since at the same time they suggested a return to the old two-child policy. Only third and higher-order births should be resolutely prevented.[127] When judicial personnel was delegated to birth-planning bureaus in 1993, and the Northeastern port city of Dalian took measures against migrants and evaders of birth control by charging 60,000 spare-time members of the Public Security Committees at the neighbourhood level with work as birth-control informants, the visions of a 'population police' came near to fulfilment. Since the mid-1990s similar arrangements and increasingly harsh surveillance measures have been introduced in other areas of the country, too.[128]

However, as opposed to the proposals mentioned above, these steps were coupled with strictness rather than leniency. Discarding a return to two-child policies and meeting the demands of the hard-liners, on 12 May 1991 the Party's Central Committee and the State Council passed a new resolution on strengthening birth planning. They opposed any vacillations, reconfirmed the general validity of the one-child norm, and emphasized again that exemptions were to be granted only for peasants 'in real difficulties'. Furthermore, the Central Committee and the State Council stipulated a tighter control of population statistics, the final introduction of a responsibility system for birth planning, as well as the strict implementation of all regulations and rules, together with the concomitant incentives and sanctions.[129]

Further reasons for the hardening of China's official population policy were furnished by the new population count of July 1990. To quote a census official, 'it served a caution to China'.[130] First trend signals of the approaching census results had already appeared, for sample surveys indicated that the sensitive cohorts of women in the age group 20–29 would increase by more than 16 per cent during the new five-year plan period. Due to this age structure, a new peak period of births was expected for the mid-1990s.[131]

Special problems for the Birth-Planning Commission have been created by the blatantly defective data of the statistical report system. This is why new attempts at improving data quality have been initiated since February 1990. These include disciplinary punishments of cadres responsible for data falsification, investigations to detect faked medical operations, the development of new information systems, random checks of report numbers, and the public display of second-child permits in order to instigate social control of applicants claiming difficulties in circumstances. Other measures were a drive for the computerized evaluation of population data and a decree of April 1991 that henceforth all lower administrative units were to report projections of their annual birth-control indicators by the middle of the year.[132] A network of anonymous informants for the surveillance of lower echelon birth-planning cadres has also been tested.

Rule by law and regulation is another core element of present strategy. Most newly revised birth-planning regulations of the 1990s have extended the permission requirement to the birth of the first child too. Between March 1990 and December 1991, six new administrative regulations on aspects of birth planning were promulgated at national level, documenting an ever tighter net of rules and procedures for the enforcement of population policy. These regulations covered birth-planning statistics (March 1990), the propagation of new contraceptive methods (July 1990), the establishment of birth-planning stations (July 1990), medical certificates for illness or disabledness of single children (September 1990), general procedures of population planning (February 1991), and special aspects of birth control among the migrant population (December 1991).[133] They were augmented by a large number of new intra-agency rules on procedural and administrative matters, plus a multitude of additional documents covering such areas as rewards and sanctions, insurance policies, fine collection or file handling at provincial, city and county level. A new joint circular of the Birth-Planning Commission and a number of other ministries, dated September 1992, was directed against the continuing high number of marriages below the legal age.[134]

Many of these regulations touch on areas characterized by a quagmire of corruption, falsification and misuse of power. It was in this context that in February 1990 Peng Peiyun mentioned faked medical operations, forged medical certificates, misuse of birth-planning appropriations, falsified statistics and unauthorized permits for second births. A joint circular of the Supreme Court and the Chief Procuracy of November 1993 added violence towards birth-planning cadres to this list and detailed the legal basis for prosecution according to criminal law.[135]

The passing of laws on the protection of children and on adoption in September and December 1991, on the protection of women's rights in April 1992, and on eugenics in October 1994, as well as the amendment of nearly all provincial birth-planning regulations between 1990 and 1997, must be seen in the same context.[136] All revisions aimed to tighten birth control by closing loopholes, raise penalties, strengthen controls, specify administrative obligations and powers, and introduce new rules for financial management. They also contained largely standardized additional passages on birth control among the migrant population and on eugenics. Already, in December 1993, a draft file was drawn up for provisions against unwanted births, banning all mentally or physically disabled persons with hereditary diseases from having 'inferior-quality births'. When a revised text was formally adopted in October 1994 under the title 'Law on Maternal and Infant Health Care', the relevant passages were reformulated in a more moderate version. But the right of the state remained to prohibit unwanted reproduction, to make marriages of affected persons dependent on prior sterilization, to introduce compulsory medical check-ups during pregnancy, and to press for an abortion in relevant cases. Recent judicial literature from China has enlarged on this topic and begun to discuss euthanasia for offspring already born but unfit to survive on their own.[137]

While such such developments signal the ascendancy of hard-line policies, other areas of legislation have seen a more flexible stance. A prominent case is the promulgation of national birth-planning regulations, which in 1990 had already passed through the stages of seven drafts before they were postponed once again by order of the Central Committee. Arguing that uniform regulations for the whole country would not adequately reflect China's regional diversity, liberal forces held their ground on this front. Since the cancellation of a birth-planning law for the People's Republic of China in 1980 and 1988, this was the third failure of attempts to amalgamate Chinese birth-planning rules. Nevertheless, attempts at pushing through more unified rules under a 'Law on Population and Birth Planning' have been stepped up in 1999. Altogether, the various initiatives for national birth-planning codification lasted for twenty-three years and produced forty different draft texts. The law was to be finally promulgated in December 2001. It stabilized present policies without relaxing or tightening them further.[138] In the same vein, it is conspicuous that a new campaign in favour of late marriage, added implementation rules for the marriage law of September 1992 and February 1994, as well as a project for revising the marriage law underway since 2000, have not raised the legal marriage age again. This has been a demand of hard-line politicians for many years.[139]

With the decision to raise the birth-planning budget from an annual 1 yuan per capita to 2 yuan by 1995, the Central Committee and State Council reacted to intensive lobbying by the Birth-Planning Commission. Starting in August 1990, Peng Peiyun and her deputy Chang Chongxuan had repeatedly urged this step in order to close gaps in birth control and to secure the financing of contraceptive measures for the large cohorts of young women.[140] The additional appropriations served to enlarge the recruitment of birth-planning personnel, to finance wage rises, bonuses and better social security benefits for birth-planning cadres. They were also used to create birth-planning bureaux in rural towns and townships and to establish institutions for contraceptive operations at the grass-roots level. Later pledges promised to raise the standard to 4 yuan per capita by 2000 and to more than 10 yuan by 2005.[141]

A major initiative has been the large-scale extension of the Birth-Planning Association, intended to close the glaring gaps in organization and funding in the villages.[142] Such problems continue to hinder the large-scale expansion of insurance payments for one-child families that are used to cover old-age security, health risks and greater liabilities in the raising of children. Until October 1992, 15.68 million persons were at least partially protected by this type of insurances. Due to efforts by the Birth-Planning Association and the Ministry of Civil Administration, their numbers had increased to 45 million in 1995 and 82 million in 1998. Similar objectives have been pursued through the attempt to involve the State Birth-Planning Commission, the ministries of agriculture, forestry and water conservancy, and five other national organizations in joint assistance schemes for one-child families. During recent years, this has been a major theme in birth-planning propaganda.[143]

Further steps have also been taken to tighten birth planning among China's national minorities, but a conference convened in June 1992 to discuss this issue had to recognize the sensitivity of the matter. Not only had the distinctly different living conditions in minority areas to be taken into account, but China's leaders also needed to consider the fact that policies adopted in emulation of the stringent regulations for Han-Chinese regions would re-enforce anti-Chinese sentiments and might provoke open rebellion. The conference therefore recommended a cautious course in consideration of specific customs and religious creeds, paying particular attention to the varying financial resources of minority areas and to the question of whether border regions or inland areas were involved. Tibet Autonomous Region constitutes the most critical case for testing this policy mix. In 1992, the region stipulated the first clear birth-planning rules for the Tibetan population at large. Although these are stricter than antecedents from 1986, the paragraphs on fertility control for Tibetans are still more favourable than most other birth-planning regulations and contain a number of escape clauses for special groups.[144]

The perfecting of responsibility systems for birth-planning cadres has occupied a particularly prominent place in present strategy. Experiments with such methods have taken place since the early 1980s. They received a further push when in December 1991 the Ministry of Personnel and the Organization Department of the Central Committee issued a joint circular that urged turning investigations of birth-control performance into an integral part of the regular cadre evaluations. Since then, a system of written commitments has been further extended. Although the precise terms of such commitments differ locally, the system always implies collective liabilities of village communities and grass-roots cadres for the birth-planning performance of private households. Parallel procedures for urban areas make enterprise managers personally accountable for birth planning among their employees. Higher cadres have also been obliged to pledge their personal responsibility for birth planning by signing written commitments. Furthermore, new organizational arrangements have been taken in order to solve problems of coordination between the birth-planning commissions and other departments. As a rule, the First Party Secretary of an administrative unit is forced to assume personal responsibility for such coordination and all work related to birth control.[145] Last but not least, cadres with non-authorized offspring are increasingly meted out disciplinary punishments in public.

While coverage of these measures in press reports and specialized journals has been more or less detailed, information on another subject has been mute. However, in studying relevant statistics and insinuations made in official statements, there can be no doubt that another campaign in favour of IUD insertions, sterilizations and abortions was waged in 1991 after the disappointing results of the fourth population census. It seems that this new campaign was decided by a birth-planning conference held in April 1991. Another meeting, convened in August 1992, confirmed that the previous year had seen the highest number of contraceptive operations and abortions since 1983. Furthermore, in 1991, the leadership did not hesitate to commit the cultural atrocity of sterilizations for couples with only one daughter. This clear tightening of the previous practice of compulsory sterilization only after the second child became particularly prevalent in Shandong, Jiangxi, Guangdong, Guizhou, Shaanxi and Gansu provinces with their high fertility levels.[146] One year later, however, the campaign appears to have fizzled out due to lack of financial resources.

There can be no doubt that these new initiatives imply a tightening of birth control since 1990. Political semantics also reveal the backsliding in hard-line positions when the slogan 'Open a small hole to close a big gap', which served as the motto of relaxed birth control in the 1980s, disappeared.[147] None the less, it has been only a qualified victory for the advocates of a strict one-child policy, who were forced to accept that the 1.2 billion population limit for the year 2000 had to be revoked. They were also unable to stage the desired roll-back of existing second-child permits. It is worth noting that in defence of their position the promoters of these permits also quote the Central Committee's and State Council's injunctions against any vacillations. Finally, the hard-liners have to live with the fact that China's academic journals continue to publish opinions drawing quite different conclusions from the 'special conditions of China': not the verdict that strict birth control is unavoidable but rather the belief that the one-child policy simply does not square with Chinese conditions.[148]

Such sentiments convey the impression that to a certain extent hard-line one-child policies are kept in suspense. Above all, concerns for domestic stability have motivated the concessions of the leadership. Speaking to a demographic symposium organized during November 1991 after the fall of the communist regimes in Eastern Europe, Peng Peiyun confessed that their demise contained the following lesson: the Party should never be divorced from the masses; only democratic procedures and educational work were permissible.[149] Innumerable studies published in China's demographic journals also hint at other factors diminishing the clout of the state: old-style controls simply do not work any more, since they are eroded by the increasing mobility within the country. Major factors contributing to this situation are the increasing number of discharges in the state sector and enterprise reforms that weaken direct chains of command, a growing population mobility, a rising number of self-employed and private-sector employees, as well as divorces, second marriages and non-registered, informal unions. Present policies therefore amount to a compromise. Flexibility and exemptions from the one-child norm are combined with strictness in the implementation of relevant regulations. Ambiguous points of the second-child rules tend to be interpreted in a narrow way, while sanctions for unauthorized births increase.

This combination of a reinforcement of birth control with a continuing de-control of economic and social affairs has produced a volatile situation. Whereas the age structure of the population and the high fertility levels of the late 1980s led politicians to expect a new wave of births in the early 1990s,[150] the birth rate in 1991 suddenly dropped conspicuously. Even more dramatic has been the abrupt decline of the more indicative total fertility rate, whose current level of supposedly 1.4 (unadjusted) to 1.8 (officially adjusted) children per woman has outperformed former calculations and reached the lowest national average ever recorded in China. Some local progress reports outdo even these calculations, and boast of a drop to 0.7 in 1993 and an average 1.0 between 1991 and 1995.[151] These unprecedented lows have been accompanied by equally unprecedented highs in the sex proportion at birth. Figures for missing infant girls have been such that in 1992 and 1993 the centre felt prompted to convene another national conference on this subject and to circulate a new round of directives prohibiting prenatal sex determination and infanticide. Even former Premier Li Peng has found it necessary to include the topic in his recent pronouncements on population policy.[152]

It is not altogether clear whether the abnormal fertility figures of recent years reflect a decreasing number of births or an increasing number of concealed deliveries. Some initial sighs of relief are heard. In 1995, the Chairman of the Birth-Planning Association, former Politburo member Song Ping, has been quoted as saying, 'the Hardship Number One Under Heaven is already not as hard any more'.[153] And yet, most ranking politicians such as Jiang Zemin, Li Peng and Peng Peiyun have thought it necessary to warn against ill-founded optimism and statistical falsification. The persisting gap between state regulations and peasant birth preferences, as well as the great regional imbalances, have given them cause for further worries. Time and again, they have spoken of an 'unstable' situation, pointing to the danger that fertility could resurge immediately once birth control slackens. This is coupled with the sober assessment that despite all public emphasis on propaganda, education and economic incentives, 'birth control in the villages is still mainly relying on forceful administrative measures'.[154]

Under these circumstances, drafting target numbers for the eighth five-year plan for the period 1991 to 1995 and for the mid-term perspective until 2000 has been demanding. Plan formulation, which commenced in 1990, was delayed until late 1991 in order to incorporate the results of the fourth population census. When target figures were transmitted to the provinces in January 1992, they conformed to Central Committee proposals of December 1990 and were based on natural increase by an average 1.25 per cent between 1991 and 2000. This corresponds to an average total fertility rate of 2.08 over the decade (falling from 2.26 in 1991 to 1.92 in 2000) and a population total of 1.294 billion at the turn of the century.[155] It remains noticeable that the raised upper limit of 1.3 billion is now accepted. But in April 1991, Party chief Jiang Zemin spoke of the real danger that even this number could be breached. One year later, the then Minister of Birth Planning Peng Peiyun repeated that it would be of great benefit if the population could be kept within this limit.[156]

Official population figures from the period 1991 to 1995, however, indicate that the last five-year plan has been overfulfilled by a wide margin. Instead of an average 1.42 per cent as planned, annual natural increase went down to 1.16 per cent. Starting in 1993, annual plan figures were continuously revised downward. Projections for the ninth five-year plan work with an average natural increase of 1.08 per cent between 1996 and 2000. Conspicuously enough, a lengthy programme for birth control in the period 1995 to 2000 contained few precise figures and did not adjust the absolute target figure for 2000.[157] This betrays continuing uneasiness about the reliability of population data.

And the leadership is not relenting. Party chief Jiang Zemin, former Premier Li Peng and ex-minister Peng Peiyun have opposed all calls for a change in policies. They have repeatedly warned against believing in a relaxation of population pressures and relying on a spontaneous decline of birth numbers in the course of economic development. All recent birth-planning symposia of the Central Committee and the State Council have been used to repeat such statements in public. In 1996 a national birth-planning conference combined them with the admonition that birth-planning cadres should prepare for a resurgence of fertility, once women forced to respect a longer birth interval started to deliver their second children.[158] Again, such statements reveal the continuing existence of a hidden dispute about the one-child campaign. At the same time, they document the treacherousness of the data situation, the paramount importance of perception and interpretation. Low population figures can be just as intractable as high ones.

Part III
Bureaucratic implementation

6 Legal norms and practice in flux

6.1 Channels, types and rhythm of birth-control norms

Since 1979, Chinese Party and state organs have issued a multitude of instructions and regulations on birth planning.[1] In many cases these build on much shorter, less systematic and less numerous rules promulgated in preceding decades. During the entire period from the beginning of the first birth-planning campaign in 1954 to the start of the one-child policy in 1979, the average province issued only some four to five documents with overall birth-planning guidelines. Whereas in the 1950s these mostly pertained to rules for contraceptive use and surgery, in the 1960s and 1970s they laid down the increasingly stringent state demands for late marriage and limited childbearing.

However, there are significant similarities between the earlier and later eras: in both periods no national birth-planning regulations for the whole of China were ever passed. Already in the 1960s the Party began to supersede state organs as the prime actor in birth-control matters, sharing the authorship of many documents with provincial governments or revolutionary committees and reserving for itself the right of approval. Another legacy which had enduring repercussions until the end of the 1980s was the informal character of most former documents, which were transmitted as directives, circulars or opinions from higher levels. Only rarely did the leadership find it suitable to issue more precise rules; it often refrained from publishing its various decrees; and it never bothered to involve legislative organs in its deliberations.

Until the late 1980s, most central directives and provincial regulations have thus been circulating in internal documentary literature only. Since then, provincial birth-planning regulations formally passed by the legislatures, plus a growing number of executive decrees, have also been publicly issued, but because many details of implementation continue to be delegated to lower levels, information on a number of aspects is patchy. Although the State Birth-Planning Commission tries to keep abreast of sub-provincial birth-planning rules, it holds no complete file of local norms for perusal. The frequent change of norms in the 1980s and 1990s has caused considerable problems. In a number of instances, alterations instigated by central government have been implemented by the provinces after a considerable time lag. On the other hand, some new policies originating at the province level have been enacted there in advance of new nationwide rulings. Crucial issues pertaining to second-child permits, the incentive system and the types of sanction applied have been the reserve of the Beijing authorities, however. It can be documented that all incisive policy changes at national level have involved decisions of the Central Committee Secretariat, with the most basic guidelines flowing right from the highest Party organ, the Standing Committee of the Politburo.

In view of their limited financial power, their lack of control and their incomplete understanding of the extremely varying local conditions, the central organs are shrewd enough to grant large margins for action to subordinate authorities. This imbues many central directives with an aura of diffuseness, ambiguity and imprecision, thereby creating wide latitude for different interpretations. Many central documents such as the Open Letter of the Central Committee of September 1980, the various circulars issued in the internal Party and government literature, the March 1988 Minutes of the Standing Committee of the Politburo, or the joint decisions of the Central Committee and the State Council of May 1991 all display these characteristics. These documents convey the 'spirit' of birth planning prevailing at the time. Its codification in exact and unified legal norms at national level has been tried in vain. Between 1978 and 1990, this led to three failed attempts to promulgate national birth-planning norms. It took another eleven years to ratify a Law on Population and Birth Planning in December 2001. Containing only broad guidelines, it once again delegates the power to pass specific rules on the one-child policy and exemptions for a second child to the provincial level.

For many years, provincial birth-planning norms were available only as 'views', provisional rules or circulars of leading bodies. This resulted in the preliminary nature and contradictory character of many rulings, once again creating widely exploited margins for interpretation. Circulating the 'views' of a provincial Party Committee in written form usually commands the force of an order. However, with the lapse of time it becomes unclear if the original 'views' are still being held or have changed. Sometimes, even the centre seems to be puzzled and ill informed. Occasional discrepancies between the record of provincial rules and their summary listing in central documents thus hint at lack of coordination or instances of disagreement between the authorities.

A further enduring characteristic of provincial documents has been the frequent co-authorship of Party and state organs. This again demonstrates the outstanding role played by the Party in birth planning not only at national but also at regional level. It is a result of the repeated admonition from Beijing that the Party's First Secretaries should be personally responsible for birth planning at all levels. In contrast to many other policy arenas in the economic and social sphere, the Party has by no means withdrawn from operational involvement in birth planning.

The highest degree of codification is evinced by the birth-planning regulations and the earlier birth-planning rules, which were promulgated largely in provisional form. The first provisional rules date from the early 1960s and 1970s. With the beginning of the one-child campaign in 1979 codification became an increasingly important affair. During the first months of that year,

Guangdong, Tianjin and Anhui provinces played a vanguard role. The centre, however, recognized only the unpublished rules from Guangdong and Tianjin as model statutes. Altogether, twenty-seven provinces are supposed to have issued birth-planning rules in 1979.[2] In comparison to later documents, these are still brief and with a low degree of legal formalism; but, compared to the earlier period they already evince an elaborate system of restrictions, incentives and sanctions that did not exist before. In this respect, they clearly betray overall guidance by the central organs in Beijing.

Only a small number of new rules was issued in the two following years. It needed yet another intervention from the centre to spur the drafting of birth-planning norms. After Document No. 11 with new birth-planning directives from the Central Committee and the State Council was transmitted in February 1982, nearly all provinces promulgated newly revised rules or regulations. Most of these date from March to June 1982, and codification activities slowed down thereafter. Document No. 7 of April 1984 ushered in a new round of activities. Again, the majority of provinces reacted to it with revised rules and regulations. In those cases where no new norms were issued, provincial circulars detailed additional clauses to original rules. The years 1985 and 1986 saw an uninterrupted series of new rules and regulations, too. Between the end of 1988 and the end of 1991, the number of provinces that had elevated their provisional documents to the stage of formal birth-planning regulations had finally grown from sixteen to twenty-eight. The presently valid birth-planning regulations were issued in 1989 at the earliest; most date from the period 1995 to 1997, when a new wave of revisions was enacted. However, further amendments since then, and projected changes for the future, indicate that codification of birth-planning standards continues to be a process without any prolonged period of normative stability.

Terminological change from birth-planning rules (*guiding*) to regulations (*tiaoli*) documents the increasing degree of legal formalism, specification and systematization. It also mirrors different procedural avenues. Most birth-planning rules of the early 1980s were issued by provincial governments, and some were also promulgated as joint directives of provincial governments and Party committees. Revolutionary Committees, which still existed in 1979, acted as responsible organs, too. Conversely, the regulations, whose promulgation started in Guangdong in 1980 and extended to other provinces during the late 1980s, have been deliberated by the provincial People's Congresses or their standing committees. Aspiring to a greater degree of legal perfection, they have to fit into the increasingly complex framework of Chinese law. This implies compatibility with a growing body of other population laws. It also raises the issue of judicability. Judicability means, first and foremost, a sufficiently clear legal basis for applying to courts for execution of birth-control measures. Since the promulgation of a law on administrative procedure in 1989, it also includes the right of citizens to sue state organs for breach of law.

Recent provincial birth-planning regulations therefore explicitly refer to the right of citizens to appeal to higher authorities and to file suits against the birth-planning organs, if they do not accept penalty decisions. During a special conference convened by the Birth-Planning Commission in May 1990 for studying the administrative procedural law, Peng Peiyun explicitly urged leading cadres to refrain from birth-control enforcement not supported by law and to prepare for the eventuality of some suits being lost. Further regulations since the mid-1990s have detailed investigation procedures and processes for demanding compensation from birth-planning authorities that have breached the law by illegally demanding fees or penalty sums, by illegally arresting or injuring citizens, by confiscating, sealing, impounding or destroying personal possessions, or causing other unwarranted losses to private property. Special procedures for tracing personal responsibilities and obligations of birth-planning personnel have also been drawn up. An ominous note, however, is the fact that some of the procedures shift the responsibility for compensation to a higher organ once the latter organ concedes an appeal against the decision of a subordinate authority.[3]

Against this background of increasing legal sophistication, birth-planning regulations pass through a much longer process of drafting and ratification. The 1988 regulations from Liaoning province serve as an example. A first draft was circulated in February 1988 to all birth-planning commissions of cities and counties, as well as to important units directly under the provincial government. A second draft dating from March 1988 circulated among the city and county birth-planning commissions only. A third draft was then formulated by legal advisers of the provincial government and was personally introduced by the Vice-Chairman of the Provincial People's Congress on a tour through various areas of the province, where it was discussed with responsible birth-planning cadres. The discussions resulted in a fourth draft presented to the Standing Committee of the Provincial People's Congress in May 1988. Two weeks later, this draft was deliberated and ratified by a plenary session of the People's Congress. Amendments from 1992 and 1997 have been ratified by the same legislative organ. Even more complicated has been the process of legislation in Sichuan. Between 1982 and 1987, ten different drafts of birth-planning regulations circulated within that province. Twice, they were circulated for commentary to all prefectures, cities and counties, as well as to some townships of the province, and three times they were discussed at work conferences of the Provincial Birth-Planning Commission. The Standing Committee of the People's Congress of Sichuan then debated them another three times before they were finally passed in July 1987.[4]

The ratification of birth-planning regulations by the standing committees of provincial people's congresses is accompanied by the issuing of further documents, among them official explanations, reports and decisions. Explanations and reports usually contain further details on the political background of the rules, the drafting process and technical aspects of the statutes. In a number of instances, the provincial legislatures have later passed detailed implementation procedures. Between 1988 and 1991, six of the thirty provincial legislatures had added such further implementation rules to the regulations. In the majority of cases, though, they had delegated the fine-tuning to authoritative interpretations by the provincial birth-planning commissions or procedural rules at prefectural, county or township level.

Rule by executive fiat can collide with the efforts to establish a coherent system of rules that have passed through the necessary stages of legislation. Because legislation of new rules and regulations is cumbersome, provincial governments have often preferred to effect short-term policy changes by way of circulars. Such circulars have contained specifications for additional types of second-child permits, more detailed definitions for eligibility, quota ceilings for the percentage of second-child permits, or changes in the system of incentives and sanctions. In addition to issuing *ad-hoc* circulars, the provincial government can also decree supplementary rules augmenting existing norms. Recent years, however, have seen a tendency to effect major changes by way of legislated amendments. A new law passed by the Standing Committee of the Guangdong Provincial People's Congress in August 2000 marks the high point of the trend towards rule by law so far. It explicitly requires all government decisions on population matters, including adjustments of fees and charges, to obtain congressional approval before becoming effective.[5]

In this process of drafting and promulgating new norms, the birth-planning commissions clearly play only a subordinate role. If they face any new problem with long-range implications, they are required to submit their views and proposals to the Party committee in charge, which then decides to accept, reject or modify such proposals. The pre-eminent role of the Party is further demonstrated by the fact that important new proposals have also been submitted on behalf of the Party cell within the Birth-Planning Commission. If such initiatives result in official documents, these are issued as circulars of the Party committee of the appropriate administrative unit. This procedure has been adopted in the case of the Central Committee Circulars No. 7/1984 and No. 13/ 1986, and it has also been practised by birth-planning commissions within the provinces. In particular, new written clauses for second-child permits have been treated as a highly sensitive subject that always requires the Party's consent.

Powers of the birth-planning commissions are largely restricted to the interpretation and implementation of rules decided at upper levels. Precise definitions of persons eligible for second-child permits, rulings on required birth intervals and specifications for the handling of material incentives or sanctions are typical instances of problems falling within the jurisdiction of birth-planning commissions. A large number of rules decreed by the State Birth-Planning Commission relate to administrative procedures for propaganda, cadre training, plan formulation, statistical reporting and management of finances or personnel. Others deal with the powers of lower-level commissions and the handling of birth planning in Sino–foreign joint ventures. During the 1990s, the list of contextual rules greatly increased, and came to include written prescriptions for the handling of various applications and birth-planning formalities, procedures for special groups of the population, requirements for the filing and approval of lower-level documents, rules for the collection and use of penalty payments, and a multitude of standardized forms and papers. A case in point is Hebei province, where such supplementary rules of the provincial birth-planning commission hit the record mark of more than forty documents by the end of the 1990s.

Some of the most voluminous guidelines issued by the birth-planning commissions concern complicated definitional questions and problems of applicability: Who is a peasant? (Whereas in Maoist China this used to be an easy question, it has developed into a highly complicated issue today.) How should adopted children be treated? Do parents of twin children also receive a one-child certificate? Which rules apply if husband and wife hail from different parts of the country or are working in different economic sectors? How should children from mixed marriages between Han-Chinese and national minorities be treated? What procedures for birth planning should be adopted for the migrant population? These are further examples of the complex problems of implementing birth-planning regulations in an era of increasing social mobility. Another problem frequently faced by the birth-planning commissions is how to handle the wide margins in fixing birth-control fines.[6]

The provincial birth-planning commissions have not always succeeded in formulating binding or consistent answers to such questions. As mentioned above, they have frequently confined themselves to transmitting their 'views' to lower levels, thereby avoiding a final decision. In cases where lower-level organs ask for instructions on specific cases, it is hard to maintain this posture. Work conferences are another instrument for internal coordination. They are convened by the birth-planning commissions when they confront complex problems or receive new instructions from superior authorities. Minutes of the proceedings are then circulated within the bureaucracy in order to communicate new guidelines. In the past, many lower-level enquiries have pertained to the increasing number of cases in doubt: marriages between peasant wives and husbands in cadre or worker positions; peasants officially transferred to urban household registration but who hold no right to urban subsidies; peasants hired in rural small-scale industries or earning from self-employed activities; persons working part-time for community institutions. Since 1986 the superior organs have tended to handle such cases restrictively, but it is difficult to follow the implementation of their guidelines by lower echelons. Nevertheless, the examples quoted above demonstrate the increasing complexity of birth planning, the large extent of ill-defined areas, and the high number of starting points for rule evasion.

Many problems transcend the power of the birth-planning commissions and require joint action with other authorities. One example is the medical definition of chronic ailments or disabledness of a first child that may entitle parents to a second-child permit. Relevant regulations are contained in a joint circular of the Birth-Planning Commission and the Ministry of Health. Other problems arise from financing material incentives for one-child families and from enforcing preferential treatment of single children. They have required explanations and rules of implementation jointly drafted by the birth-planning commissions, departments of finance, the People's Bank, and the departments of labour and personnel. Inter-departmental issues of particular importance are ruled by way of State Council regulations, which are directly promulgated at this higher level.

The three autonomous districts for the national minorities of Sichuan Province with their specific birth-planning rules constitute an example of the extent of special regulations at lower levels. These rules were circulated by way of minutes from a symposium on birth planning in the autonomous districts of Garzi, Aba and Liangshan, staged in October 1988. They were submitted to the provincial birth-planning commission, which endorsed and issued them by way of a circular. Up until the early 1990s, some backward areas with a high degree of ethnic fragmentation, such as Yunnan province, promulgated detailed birth-planning regulations at prefectural level only. In these cases, province-level regulations remained rather imprecise.

Besides provinces, prefectures and municipal regions, cities and counties may also enact additional rules and guidelines for implementing birth planning. Many birth-planning regulations explicitly concede to them the right to promulgate concrete rules of implementation in accordance with provincial regulations and specific conditions in their area of jurisdiction. A number of provinces make no stipulations in this regard, while others confine the right to issue local regulations to autonomous areas. But even if provincial regulations do not contain pertinent references, additional rules are widespread at the lower levels. In most cases, current provincial birth-planning regulations require lower levels to submit their additional rules for approval. Information on lower-level birth-planning norms is extremely limited. The few available reports and materials indicate that they largely specify economic and administrative rewards and sanctions.[7] Other areas governed by city and county regulations are procedures for birth applications and authorizations, medical certificates and other relevant documents, prescriptions as to the precise nature of compulsory contraceptive measures, time limits for pregnancy tests and abortions, as well as collective liabilities of the units concerned. City districts and individual units within the cities may augment and specify city regulations still further. Their pertinent rules are then embodied in 'Regulations for Workers and Staff', which can spell out detailed requirements for periodic gynaecological checkups and pregnancy tests for female employees, monthly propaganda sessions, or the establishment of a filing-card system. 'Township Covenants' and village statutes may contain similar provisions for the rural areas.

The ramifications of executive powers and the continuous delegation of duties to lower levels make up the essence of Chinese state administration. They explain the secret of how to govern a huge, highly diversified and still largely backward country such as China within the framework of a unitary state. At the same time, they also give an inkling of the bureaucratic life generated by a birth-control apparatus with up to six vertical echelons, three directly and some twenty indirectly involved state commissions, ministries and national organizations, a host of subordinate institutions, and a parallel structure of Party committees guiding this administrative edifice from behind the scenes.

This set-up creates the specific Chinese mixture of uniformity and diversity that is so bewildering to the outsider. As demonstrated by many far-reaching initiatives for birth planning, the central Party and government institutions are able to muster sufficient power to decree directives for the whole country and to transmit them to lower levels through a highly stratified, hierarchical bureaucracy. In most cases, these directives are rather general in character, but they also contain specific details in case of need. Central directives may be modified by ever-new layers of implementation guidelines promulgated by lower administrative levels, so that control of actual rules prevailing at grass-roots level is easily lost.

In theory, the vertical nature of command chains is supposed to guarantee an efficient administration from the top-down as well as exhaustive information from the bottom-up. In practice, however, upper levels often lack information about grass-roots conditions, while lower levels constantly modify central directives by claiming 'special circumstances' and 'necessary adjustments'. In theory, supplementary rules for implementation should be of a subsidiary nature only and be in full accord with norms promulgated at upper levels. In practice, however, there is often tension between upper- and lower-level norms. A major area of local latitude is the interpretation of 'real difficulties' that have to be proven in order to obtain a second-child permit. Greater local deviations also exist in the handling of material incentives and sanctions with regard to differently implemented rules for contraceptive methods, or in the detailed procedures for application and control formalities in birth planning.

In recognition of such difficulties, the centre has undertaken some steps to harmonize regional and local rules. In May 1989, a circular asked all provincial governments to secure the opinion of the State Birth-Planning Commission before promulgating new regional birth-planning regulations. A similar role for unifying local regulations has been played by the existence of national birth-planning norms in draft form, and by the introduction of ever more detailed national rules, regulations and laws for contextual matters.[8] In recent years, a number of conferences on birth-planning legislation have succeeded in introducing a largely uniform structure into the provincial regulations. Requirements for approval of local rules are handled more strictly, and fixed procedures apply for handling administrative decrees (*guizhang*) not subject to legislation. Some provinces have curtailed the power of subordinate administrations to promulgate additional rules, and county-level birth-planning commissions insist that all township permits for second and higher order births be approved by them.

Even so, local regulations inventing new policies in violation of higher level regulations have remained a source of irritation. This is why in 1995 the State Birth-Planning Commission launched a nationwide campaign to rectify local birth-planning norms. In this campaign, the materials scrutinized for conformity with national and provincial stipulations, and for compliance with promulgation and filing procedures, show the intricate nature of normative birth control: in the seventeen provinces in which the drive began, more than 50,000 documents were handled. They included decisions, ordinances, announcements, circulars, explanations, township covenants, open letters and various certificates. Fourteen thousand of these documents were either revised or revoked. Political slogans and more than 260,000 birth-planning contracts were also checked. According to the official report, the most frequently encountered problems were illegal fines and fees, improper guarantee payments or excess penalty sums, as well as unwarranted extra rules such as refusal of marriage registration before reaching the late-marriage age or compulsory sterilization of divorce applicants.[9] It may be speculated that this is a rather incomplete list.

6.2 Late marriage, late birth and birth spacing

Universal marriage, family values and the securing of male offspring for ritual, social and economic purposes rank among the pillars of Chinese culture. A weighty traditional literature recommends early marriage at 14 to 15 years of age for women and 16 to 17 years for men. Although in practice the majority of marriages seem to have been concluded somewhat later, and erosion of traditional family norms had already begun in the first half of the twentieth century, early marriage continued to be a time-honoured, widespread custom. It continued despite the introduction of legal age limits, first in the 1931 civil code of Guomindang China (16 years of age for women, 18 years for men) and later in the 1950 marriage law of the People's Republic (18 years for women, 20 years for men). Enforcement of these limits has always been delayed. The difficulties have been such that influential experts have repeatedly warned against raising the age limit still further, since this step would widen the gap between law and practice even more. Instead, they have counselled for indirectly raising the marriage age by relying on education, propaganda and supportive social policies.[10]

Debate on this issue began in 1957, when various proposals called for raising legal age limits to 20 to 25 years for women and 22 to 30 years for men. These proposals were taken up in the birth-planning campaigns of the 1960s and 1970s, which placed heavy emphasis on the instrument of late marriage. In view of the difficulties of law enforcement, the marriage law of 1950 was never formally revoked, but numerous administrative regulations and the requirement for prospective marriage partners to obtain written approval from their work unit effectively raised the marriage age. Some areas, such as Zhejiang or Hainan, aimed at rather high age limits of 25 years for women and 30 years for men in the early 1960s. More prevalent, however, were rules instituted in Jiangsu during 1964. In accord with recommendations of the central work conference of September 1963, they stipulated 23 years for women and 25 years for men as the minimum age for marriage in the rural areas; in urban areas, they even went further, and raised the limits to 25 years and 28 years, respectively. Marriage registration offices were instructed to withhold registration for couples under the desired age limits, thereby effectively abolishing the stipulations of the marriage law. A decade later, such practices had spread to the Han-Chinese population in all other provinces. Although ways to circumvent the rules persisted in the countryside, the planned delay of marriage proved to be an effective measure of birth control.[11]

The regulations for late marriage have always been unpopular. They could only be promoted by the high degree of political pressure, state regulation of economic life and social control within collective units during the Cultural Revolution. When a new marriage law was passed in 1980, the barriers to wedlock at a younger age fell. Opponents of late marriage argued that the price paid for it was too high: such barriers to marriage would lead to discontent of young people, which would foster informal cohabitation and illegitimate births, disturb social peace, raise crime rates and bring about a decline in public order in urban areas. The critics also voiced doubts about the validity of demographic arguments in favour of late marriage. They pointed out that even a late marriage could still produce a high number of children.[12] Although such arguments were not convincing in a demographic sense, the pressure to lower the marriage age was strong enough to move a Party craving popularity to comply with popular demands. The new marriage law of September 1980 stipulated a minimum marriage age of 22 years for men and 20 years for women. With regard to late marriage and late birth, the new law only mentioned 'encouraging' them. Special rules for the national minorities of Inner Mongolia, Tibet, Ningxia, Qinghai, Xinjiang and parts of Yunnan lowered the minimum age requirement by a further two years.

The lack of enforcement of the late-marriage recommendation has been reported from Shaanxi province,[13] and may also be inferred from other regional birth-planning regulations. Birth-planning rules from Liaoning and Jiangsu continued to adopt the former differentiation between rural and urban norms for late marriage in 1979. While the former amounted to 23 years for women and 25 years for men, the latter increased to 24 years for women and 26 years for men. Only the Shanghai regulations of 1981 continued to stipulate higher age limits, with 25 years for women and 27 years for men.

But the process of lowering former age limits had already begun. In later years, all provinces, including the three centrally administered municipalities, eliminated the differentiation between rural and urban late-marriage criteria. Instead, they adopted a uniform standard of 23 years for women and 25 years for men as the minimum age for late marriage. Incentives for delaying wedlock remain weak. They range from an additional three or five days (as stipulated in the 1988 norms for Xinjiang and Tianjin[14]) up to a maximum of thirty additional days of marriage leave (as proclaimed in the 1986 rules for Shanxi). Most provinces provide one to two weeks of additional marriage leave in the case of a late marriage. It is conspicuous that additional leave decreases if regulations are issued for backward areas, where work units complain about the added burden. But advanced regions such as Tianjin, Liaoning or Guangdong also provide only minimal incentives of four to ten additional days of marriage leave without prolonging this period in later regulations. One cannot escape the conclusion that the instrument of late marriage was largely discarded in the 1980s. This was also the conclusion reached by Chinese population experts and politicians, who kindled a lively debate on this issue at the end of the decade.

Since then, new supplementary rules have revived the emphasis on this instrument of birth planning. Changping town in the hinterland of Beijing serves as an example. Already, in October 1987, it introduced the new requirement that women applying for a first-child quota had to be aged at least 23 years and 3 months. Together with their application, they had to present their marriage certificate, their household book and a letter of confirmation from their work unit. Harbin City began to implement even tighter policies.

In its birth-planning regulations of January 1988, the city stressed its commitment to late marriage. Anyone who continued to insist on earlier wedlock within the legal age limit was required not to give birth to a child before reaching 25 years of age. Since that time, many cities have required all young wives under 24 years of age to sign a 'statement of compliance with late-birth requirements'. This amounts to a toleration of marriages at ages 20 to 23 provided no offspring is produced. Similar measures were taken in a number of rural areas, which saw the reintroduction of late-marriage propaganda, written pledges, deposits and fines for respecting the late-birth requirement. In the late 1990s, some counties went even further and made compliance with late-marriage regulations for urban dwellers on state payroll compulsory. Such instances effectively cancel the stipulations of the marriage law.[15]

Chinese politicians have always pleaded for a longer interval between marriage and the birth of the first child, but such pleas have proved extremely hard to realize. In many cases the interval was not defined in birth-planning norms. It is only in recent years that some provinces have laid down a late-birth requirement of at least 24 years. Regulations as to the spacing between the first and second child have vacillated between a three-year rule, as recommended by a birth-planning conference in 1979,[16] and a four-year requirement in later years. This is also the standard of most present birth-planning norms, which stipulate birth spacing of four years or 'more than three years'. Some provinces, such as Guizhou and Jiangsu, adhered to the lower spacing requirement until 1986; later, many prolonged it to five or six years. In January 1985, Jiangxi province decreed a graded method of birth spacing in accord with changes in the age structure of the population. Until 1990, the interval between the first and second birth was to amount to five years, it was to decrease to four years between 1991 and 1995 and to three years in 1996. Implementation of these rules would signify an intelligent form of birth planning in conformity with changing demographic conditions. In a number of instances, different birth intervals have been coupled with the various types of circumstances under which second children are permitted. Flexibility is also signalled by a stipulation in some newly revised regulations of the late 1980s and early 1990s that empowers sub-provincial administrations to set the required birth interval in accordance with local conditions.[17]

It seems that spacing requirements, too, were only weakly implemented in the 1980s. In her study of birth planning in three villages of Shaanxi province in 1985, Greenhalgh reported that non-compliance of spacing requirements was no longer penalized.[18] However, just as in the case of the late-marriage recommendation, the 1990s have witnessed determined efforts at stricter enforcement. In 1993 to 1994 a new campaign against early marriages with threats of hefty penalty payments swept through the villages. A year later, the provinces started to make compliance with marriage regulations an integral part of annual evaluations, and decreed that henceforth no second-child permits would be granted to violators of the minimum age requirement. Births after premarital conceptions were summarily prohibited.[19]

6.3 Procedures for birth permits

Since the beginning of formalized birth planning in the 1980s, the procedures for birth permits have usually been fixed below the provincial level. Although precise information is available for only a few areas, it may be assumed that the basic outline of procedures in big cities is similar. Different conditions prevail in small towns and rural townships, however. Since many of them cannot afford costly procedures such as compulsory marriage guidance and maternity courses, their list of formalities tends to be shorter.

Earlier birth-planning rules did not make any prescriptions as to the birth of the first child. Since the tightening of the one-child campaign in the late 1980s and early 1990s, however, almost all newly revised birth-planning regulations have introduced formalities for the birth of the first child, too. As in the case of second children, these require written applications by the prospective parents as well as comment, examination and approval from the authorities concerned. The right to grant permits for first births is usually the domain of the birth-planning bureaus of rural townships and towns or the urban street committee offices.

Second births have to be authorized by the birth-planning bureaux of counties, cities or city districts. Further permissions or cases not covered by detailed clauses used to require the consent of the birth-planning commission of a prefecture or municipal region; nowadays they are even forwarded to the province level. This is the present state of affairs as it should be. In the past, second-child permits have frequently been issued by towns and townships, too. In order to tighten controls, recent years have seen the introduction of the rule that all birth permits expire after the planning year and must be renewed. Furthermore, detailed instructions for the printing, signing, sealing, checking and filing of documents have been decreed. In case of second births, they involve two or even three echelons of the birth-planning bureaucracy.

Comprehensive procedures, which are largely similar and serve as models for Chinese birth planning, were adopted in Guangzhou and Beijing at the beginning of the 1990s.[20] In many respects they amount to a hardening of birth-control rules. According to these regulations, the procedures for obtaining a birth permit are as follows.

Women under the late-marriage age have to sign a 'Statement of Compliance with the Late-Birth Requirement' at the birth-planning office of their street committee before registering their marriage. Another requirement for marriage registration is a form certifying that both applicants have undergone a medical examination to check for eugenic indications. Since promulgation of the Law on Maternal and Infant Health Care in October 1994, relevant passages have been introduced into all recent birth-control regulations. In critical cases, they serve as the basis for proscribing childbearing and requiring sterilization before marriage registration. Under ordinary circumstances women may immediately apply for a birth permit at the birth-planning office of their street committee once they produce marriage registration and have reached the late-birth age of 24 years. Births always require permission, even if they conform with all relevant laws and regulations. The following documents have to be attached to the written application: a stamped form certifying attendance of a marriage guidance course, a statement from the work units of both spouses, and a statement of the responsible neighbourhood committee. Women may become pregnant only after having obtained the written 'Birth Planning Certificate' issued by the birth-planning office of their street committee.

All pregnancies have to be registered in a hospital within two months after conception. The hospital's written registration has to be presented to the street committee, which then assigns the women to a maternity course. At the end of the course, pregnant women are required to obtain a 'Statement of Guarantee for Contraceptive Measures After Delivery' from their work unit. This statement of guarantee is then presented to the street committee, where again a 'Statement of Compliance With the One-Child Norm' is signed. Together with the 'Statement of Guarantee', household registration documents, the marriage registration form, the Certificate of Attendance for the maternity course, as well as two photographs of the pregnant woman, it then has to be submitted to the work unit four months after the beginning of pregnancy. A deposit for the risk of contraceptive failure must be paid in case oral contraceptives are preferred over IUD insertion. The relevant receipt has to be presented to the street committee.

Second-child permits require special exemptions from the one-child rule. At the earliest, they can be granted four years after the birth of the first child. Conformity with regulations for second-child permits has to be proven by official certificates. Further procedures for second-child permits are similar to those for a first birth.

These regulations, dating from 1991 and 1992, mark the reach of Chinese bureaucracy. Altogether, they add up to the astonishing number of twelve forms requisite for giving birth to a first child. In essence, they transform the late-birth recommendation into a requirement, and block all illegitimate childbearing. Furthermore, the procedures introduce many additional formalities not outlined in the provincial regulations.

It remains to be seen, however, if this tight monitoring network can be forged in all rural areas. In view of the lack of personnel and finances, and the resulting gaps in control and sanctions, such procedures are frequently unmanageable. It is therefore hard to realize the late-birth recommendation and strict permission requirements in the villages. In many cases, birth permits will have been handled as mere formalities as long as second-child criteria were respected. This is why birth permits in rural areas were often handed out only after delivery.

The late 1990s, however, have seen attempts to establish similar formalized application procedures for any type of birth in rural areas, too. Many provincial birth-planning regulations of recent years explicitly require premarital check-ups for eugenic indications, personal birth applications from both spouses, written comments from village committees, neighbourhood committees or work units, and written approval from township (town) governments. If the birth of a second child is involved, the applications are forwarded to the county birth-planning commission for final approval; if they concern state employees, the municipal birth-planning commission has the final say. Often, implementation procedures also demand a public posting of name lists with birth quotas and the personal receipt of a 'Birth Quota Notice' before a birth is allowed to take place; they also make the issuing of a final 'Birth Permit' dependent on medical examination four to six months after conception. In other cases, tightened rules of the late 1990s have introduced written check-lists for all birth permit requirements, additional birth permit proof lodged with the authorities, and a multitude of standardized forms for various certificates, reviews, permits and official statements needed in the application process.[21]

6.4 Second-child permits

No fixed birth limits were imposed in the first and second birth-planning campaigns of the 1950s and 1960s. Although Chen Yun, one of the foremost Party leaders, and economic planning chief and member of the Standing Committee of the Politburo, started to call for a maximum of two children for Party members in August 1957, no legislation or Party directives were passed to that effect. Beginning in 1963 and restarting in 1971, an average number of two children per couple was propagated among the populace at large, but central guidelines emphasized flexibility, and insisted on broadly defined ceilings for natural population increase only. It was left to the discretion of lower-level units to translate these into more precise rules. In practice, this meant increasing pressures first for state employees, then for all other urban inhabitants, and finally for the peasant population. There are indications that in 1973 the provinces began to tighten the two-child recommendation by requiring permissions for third children from all employees listed as workers and staff. But even if pressures against having more children grew successively, higher-order births were still tolerated in many cases, most notably among the national minorities.[22]

After China's two-child policy started to move to the one-child norm in late 1979, the Open Letter of the Central Committee of September 1980 has been regarded as the final public proclamation of the new line. Since the main emphasis of the letter was on the propagation of the one-child family, this was undoubtedly correct. Nevertheless, the two-and-a-half pages of the Chinese document contain a formula that served as a break-through for the partial return to two-child policies in subsequent years: 'If members of the masses are in real difficulties defined by regulations, they can be permitted to give birth to a second child.'[23] During the first years, when all public attention was focused on the propagation of the new one-child norm, this sentence was hardly noticed. But it continued to exist as one of those elastic clauses that help the leadership to evade precise commitments and to demonstrate flexibility. This flexibility is necessary for a large country such as China, but it can also be used to bend directives so that they deviate from original intentions. As with similar cases, this seems to have happened with the second-child permits.

At first, the brief clause of the Open Letter did not evoke any further comments. The joint directive of the Central Committee and the State Council on birth planning of February 1982 only repeated the formula without adding further explanations, but the first authoritative interpretation at national level must have been drawn up by the Birth-Planning Commission shortly after. The uniformity of official criteria for second-child permits issued by most provinces in 1982 is apparent: these were allowances for couples whose first child was disabled; who had entered a second marriage with one spouse being childless while the other brought a child with them; or who had adopted a child after long years of childless marriage but became pregnant later on. The special clauses for second children are in Table 2. Although the list of birth-control norms is incomplete, it still demonstrates that, starting in 1982, these three types of cases are mentioned everywhere. In Shanghai and Shaanxi they even show up a year earlier. Provinces with a tight policy restrict themselves to these norms, while regions with a more relaxed policy include other criteria.

In this early period Guangdong province served as the front-runner of a policy revision. In its birth-planning regulations of February 1980 the province continued to concede a global second-child permit to all citizens. When it was later forced to modify this clause, it continued to grant second-child permists to persons living in poor mountainous or coastal areas with a lack of manpower. Still more important was the concession of a provincial work conference in 1981 to grant second-child permits, if the first born was a girl. Later versions of the Guangdong birth-planning regulations were worded in such a way that they amounted to global permission for second births to all peasants who adhered to a four-year birth interval. Second-child permits on the basis of such criteria have only been conceded to the rural population with agricultural household registration. The strict differentiation between agricultural and non-agricultural population is a characteristic of all other norms, too. Although peasants enjoy a wider array of valid reasons for obtaining a second-child permit, the conditions for the urban population continue to be much more restricted.

It will be seen from Table 2 that the extension of second-child conditions beyond the criteria 1 to 3 was due to regional initiatives. Provinces such as Hebei, Henan, Guangdong or Shaanxi were in the forefront of such moves during 1981 and early 1982. The Beijing leadership sanctioned the additional items only at a national work conference for birth planning in August 1982. Here, the criteria 4, 6–7 and 10–13 contained in Table 2 were endorsed.[24] The conference did not mention the continuing practice of global second-child permits for large parts of the population in Yunnan, Tibet, Qinghai, Ningxia and Xinjiang. Nor did it specifically consent to the Guangdong rule of second-child permits for all peasant families with only one daughter or a sufficiently long birth interval. Nevertheless, Guangdong upheld its provincial regulations[25] – another signal of the loss of central control and the unwilling toleration of wide regional deviations. When central guidelines were further relaxed in 1985, other provinces such as Inner Mongolia, Liaoning, Jiangsu, Jiangxi, Guangxi and Gansu followed the lead of South China and granted second-child privileges for peasants with one daughter. Guangdong has pointed to the ever-

Table 2 Provincial birth-planning rules: conditions for second-child permits 1979–99
and implied total fertility rate (children per woman) 1990

	Date	Urban	Rural (additional)	Implied TFR 1990
Beijing	6-12-82	1-5	7,10,12,13	
	15-1-91	1-5,15	6,(7),12,13,(16)	1.33
Tianjin	14-10-82		1-3,6,10,12,15	
	2-11-88	1-4,(5),10	6,12,13,(16)	1.35
	9-3-93			
	15-4-94			
	30-1-97	1-4,(5),10	6,12,13,(16)	
Hebei	5-4-82	1-3	5,7,8,10,12,13	
	28-2-86	1-3,9	5,7,8,10,12,13	
	14-3-89	1-6,9,10,15	(7),8,13,(16)	1.67
	2-9-94	1-6,9,10,15	(7),8,13,(16)	
	3-9-97	1-6,9,10,15	(7),8,13,(16)	
Shanxi	29-6-82	1-5	6,7,10,12-14	
	28-12-86	1-3,15	10,12,13	
	22-9-89	1-6	7,(12),13,(16)	1.69
Inner Mongolia	15-6-82	1-3,5	15	
	15-1-85	1-5,9,10,15	6,7,12,13,16	
	1-12-88	1-5,9	6,7,12,13,16	
	12-10-90	1-3,5,9,15	6,16	1.80
	7-11-95	1-3,5,9,15	6,16	
Liaoning	16-6-79	17		
	3-4-80	1,3		
	24-6-82	1,3	5	
	9-84	1-3,10	5,8,12,13	
	1-10-85	1-3,10	5,8,12,13,(16)	
	28-5-88	1-3,(5),10,15	5,6,8,12,13,16	1.50
	25-9-92	1,3,(5),10,15	5,6,8,12,13,16	
	27-9-97	1,3,(5),10,15	5,6,8,12,13,16	
Jilin	21-7-88	1-5,10,15	6,11,12,16	1.50
	11-9-93	1-5,10	(6),12,(16)	
	14-11-97	1-5,10,15	(6),12,(16)	
Heilongjiang	9-79	1,17		
	31-1-83	1-3,5	10,12,13	
	13-12-89	1-6,10	12,13,16	1.44
	21-5-94	1-5,15	7,10,12,16	
	18-12-99	1-5,10,15	7,16	
Shanghai	28-7-81	1-3		
	3-6-82			
	16-10-84	1,2	3,6,10,12,13	
	30-5-87	1-4,9	5,6,8,10,12-14	1.28
	17-10-92	1-4,(5),10,15	6,(8),(13)	
	16-6-95	1-4,(5),10,15	6,(8),(13)	
	10-12-97	1-4,(5),10,15	6,(8),(13)	

	Date	Urban	Rural (additional)	Implied TFR 1990
Jiangsu	31-7-79	1,17		
	24-6-82	1-3	10,12	
	9-85	1-4,8-10,14,15	7,12,13	
	28-10-90	1-4,(8),(9),10,11,14,15	7,12,13,(16)	1.52
	16-6-95	1-4,(9),10,11,14,15	7,(8),12,13,(16)	
	31-7-97	1-4,(9),10,11,14,15	7,(8),12,13,(16)	
Zhejiang	4-3-82	1-3,5	(15)	
	4-2-85	1-5,9,10,14,15	6,(7),(8),12,13,(15)	
	29-12-89	1-5,(9),10,14,15	(7),(8),11,13,(16)	1.54
	28-9-95	1-5,(9),10,14,15	(7),(8),11,13,(16)	
Anhui	1-4-79	17		
	9-5-81	1-3,5		
	17-8-84	1-6,9,10	7,12,13	
	31-10-88	1-6,9,10,12	13,16	1.61
	30-8-92	1-6,(9),10,12	13,16	
	24-4-95	1-6,(9),10,12	13,16	
Fujian	28-5-82	1-3,5	13,15	
	29-4-88	1-6,8,9,14	7,10,12,13	1.61
	28-6-91	(1-6,8-10,14)	7,11-13	
	25-10-97	(1-6,8-10,14)	7,11-13	
Jiangxi	18-1-83	1-3	7,10,12,13	
	4-1-85	1-5,9,10	7,10,12,13,16	
	16-6-90	1-4,(5),(9),14,15	11,12,(13),16	1.52
	30-6-95			
	20-6-97	1-4,(5),(9),14,15	11,12,(13),16	
Shandong	29-7-82	1-3	10,12-14	
	20-7-88	1-5,(6),8,(9),15	8,12-14,16	1.55
	14-10-96	1-5,(6),8,(9),10,15	8,12-14,16	
Henan	15-6-82	1-3,7,12		
	11-12-85	1-6,9,10,14,15	7,11-13	
	23-8-87		(16)	
	12-4-90	1-4,(9),14	5,(7),13,16	1.56
Hubei	27-9-79			
	19-12-87	1,2,4	6,10,13,16	1.55
	1-12-91	1-4	6,11,13,16	
	28-3-97	1-4	6,11,13,16	
Hunan	6-79	(17)		
	10-5-82	1-4	(15)	
	3-12-89	1-5,10	11-14,(16)	1.64
Guangdong	2-2-80	(17)		
	81	1,8,9	3,7,16	
	17-5-86	1-5,9,10	(16,17)	1.85
	28-11-92	1-3,(4),(5),9,10	(17)	
	1-12-97			
	18-9-98	1-3,(4),(5),9,10	16	
Guangxi	25-11-82	1-3,6	5,15	
	4-85	1,5,6,9,10	7,13,16	
	17-9-88	1-3,5,6,10,14	7,12,13,16	1.57
	26-11-94	1-3,5,6,10,14	7,12,13,16	

	Date	Urban	Rural (additional)	Implied TFR 1990
Hainan	12-6-84	1-3,9,10	7,8,16	
	85	1-3,9,10	16	
	11-3-89	1-5,(6),(9),(14)	15	1.97
	27-10-95	1-5,15		
Chongqing	13-9-97	1-4,10	6,7,11-14,(16)	
Sichuan	29-4-82	1-4,15	15	
	5-84		6,7,12-14,(16)	
	2-7-87	1-4,10	6,7,11-14,(16)	1.57
	15-12-93			
	17-10-97	1-4,10	6,11-13,(16)	
Guizhou	6-79	17		
	15-3-82	1-3	5,15	
	27-7-84	1-3,5,6,10	11-13,15	
	16-7-87	1-5,10	13,15	1.74
	24-7-98	1-4,10	13	
Yunnan	86	1-5,(6),10,13	5,7,17	
	22-12-90	1-4,(6),10	(5),(7),15	2.13
	3-12-97	1-4,(6),10	(5),(7),15	
Tibet	20-12-79	5		
	15-4-80	5		
	3-83	5		
	28-3-85	1-3,5,10		
	1-5-86	1-3,5,10		see note
	8-5-92	1-3,(5),(6),10	17	
Shaanxi	6-79	17		
	30-4-81	1-3,5,7		
	1-10-82	1-5	7	
	1-85	1-6	7,11-13	
	25-7-86	1-5,10,15	6,7,12,13	
	5-11-88	15	(7),(16)	1.64
	3-3-91	1-5,10	6,7,13,16	
	2-8-97	1-5,10	6,7,13,16	
Gansu	16-3-82	1-3	15	
	15-6-85	1-3	15,16	
	28-11-89	1-3	5,13,(7+16)	1.58
	29-9-97	1-4	5,13,16	
Qinghai	5-6-82	3,15		
	9-85	3,4,6,10		
	17-4-86	1-6,10	15,17	2.08
	28-2-92	1-6,10	15,17	
Ningxia	6-1980	17		
	2-9-82	1-3	17	
	28-8-86	1-6,9,10,15	17	
	28-12-90	1-5,9,10	17	2.06
Xinjiang	4-4-81	5		
	30-4-88	5		
	15-8-91	1,3-6,9,10	(17)	2.40

Conditions for second births:

1 first child is disabled or dead
2 pregnancy after long years of childless marriage and a subsequent adoption
3 in a remarriage one spouse has been childless, the other spouse already has had one child or two children
4 one spouse or both Chinese spouses returned from overseas, Hongkong or Taiwan
5 one spouse or both spouses belong to a national minority with less than 10 million members
6 one spouse is disabled and cannot work
7 a peasant couple lives in sparsely settled mountain, reclamation or border areas
8 one spouse is a deep-sea fisherman
9 one spouse has been constantly working in underground mining for more than 5 years
10 one spouse or both spouses are single children
11 only one child or one son has been born to a family for two generations
12 among brothers, only one is able to produce children
13 husband settles in the family of his wife which has daughters and no sons
14 one spouse is the (single) child of a revolutionary martyr
15 couple has real (economic) difficulties or claims other peculiar reasons
16 first child is a girl (and couple has real difficulties)
17 three, four, or five years after birth of first child

Notes: Documents are listed by date of ratification. Conditions for clauses 4–6 and 10 vary as to the question whether one or both spouses have to meet the requirement. The required interval between the first and second birth varies, too. Types of cases in brackets have to comply with additional conditions. Many birth-planning regulations contain further qualifications of specific clauses. Regulations from a number of autonomous minority areas also specify conditions for bearing three or even more children; see chapter 6.9.1. Because of the fluid nature and the weak organization of birth planning in Tibet, the State Birth-Planning Commission did not calculate an implied TFR for the Autonomous Region in 1990.

Sources for the birth-planning rules: Anhui jingji nianjian 1985; FBIS, 20 April 1979; ZJSN 1986–; PDR, No. 3/1983; *Sichuan ribao*, 4 July 1987; White 1985, 301–314; Greenhalgh 1986; Greenhalgh 1990; Kessler 1990; Tien 1991, 119; Peng Xizhe 1991, 48; ZRGDFH; ZRGFFQ 1994; ZRGFFQ 1996; Xu Xifa 1995; *Xinhua ribao*, 28 June 1995; ZJSQ; Hebei sheng renkou diaocha dui 1996; www.cpirc.org.cn/policyfp.htm; field research. For German translations of rules from Inner Mongolia, Heilongjiang, Jiangsu, Fujian, Guangdong and Shaanxi in the 1980–90 period compare: Scharping and Heuser 1995; for English translations of Liaoning, Zhejiang and Tibet documents in the 1954–97 period: Scharping 2000a and Scharping 2000b.

Source for the implied TFRs: official estimates of the State Birth-Planning Commission according to Zeng Yi 1997, p. 1409

increasing links with Hongkong and to the strong influence of overseas Chinese to justify its special policies. Notwithstanding these arguments, the province has been suffering continuous criticism of its high birth rates. In September 1998, the centre finally prevailed in its long-standing efforts to force an abolishment of the general second-child clause for Guangdong peasants. The new provincial birth-planning regulations passed at that time are among the most uncompromising.[26]

The regional birth-planning rules testify to the fact that the years between 1984 and 1986 saw the high tide of regional diversification in birth-control policies. The patterns evolving at that time clearly reflect the different natural, economic and demographic endowment of China's regions. Densely populated provinces in the coastal areas and large plains granted only some second-child permits under restricted conditions. A global second-child permit policy for the agricultural population was practised in minority and border areas such as the provinces or autonomous regions of Ningxia, Qinghai and Xinjiang. Other provinces adopted special rules only for experimental counties and areas with a lack of manpower. Different procedures are followed if the regulations vary between plains, hilly country and mountainous areas within a province. Such diversified birth-planning rules have been enacted in Beijing, Hebei, Zhejiang, Sichuan, Yunnan, Shaanxi and Gansu. These are all provinces with a high degree of geographic, economic, and social fragmentation. At the same time, some experimental areas have also linked the granting of second-child permits to a decline in numbers for higher-order births. Yet other experimental areas have experimented with a global second-child permit for late marriages.[27]

Despite the attempts of the Central Committee to check the ever-increasing trend towards second-child permits, the further extension of special second-child criteria continued unabated. During autumn of 1986 global second-child permits for the peasant population or even wider privileges for minority nationals were introduced or continued to be granted in Guangdong, Hainan, Yunnan, Tibet, Qinghai, Ningxia and Xinjiang. Second-child permits for peasants with only one daughter had spread to the whole of the Northeast (Liaoning, Jilin, Heilongjiang), parts of the East (Zhejiang, Jiangxi, Shandong), as well as to parts of the Southwest (Guangxi, Guizhou) and the Northwestern province of Shaanxi. More restricted second-child permits with a ceiling of 30 per cent of all current births were handed out in Anhui, Fujian, Hubei and Sichuan provinces. The most restrictive second-child rules applied to the densely populated provinces of Jiangsu and Henan, as well as to the three centrally administered municipalities of Beijing, Tianjin and Shanghai.[28] Table 2 contains exactly twenty birth-planning regulations that were passed in the period between the issuing of Document No. 13 in June 1986 and the fall of Zhao Ziyang in June 1989. There is not a single case in which the highly critical criteria No. 15 (second-child permits for families in difficulties or claiming other peculiar reasons), No. 16 (second-child permits for peasant families with only one daughter) and no. 17 (global second-child permits for peasants with four years of birth spacing) were completely abolished. In a few instances, however, the applicability of the rules was confined by changing clause No. 15 to clause No.16 or by excluding certain groups of the peasantry from the privilege.

According to contemporary sources, in 1988 some 12 per cent of the total Chinese population lived in areas with global second-child permission. Some further 50 per cent lived in provinces extending a second-child permit to peasant households with only one daughter. A restrictive second-child policy with special regulations for a small number of hardship cases was followed in provinces with 28 per cent of China's population.[29] Detailed information on the relative importance of different second-child criteria is available from Hebei, which belonged to this latter group. Between 1980 and 1988 about 33 per cent of all second-child permits in this province were granted for couples claiming death or disability of their first child. This figure increased to 56 per cent among workers. The second largest number of second-child permits were handed out to persons living in remote mountainous areas (17 per cent for both peasants and workers). Indicative of the fluid character of policy implementation, 14 per cent of the permits were granted to cases claiming certain reasons not covered by regulations. Couples with only one son in two generations made up 10 per cent of all cases. A further 9 per cent comprised minority nationals, disabled persons, miners, fishermen or returned overseas Chinese, 7 per cent remarried persons, 6 per cent uxorilocal marriages and 5 per cent brothers without male offspring. During the period in question Hebei did not specifically stipulate exemptions from the one-child rule for families with only one daughter, so that such cases made up just 1 per cent of all permits.[30]

As shown in Table 2, patterns of second-child exemptions changed only slightly after the Tian'anmen crisis and the fall of Zhao Ziyang. During 1989 and 1990 a number of newly revised provincial regulations thus continued the trend to an ever-wider prevalence of second-child permits for peasant families. New Hainan regulations passed in October 1989 and following the model of Guangdong, extended a global second-child permission for most peasants respecting proper birth spacing; Heilongjiang regulations dating from December of that year for the first time made peasants with only one daughter eligible for second-child permits. In all other cases, however, the provinces proceeded more cautiously: Shanxi and Zhejiang province introduced the second-child privilege for one-daughter peasant households, with the rider that all counties should demonstrate prior control of above-quota births. The Hunan and Henan regulations of 1989 and 1990 contained the addendum that one-daughter families in rural areas had to prove real hardship before applying for a second-child permit, while Jiangsu restricted the newly introduced rule to deep-sea fishermen or inhabitants of sparsely settled reclamation areas.

Today, most two-child policies conceded in earlier years continue to be in force. They have even become extended in some instances. Examples are Heilongjiang province, where revised regulations of December 1999 extended the second-child permit for spouses who were themselves single children to the urban population, and Gansu, where restrictions on second-child permits for peasant households with only one daughter were lifted. In the vast majority of cases, however, a tendency to reject further extensions of second-child permits became evident in the 1990s. Moves to introduce global second-child permits to the peasant population of Guangxi, Guizhou and Shaanxi provinces thus did not materialize in later years. Jilin raised additional barriers for peasant families claiming a second-child permit according to criterion No. 16; other provinces such as Liaoning, Zhejiang and Guizhou deleted individual clauses in the list of conditions for second-child permits. In 1998 Guangdong withdrew global second-child permits for all peasants with sufficiently long birth intervals. Conditions for remarried couples have also become more restricted. Xinjiang and Tibet Autonomous Regions saw a tightening of regulations by introducing a moderate form of birth planning for their minority population at the beginning of the 1990s. Moreover, since 1993 a growing number of provinces have introduced a far-reaching change by initiating hefty fees for second-child permits.[31] A hardening of second-child conditions has also been noticeable as far as precise definitions of 'peasant' status are concerned. Many current regulations explicitly exclude from this category those with rural registration who work in small-scale industries, in commerce, small enterprises, or urban areas. Peasants with urban registration are not entitled to second-child permits as well. These changes more or less replicate internal implementation rules that were promulgated earlier without a convincing degree of success.

Grouping the provinces by their current approach towards birth control, the following pattern emerges: A strict one-child policy with few exemptions is implemented in the three centrally administered municipalities of Beijing, Tianjin and Shanghai, as well as in Jiangsu and Fujian provinces, and in the greater part of Sichuan. A moderate policy with extended second-child permits for the peasant population has been adopted by the majority of provinces: Hebei, Shanxi and Inner Mongolia in North China, Liaoning, Jilin and Heilongjiang in the Northeast, Zhejiang, Anhui, Jiangxi, Shandong, Henan, Hubei, Hunan, Guangdong, Guangxi, Guizhou and Shaanxi in the East, the Central-South, Southwest and Northwest regions of the country. A global or widely defined second-child permit policy for peasants has been implemented by Hainan, Yunnan, Tibet, Qinghai, Ningxia and Xinjiang. These regions grant privileges for even higher birth orders for some groups of their population.[32]

Nowadays, the conditions for obtaining second-child permits have become extremely complicated, so it is difficult to calculate even a rough estimate of the number of eligible persons. A crude approximation on the basis of the rules summed up in Table 2 would result in approximately 60 per cent of the Chinese peasant population and some 5 per cent of the urban population. This would conform with the various implied fertility rates in Table 2 and the calculation that in 1990 a total fertility rate of 1.63 would have ensued at the national level had all regulations been carried out meticulously. It is probable that the subsequent narrower interpretation of the rules again has reduced the percentage of eligible couples and thereby lowered the implied total fertility rate to below 1.50 in the 1990s. In recent years, some specialist literature from China estimates that about 40 per cent of all one-child families enjoy the right to another birth.[33] If the high number of unauthorized second births is added to this percentage, an extremely ambiguous situation results, for, while the one-child norm continues to be propagated in all political statements on birth control, two-child policies have been adopted in many rural areas. Whether this is sufficient or excessive, remains a bone of contention.

Looking at the conditions for second-child privileges from another angle, some interesting conclusions emerge. Among the various types of conditions for second-child births, manpower shortage emerges as an important and acknowledged reason for obtaining permission. This applies to the great majority of cases bracketed under numbers 1, 6–12 and 15–17 in Table 2. The insistence on blood relationship also plays a major role and has been recognized as a legitimate reason for second-child permits in the types of cases bracketed under numbers 2 and 3. Foreign or domestic policy considerations apply in cases listed under numbers 4 and 5. They involve state interest in attracting overseas Chinese capital into China and in mollifying the discontent of national minorities. Special regard has also been paid to the widespread fear of lack of old-age support and discontinuation of ancestor worship. The types of cases listed under numbers 1, 10–13 and 16 take these anxieties into account. Cases in group 10 may serve as a gateway to a future resurgence of birth numbers. In particular, this applies to those provinces where it is sufficient to prove that one parent was an only child (Tianjin, Shanxi, Liaoning, Jilin, Shanghai, Jiangsu, Anhui). Finally, condition number 15 functions as an escape clause for all peculiar circumstances not covered by other regulations.

6.5 Contraceptive measures

Birth control was a highly controversial subject in the early 1950s. When it began to gain acceptance after 1954, Chinese newspapers published traditional contraceptive methods, among them the swallowing of tadpoles widely noted in contemporary press reports. From July to October 1956 there was a flurry of such reports. It may be speculated whether these methods had been circulated and used among the population in the past; some appear to have come out of the former brothels of Shanghai. Although it is hard to judge their effectiveness and the extent of their earlier use, contraceptive prescriptions, abortifacients, abstention, and sexual techniques favouring contraception were known in Chinese social history. Self-induced and back-street abortions were also practised, even if the subject was largely taboo in public discourse.[34]

Production of modern contraceptives began in 1956. The first plans for the next few years were to supply 10 per cent of all married couples of reproductive age with various contraceptive devices. Since only the urban population was targeted, the projected production figures were low. But, even in the cities less than one-third of men and women of reproductive age would have had access to contraceptives. It is doubtful whether this goal was realized. The 1965 estimate for the rate of contraceptive use, including sterilizations and the newly available IUD insertions, does not exceed the maximum of 10 per cent mentioned above. During the heyday of the Cultural Revolution it is likely that there was a drop in this figure due to the disruption of production, transportation, distribution and administration. However, mass production of the pill, which began after 1967, may have stabilized the situation. An overall rate of 13.5 per cent, rising to 29.3 per cent in the cities and falling to 9.6 per cent in the villages is given for 1970. In a big city such as Beijing and its rural counties, figures rose to 70 per cent and 40 per cent, respectively. The third birth-planning campaign managed to turn this advanced level into an average for the whole country. Starting in 1971, the overall rate of contraceptive prevalence increased annually by approximately 5 percentage points until it reached 50 per cent in 1978.[35] An overview is provided in Table 7 in the following section.

These developments indicate the fast pace of an intensifying campaign, crossing the threshold from optional to recommended birth prevention. Although social and political pressures to comply with government wishes were formidable in the Cultural Revolution, in a strict sense contraception had not yet become mandatory. The great inner diversity of an uncharted country, the lack of accountability of an administrative system in disarray and the manifold ways of circumventing directives acted as powerful counter-forces against the increasing pressures. The time series on contraceptive operations in

Table 7 confirms this assessment. It shows three distinct turning points which coincide with the onset of the second birth-planning campaign in 1963, the beginning of the third in 1971, and the start of one-child policies in 1979. The figures for these three years see sharp increases. A further peak is marked by the year 1975, when sterilizations and IUD insertions reach record proportions that were surpassed only in 1983. Extremely high numbers can also be observed between 1989 and 1996. The true extent of contraceptive operations in the 1990s is in doubt, however, since sterilizations and IUD insertions reported by the Birth-Planning Commission exceed numbers from the Ministry of Health by 40 per cent to 60 per cent.[36] It is probable that, different systems of record-keeping and the desire to report high figures for plan fulfilment and financial purposes are the major reasons behind the divergences.

No figures are available for the 1950s, but the few fragmentary pieces of evidence indicate that social conventions, political circumstances and legal provisions, and the lack of medical facilities and production plants for contraceptives all combined to keep the earlier numbers low. The same may be said for the second half of the 1960s, when central government control broke down. Compulsory contraception was introduced with the birth-planning regulations of the one-child campaign. The first relevant rules were decreed by the Guangdong Revolutionary Committee in January 1979, which ordered IUD insertions for all peasant women three months after the birth of their first child.[37] IUD insertions after the birth of the first child were also advocated by the then minister of the Birth-Planning Commission in late 1982 and early 1983.[38] They began to be widely enforced during the shock campaign of early 1983. It is noteworthy that until the mid-1980s birth-planning norms did not explicitly demand IUD use. Many regulations after 1986 referred to the 'advocacy (*tichang*)' of this contraceptive measure.

Practices in the 1990s have varied. Whereas regulations from Shanghai and other provinces continue to refrain from specifying a particular contraceptive method after the first birth, a number of provinces raised IUD use after the first child to the level of a measure that 'shall (*ying*)' be taken. Henan's birth-planning regulations of April 1990 furnish a relevant example. Guangdong province first introduced a clear-cut IUD requirement in 1992, only to change it six years later to the convoluted prescription that 'women of reproductive age who already have one child shall primarily choose to use intra-uterine devices'. A year later, Heilongjiang province displayed mastery of international birth-planning jargon by calling for 'gradual promotion of informed choice of methods for birth planning, contraception, and birth prevention'.[39] This confirms the impression that Chinese birth planning has vacillated over time. Although there have been periods of hard-line policies where campaigns for IUD insertion or even sterilization after the birth of the first child have predominated, pressures have eased at other times. Actual practices are left to the regional authorities in charge, who are torn between the demands to guarantee both contraceptive choice and contraceptive efficiency.

From the point of view of the birth-planning authorities, IUD insertion is a simple-to-use, economical, long-term measure requiring no hospitalization.

Conversely, oral contraceptives are more expensive. Moreover, many peasant women do not take them with the necessary degree of regularity, creating the problem of how to enforce use. Medical considerations have argued against the use of IUDs, however. In the past, most devices produced in China were stainless steel rings; they provoked menstrual bleeding, and led to expulsion and failure rates of more than 30 per cent two years after insertion. A new generation of copper devices introduced from abroad in the 1990s has reduced these problems without totally solving them.[40] However, acceptance of IUDs is generally good, because they imply temporary contraception without excluding the option of another pregnancy.

Because IUDs may be removed, their use cannot be completely controlled by the birth-planning authorities. Chinese press articles have repeatedly reported the widespread practice of secret IUD removals at the request of the women concerned.[41] In April 1981, the Ministry of Justice ruled in a leading case that unauthorized IUD removals would be treated as fraud, bodily harm, and – in case of quack operations with lethal results – manslaughter. When this ruling was confirmed two years later, breach of public order and hooliganism were added to the list of crimes liable to prosecution in connection with IUD removals.[42] Press reports on illegal IUD removals in the countryside have infuriated the late Politburo member Hu Qiaomu, who in a letter of July 1981 to the then Minister of Birth Planning Chen Muhua urged new regulations against such actions.[43] In practice, the effectiveness of IUDs and other contraceptive measures is checked by compulsory gynaecological tests. In urban areas, such check-ups are regularly organized by the work unit; in the countryside or among the migrant population, similar tests are usually enforced in January and February before the Chinese New Year Festival when conception is particularly high. In the mid-1990s controls have become tighter, with some supplementary regulations at county level stipulating two check-ups per year. At the end of the decade, this was raised to quarterly controls wherever possible. As witnessed by amendments to a number of birth-planning regulations in the late 1990s, prescribed regular pregnancy tests and IUD check-ups have also begun to appear in provincial documents.[44]

Although legal requirements are often not clear-cut, in many cases IUD use has become more or less compulsory. Oral contraceptives or condoms are not produced in sufficient numbers for the countryside and results have been unsatisfactory. In the urban and rural areas of Hebei, Shanghai and Shaanxi, the in-depth fertility survey of 1985 revealed failure rates of 23 per cent for condoms and 27 per cent for pills compared to between 8 per cent and 14 per cent for IUDs. Other investigations from the late 1980s resulted in still higher averages of 37 per cent, 33 per cent and 29 per cent, respectively, with rural areas significantly above these levels. The 1988 national fertility survey produced figures of 26 per cent, 17 per cent and 9 per cent for women practising the three contraceptive methods who had to undergo an abortion. Traditional methods led to even higher failure rates. By international standards for developing countries, the effectiveness of short-term contraceptives in China is low – a fact which highlights the unpopularity of birth control and the lack of cooperation on behalf of users.[45]

. Hence there is a general reluctance to rely on short-term methods in the countryside. Replacing them with IUDs or sterilizations, which cannot be reversed by the women themselves, amounts to substituting personal freedom with state control of fertility decisions. Because of easier birth-control enforcement and the improved supply situation in the cities, urban authorities have been more willing to permit the use of oral contraceptives or condoms there.[46] Since the late 1980s they have frequently demanded the payment of a deposit in order to guarantee the use and efficacy of these alternative methods.

Cost-free sterilizations with five to seven days of leave for vasectomies or twenty days for tubal ligations were introduced in September 1963.[47] Later rules for sterilizations convey the same picture as in the case of IUD insertions. The birth-planning regulations vacillate again between a general call for 'reliable', 'long-term', 'comprehensive' or 'effective' measures of contraception, the more precise stipulation to 'advocate (*tichang*)' or 'mobilize for (*dongyuan*)' sterilizations after the second child, and the formulation that they 'shall (*ying*)' or even 'must (*bixu*)' be practised at that point. The latter formulations have been used increasingly in the late 1980s and early 1990s, while in the preceding period the majority of rules contained the more moderate versions. Although since 1993 the pendulum has swung back to more contraceptive choice, this principle remains far from being an accomplished fact in the countryside. A number of provinces also continue to insist unequivocally on sterilization after the second child.

Just like IUD use, sterilizations on a mass scale have been closely associated with special campaigns. The degree of coercion used during these movements has again differed to quite a large degree. While in his village study of 1979 and 1980 Mosher is clearly referring to coercive sterilizations after the second birth, Potter and Potter in their field research on rural areas of Dongguan county note such measures only in case of illegitimate pregnancies, non-use of contraceptives, non-compliance with birth-spacing rules and prior abortion. These authors also mention that sterilizations after a second birth were not performed if women consented to other effective methods of contraception. Even after the birth of a third child, no married woman without a son was sterilized, provided she paid the prescribed penalty sum. Between December 1984 and June 1985, the village studied still permitted fourth pregnancies if women agreed to a sterilization afterwards.[48]

Coercive sterilization has always been disputed within the Chinese birth-planning bureaucracy. At one end of the spectrum is the shock campaign in February 1983, which included a massive sterilization drive promoted by the then Minister of the Birth-Planning Commission. He was assisted by the Vice-Governor of Guangdong, who supported sterilizations as an effective, cheap and long-term method preferable to other forms of contraception.[49] The extraordinarily high figure of more than 16 million sterilizations in 1983 – four to five times as many as in most other years of the decade – is telling. A year later, though, the tide had turned, and Weinan prefecture in the south of Shaanxi province was criticized by the centre for enforcing coercive sterilizations.[50] Most reports, though, leave little doubt that more or less forced sterilizations in rural areas continued. This situation has prompted Chinese demographers and birth-planning cadres to propose using second-child permits as an incentive in order to gain the consent of the women concerned.

In January 1990, the hard-liners reacted to the ambivalent policies of the 1980s with the call for devising clear-cut rules for IUD use and sterilization in the future. It is due to their influence that in the early 1990s the number of provinces laying down a more or less explicit rule of sterilization after the second child grew to sixteen.[51] Moreover, an increasing number of women had already been sterilized after the birth of their first child, even if this child was a daughter. In recent years, sterilizations have also been performed in accord with fixed annual plan targets. An example of tightened rules is Qingtian county in Zhejiang province, which in 1996 prescribed sterilization of women in the maternity ward right after delivery of their second child.[52] However, although they threaten increasingly stiff penalties for non-contraception and unauthorized births, the various provincial regulations stop short of straight compulsion. As with forced abortions, forced sterilizations in the sense of direct physical coercion have been repeatedly condemned and prohibited by the government.

Moreover, recent developments have seen some backtracking from the harsh position of the early 1990s. Policy statements of the State Birth-Planning Commission from 1994 and 1996 stress respect for citizens' rights and contraceptive choice; they unequivocally call for a revision of some provincial birth-planning regulations and a return to the earlier principle of merely demanding 'safe and reliable' contraception. Relevant amendments were enacted in fifteen provinces between 1993 and 1997.[53] In some cases, though, such changes have not been made or, if they have, they have been more or less cosmetic. An example is Hebei province, which effected the above-mentioned change in the revised provincial birth-planning regulations of 1994 and 1997, while upholding implementation procedures that unequivocally demand an IUD insertion after the first child and a sterilization after the second. Inner Mongolia, Shandong, Guangxi, Gansu and other regions continue to reiterate this principle in their provincial regulations. In the late 1990s, Guizhou and Shaanxi even bolstered it by limiting some one-child privileges to sterilized persons. Other provinces such as Zhejiang show up in public listings of regions with contraceptive choice. However, they delegate the precise handling of contraceptive requirements to the county and city level, where some administrations take drastic action.

The legal basis for some of these procedures is not altogether clear, since the centre has also affirmed the unity of law and the principle that rules of implementation should not be stricter than the regulations on which they are based. There are thus continuing strains and tensions between legal stipulations and actual practice. Although some Chinese authors point to an 'unsettled debt' of approximately 25 per cent of all persons who should have undergone IUD insertion or sterilization but have not done so, others openly criticize continuing cases of forced sterilization.[54]

If birth-planning rules and practices have specifically urged the sterilization of one spouse instead of just calling for 'effective contraceptive measures', they have not laid down a preference for female sterilizations (tubal ligations) or male ones (vasectomies). As shown in Table 3, 21 per cent of the married women of reproductive age were sterilized in 1981, while only 8 per cent of married men consented to vasectomies. These percentages rose steeply in the early 1980s, stabilized or fell back slightly during mid-decade, and began to climb again in 1989. In 1997 they reached 39 per cent and 10 per cent, respectively, before sliding back again.[55] Applying a method developed in Sichuan during the late 1950s, male sterilizations frequently avoid severing the seminal ducts. Instead, a supposedly reversible instillation of the vas is performed. Chemical occlusion of tubes is more difficult. Therefore, the reversibility of female sterilizations is in doubt, impairing their acceptance by women.[56] Overall, China has the highest percentage of sterilized men worldwide. The same applies to tubal ligations for women. With the exception of long-term injected contraceptives, which have been a focus of Chinese medical research for many years, usage of other methods in China, such as condoms and oral contraceptives, is way below the international average. This has to do with the temporary nature of pill and condom use, financial difficulties and the other problems connected with them.[57]

Between 1979 and 1999, the percentage of women of reproductive age who practised contraception or underwent contraceptive surgery rose from between 60 and 70 per cent to between 80 and 90 per cent. Once again, these are the highest rates in the world. Table 3 also allows the comparison of provincial averages. The figures hail from the report system of the birth-planning

Table 3 Contraceptive rates by methods and provinces 1981, 1999 (persons using contraceptive methods/married women in reproductive age, %)

	Total	Male sterilization	Female sterilization	IUD	Oral pill, injection, implant	Condom	Diaphragm	Others
1981								
Beijing	84.6	1.4	11.3	20.8	29.5	14.3	2.0	5.3
Tianjin	82.0	2.1	10.6	29.4	21.4	13.9	1.3	3.3
Hebei	80.4	1.9	8.5	56.9	7.6	3.5	0.5	1.5
Shanxi	81.3	0.4	17.3	52.3	7.1	2.7	0.4	1.1
Inner Mongolia	74.3	0.5	21.3	30.8	16.7	3.1	0.4	1.5
Liaoning	86.6	1.0	30.4	42.9	5.6	5.6	1.0	0.1
Jilin	85.7	0.4	25.4	51.2	4.1	3.3	0.4	0.9
Heilongjiang	88.0	1.1	30.7	48.8	3.4	3.3	0.6	0.1
Shanghai	84.4	3.8	22.7	24.0	23.0	7.9	0.1	2.8
Jiangsu	86.1	5.2	25.9	43.1	9.2	0.9	0.6	1.1
Zhejiang	78.5	3.0	31.4	27.8	11.4	1.8	0.6	2.5
Anhui	81.8	7.1	18.8	46.1	7.6	1.3	0.2	0.7
Fujian	81.5	9.9	25.9	41.5	1.3	1.7	0.1	1.1
Jiangxi	78.8	1.3	31.1	41.8	2.8	0.7	0.3	0.8
Shandong	78.2	15.5	23.1	35.3	2.4	1.4		0.6
Henan	81.7	7.4	27.5	42.1	1.9	1.6	0.3	0.8
Hubei	81.3	5.3	22.6	43.7	6.5	1.4	0.4	1.5

	Total	Male sterilization	Female sterilization	IUD	Oral pill, injection, implant	Condom	Diaphragm	Others
Hunan	78.1	9.7	34.1	28.4	2.9	1.5	0.5	1.1
Guangdong	75.5	8.0	20.2	41.4	2.6	1.7	0.4	1.3
Guangxi	60.2	1.5	5.1	39.1	8.4	1.4	0.6	4.1
Hainan								
Sichuan	81.3	30.7	9.0	35.4	3.0	1.6	0.4	1.3
Guizhou	66.4	8.4	8.8	45.4	1.8	1.0	0.2	0.9
Yunnan	58.2	4.2	9.4	35.6	4.8	1.8	0.2	2.3
Tibet								
Shaanxi	82.7	1.2	11.8	60.1	5.0	2.4	0.5	1.5
Gansu	82.1	0.6	34.4	41.1	3.3	1.6	0.2	1.0
Qinghai	53.7	0.1	7.8	21.5	20.4	1.7	0.5	1.7
Ningxia	62.1	0.2	15.1	18.4	23.0	1.7	0.8	2.9
Xinjiang	73.6	0.7	24.0	15.9	23.7	6.2	2.3	0.8
China	79.6	8.0	20.8	40.8	6.0	2.3	0.4	1.3
1999								
Beijing	88.8	0.2	6.9	55.0	6.4	19.2	0.3	0.8
Tianjin	91.2	0.3	13.2	52.8	4.2	20.3	0.3	0.0
Hebei	91.6	6.9	46.5	33.2	2.4	3.0	0.1	0.2
Shanxi	89.0	1.0	51.3	33.4	2.0	0.9	0.2	0.2
Inner Mongolia	92.7	0.3	39.8	48.1	2.3	2.1	0.1	0.0
Liaoning	91.4	0.1	17.9	64.9	2.3	6.0	0.3	0.0
Jilin	91.0	0.0	27.0	57.4	2.7	3.4	0.3	0.0
Heilongjiang	92.8	0.1	28.7	57.2	2.4	4.1	0.1	0.1
Shanghai	90.8	0.4	4.0	67.9	5.1	10.5	0.5	2.5
Jiangsu	92.3	3.8	23.2	59.9	3.0	1.8	0.2	0.1
Zhejiang	91.4	1.0	37.8	45.5	3.0	3.8	0.2	0.1
Anhui	91.3	6.1	46.9	34.2	2.5	1.3	0.1	0.2
Fujian	90.5	8.0	49.9	25.4	2.6	4.1	0.3	0.3
Jiangxi	89.8	0.5	54.7	28.7	2.3	3.2	0.3	0.1
Shandong	90.8	16.4	26.7	42.1	0.9	4.3	0.2	0.2
Henan	90.7	13.1	42.7	30.3	1.1	3.3	0.2	0.1
Hubei	89.2	6.1	42.2	36.0	2.2	2.4	0.3	0.0
Hunan	91.8	8.1	44.5	33.2	1.4	4.6	0.4	0.0
Guangdong	89.4	12.6	47.7	24.9	0.8	2.6	0.4	0.2
Guangxi	89.4	14.1	36.4	33.3	2.6	2.0	0.6	0.2
Hainan	85.4	2.6	52.2	26.6	1.2	1.8	0.4	0.6
Sichuan	92.4	23.9	5.9	56.5	2.2	3.4	0.3	0.2
Guizhou	91.0	18.1	39.8	25.2	2.9	3.2	0.4	0.1
Yunnan	86.1	5.2	24.9	50.2	3.5	1.6	0.3	0.3
Tibet	67.1	0.0	12.5	14.6	37.0	1.9	0.3	0.8
Shaanxi	90.2	3.8	50.0	29.3	2.8	3.7	0.6	0.1
Gansu	88.0	0.2	61.3	23.7	1.2	1.2	0.3	0.0
Qinghai	86.5	0.1	40.1	34.4	7.9	2.7	0.7	0.2
Ningxia	89.9	0.0	36.5	38.1	9.1	5.2	0.7	0.1
Xinjiang	82.5	0.6	11.4	57.5	4.8	6.7	0.9	0.6
China	90.6	8.4	34.6	41.2	2.3	3.5	0.3	0.2

Sources: Own calculations from birth-planning report data in ZJSN 1986; ZRTN 2000

commissions and show a tendency to over-report compared with rival data from fertility surveys in Table 7. The total rate of contraceptive prevalence as enumerated in the surveys of 1982, 1988, 1992 and 1997 was 12, 16, 8 and 7 percentage points less than according to the report figures for the respective years. Figures for 1982 yielded by the fertility surveys of 1982 and 1988 also differ. Because of the increased political pressures and the continuing falsification of statistics, both report and survey figures from the 1990s are particularly vulnerable to bias. Later adjustments are therefore likely.

Nevertheless, the data are valid for analysing general trends in regional and temporal differentials. As report figures for the individual provinces span a greater length of time than do survey results, they are preferred. The provincial data demonstrate that over the years the large gap between contraceptive rates in the eastern and western half of the country has gradually reduced. In the main, this is the result of tightened birth planning in the 1990s. Progress in the 1980s was much slower. The highest rises in contraceptive rates have occurred in backward rural areas and minority regions, which were formerly largely exempt from birth control. However, minority regions such as Hainan, Yunnan, Qinghai and Xinjiang continue to trail behind the national average by some 5 to 10 percentage points. The biggest deviant case is Tibet, the last region to implement birth control, where the total contraceptive rate is nearly 25 percentage points below the national average.

Among the various contraceptive methods, female sterilizations score the greatest increases; extension to the rural areas of high-fertility provinces such as Anhui, Fujian and Jiangxi, Guangdong, Guangxi and Shaanxi plus all minority regions has been massive. There are marked differences in the prevalence of either female or male sterilization. In the North, Northeast and Northwest of the country vasectomy is almost non-existent, and even less so in the Muslim regions. Its use increases markedly in Shandong and the provinces of the Center-South, and has become widespread in the Southwest. With four times as many cases of vasectomy as cases of tubal ligation, Sichuan is the only province where male sterilizations outnumber female ones. In all other cases, the onus of contraception falls largely on women.

There are complicated reasons for regional differences. Essentially, contraceptive mix is a policy choice of regional authorities. It may be assumed that their policy choices in turn are conditioned by the extent of population pressures, political and organizational clout, cultural sensibilities, financial considerations and the availability of specific medical techniques. A fear that some methods could have side-effects bearing on the sex-specific division of peasant labour may also play a role. Finally, the contraceptive mix is also contingent on the composition of women of reproductive age, in particular on the percentages for newly married women and women with second-child permits. Many of these factors combine in Sichuan, where a strict birth-control programme operates. It applies low-cost vasectomy in a social environment characterized by involvement of women in heavy agricultural labour, extremely high population numbers and consequently high financial pressures to economize.

In contrast to sterilization and IUDs, national averages for the use of pills, injections, and implants have declined. Again, this reflects conscious policy choices over the past two decades. While today about 40 per cent of women of reproductive age are supposed to be using IUDs, the percentages for pills, implants and condoms amount to only 2 to 4 per cent, respectively. For diaphragms and other methods, they make up less than 1 per cent each. Even the three municipal regions, where percentages for condoms and pills rose to between 30 and 40 per cent in the past, have largely substituted these methods with more long-term techniques of birth control. In the Muslim areas of the Northwest, where the more easily acceptable pills and condoms served to mollify resistance to long-term contraception, they have also been phased out to a large degree. Only Tibet remains as a case of primary reliance on the pill. Judging from past experience in other minority regions, this will be a temporary compromise only.

Data from the national fertility surveys of married women in 1982, 1988 and 1992 permit more sophisticated analyses. The latter investigation has been particularly ambitious. Along with the usual set of individual items, it collected a number of community variables such as accessibility of health, educational or administrative institutions, but it remains a yet unresolved riddle why all attempts to analyse these figures for linkages to contraceptive use fail.[58] Other figures deliver clear messages, though. In interpreting contraceptive rates for the influence of the number and sex of children already born, the following patterns emerged.

According to the 1992 survey results, contraceptive prevalence for childless women was minuscule and remained at around 6 per cent (1988: 4 per cent, 1982: 2 per cent). It became prevalent after the birth of the first child only, after which more than 70 per cent (1988: 55 per cent, 1982: 44 per cent) of women resorted to IUDs. This percentage declined to 18 per cent (1988: 26 per cent, 1982: 44 per cent) after the second child. Less than 2 per cent of married men or women with one child were sterilized. After the second child the figure increased to 58 per cent (1988: 39 per cent, 1982: 19 per cent) for tubal ligations and 14 per cent (1988: 11 per cent, 1982: 7 per cent) for vasectomies. While in 1992 female sterilizations after higher-parity births remained at this high level (1988: 43 per cent, 1982: 28 per cent), vasectomies grew to 19 per cent (1988: 15 per cent, 1982: 11 per cent) – a telling indicator of the pressures exerted, since most Chinese men are no exception to the worldwide antipathy of males to being sterilized. The comparison of figures documents the general shift to long-term contraception since the beginning of the one-child campaign and the extent to which even IUD use after the second child has become substituted by the still more reliable sterilization.

In the survey of 1988, which also furnished detailed sex-specific data, acceptance of IUDs among mothers of boys was noticeably higher than among mothers of girls. This differed from the situation for pills and condoms, which offer the greatest freedom of personal fertility decisions and showed no sex-specific differences. After the birth of a second child, rates for IUD use declined to around 25 per cent, again with the expected sex-specific difference. Instead of

IUDs, sterilizations became the main contraceptive method at this stage. If there was at least one son among two children or more, over 60 per cent of all couples underwent either tubal ligations or vasectomies. If not, this percentage shrank to about 40 per cent.

The same pattern also underlies the age-specific figures in Table 4, which show IUD use decreasing and sterilization increasing until the late stages of the reproductive period. Understandably, the lowest percentages for any type of contraceptive use are always recorded for women in the youngest and oldest age groups, who are either awaiting pregnancy or show growing instances of infertility. Between the ages 20 to 39, total contraceptive rates invariably rise – reflecting the increasingly strict birth-control demands after one or two births.

Table 4 Contraceptive rates by methods, age groups and residence 1982, 1988, 1992 (Persons using contraceptive methods / married women in reproductive age, %)

	Total	Male sterilization	Female sterilization	IUD	Oral pill, injection	Condom	Supposi- tories	Others
1982								
China	69.7	6.9	17.7	34.9	5.9	1.4	0.2	2.7
15–19	10.0	0.0	0.2	6.6	2.0	0.1	0.0	1.1
20–24	30.5	0.4	1.7	21.5	4.1	0.6	0.1	2.2
25–29	68.2	3.8	10.5	41.4	8.0	1.5	0.2	2.8
30–34	87.5	8.6	26.0	42.0	7.2	1.5	0.2	2.0
35–39	89.0	11.0	31.3	37.3	5.9	1.5	0.1	2.0
40–44	82.0	10.8	24.5	36.0	5.3	1.9	0.2	3.3
45–49	52.9	8.3	12.9	23.3	2.5	1.4	0.1	4.6
urban	74.1	2.1	15.0	29.0	13.9	7.1	0.7	6.2
rural	68.9	7.8	18.2	36.0	4.3	0.3	0.1	2.1
1988								
China	72.1	7.9	27.6	29.9	3.5	1.9	0.3	0.9
15–19	11.3	0.1	0.3	9.0	1.4	0.3	0.1	0.2
20–24	38.2	1.2	4.3	27.4	3.1	1.5	0.3	0.4
25–29	70.9	4.3	17.6	39.9	5.0	2.7	0.5	0.9
30–34	88.2	10.2	36.2	34.1	4.0	2.3	0.4	1.0
35–39	92.5	13.3	46.7	26.5	3.3	1.6	0.2	1.0
40–44	86.4	12.5	41.0	26.7	3.2	1.5	0.2	1.3
45–49	54.5	7.2	21.3	20.8	2.1	1.6	0.1	1.4
cities	76.6	3.6	19.3	38.8	5.1	6.5	0.8	2.6
rural	71.0	9.0	29.6	27.7	3.2	0.8	0.2	0.5
1992								
China	83.4	9.8	34.7	33.5	3.1	1.5	0.2	0.5
15–19	27.8	0.6	1.0	21.1	3.0	1.3	0.6	0.2
20–24	53.8	1.7	7.6	38.9	3.3	1.7	0.3	0.2
25–29	84.2	8.0	26.2	44.1	3.5	1.8	0.3	0.4
30–34	93.0	10.9	40.4	36.1	3.2	1.8	0.2	0.4
35–39	95.5	13.6	48.6	28.2	3.1	1.4	0.2	0.5
40–44	94.2	14.6	51.5	23.1	3.1	1.1	0.2	0.7
45–49	79.6	12.6	43.0	20.0	1.9	0.9	0.1	1.1
non-agricult	83.8	2.4	16.2	52.6	5.5	5.1	0.7	1.2
agricult.	83.3	11.7	39.4	28.7	2.5	0.6	0.1	0.3

Sources: Data from the 1982, 1988 and 1992 fertility surveys in: ZJSN 1986; Liang Jimin and Chen Shengli 1993, Vol. 3; Jiang Zhenghua 1995

Case numbers for very young women are small, so that the survey results for the age group 15 to 19 may be spurious. Moreover, they are slanted by the fact that only the extremely small number of married women under age 20 are documented. However, it is also plausible that between 1988 and 1992 the percentage of very young women who practised contraception increased. A closer look at provincial data reveals that again this seems to involve mostly agrarian provinces and minority regions with high levels of fertility and early marriage. Some provinces such as Liaoning and Jilin, Zhejiang, Anhui and Jiangxi seem to have pushed IUD use specifically for very young women under the legal marriage age. Some county regulations offer a clue to the mechanisms involved. They threaten immediate sterilization to all couples with early marriages and early births who do not consent to sign a 'Contract for Not Having Another Birth'.

The recent push to extend contraception in the countryside has left other marks, too. As far as the totals for contraceptive rates are concerned, although the urban–rural gap continued to be wide between 1982 and 1988, it is supposed to have almost closed between 1988 and 1992. The figures for the specific methods of contraception, however, show a continued existence of urban-rural differences in the contraceptive mix. Widespread sterilization is increasingly becoming a rural phenomenon, while urban areas resort to IUDs.[59] This is the price exacted by the state for granting second-child permits in the countryside.

It is a price that is often paid only grudgingly. The figures in Table 5 come from a backward and impoverished rural area of Northern Anhui which is conspicuous for its traditionally high fertility and mortality level. They hail from a province that has decreed compulsory abortions of unauthorized pregnancies and from a county claiming successful birth control due to effective responsibility and evaluation schemes.[60] The data are restricted to women under age 35 who underwent sterilization after their second child, or to women under age 40 who consented to sterilization after a third or higher-order birth. As shown in the table, less than 40 per cent did this of their own volition. The rest indicated directly or indirectly that they were to various degrees pressured into complying with policy. It is noteworthy in this respect that the fear of penalties ranked much lower than resignation to the situation. This points to the realization that non-acceptance of sterilization would not offer any advantage, since compulsory abortion would follow anyway.

Table 5 Motives of women for final acceptance of sterilization: survey from Fengyang County, Anhui, 1992 (% checked)

No reply	8.8
Follow the mainstream	5.7
No use refusing	35.5
Fear of penalty for extra birth	1.4
Own wish	37.9
Follow policy proclamations	10.0
Set example as cadre family	0.7

Source: Peng Xizhe and Dai Xingyi 1996, 242

The Anhui figures may not be representative, since they come from a poor region. Furthermore, they are restricted to women who finally accepted long-term contraception. This is why Table 6, which shows larger samples from the whole of China, looks at the reasons given by the 30 per cent (1982) to 17 per cent (1992) of women who did not practise contraception. In order to ensure comparability, some categories in the surveys underlying this table were compressed into one entry.

Illness, sterility or cessation of menstruation, pregnancy or expectancy of it are self-explainatory reasons amenable to validation. Together they comprise about 60 per cent of all cases covered in Table 6, showing convincing patterns

Table 6 Reasons for no contraceptive use 1982, 1988, 1992 (reasons / married women not using contraceptive methods, %)

	Don't know how	Inconvenient	Breast-feeding	Ill, no menses, sterile	Fear of side-effects	Awaiting pregnancy, pregnant	Spouse absent, others
1982, first marriages							
China				20.3		37.1	42.6
15–19				0.1		76.6	23.3
20–24				0.7		66.8	32.7
25–29				3.0		40.2	56.8
30–34				14.2		15.5	70.2
35–39				23.8		8.5	67.7
40–44				46.3		3.3	50.4
45–49				78.5		0.7	20.7
urban				29.5		51.8	18.7
rural				18.9		34.8	46.3
1988							
China	0.3	0.1	20.4	23.6	1.6	39.1	15.0
15–19	0.2	0.1	20.5	0.3	0.3	71.3	7.3
20–24	0.2	0.1	28.2	2.1	0.7	59.8	8.8
25–29	0.3	0.1	30.0	6.4	2.1	43.8	17.4
30–34	0.5	0.2	22.4	16.7	3.2	31.7	25.4
35–39	0.9	0.3	10.2	34.3	3.8	15.5	35.1
40–44	0.8	0.1	2.0	63.2	3.0	3.4	27.5
45–49	0.2	0.1	0.2	84.9	1.2	0.5	12.9
cities	0.2	0.1	18.0	27.7	1.4	47.9	14.7
rural	0.3	0.1	20.9	22.7	1.6	39.3	15.1
1992							
China			17.9	14.9		40.7	26.7
15–19			18.0	0.4		47.6	34.0
20–24			23.8	1.1		60.0	15.1
25–29			23.9	10.6		43.2	26.8
30–34			13.2	18.8		27.7	40.4
35–39			5.6	32.7		12.0	49.8
40–44			1.5	44.4		2.1	52.1
45–49			0.1	61.7		0.4	37.6
non-agricult.			16.6	17.4		38.5	27.6
agricult.			18.2	14.2		41.1	26.4

Sources: Data from the 1982, 1988 and 1992 fertility surveys in: ZJSN 1986; Liang Jimin and Chen Shengli 1993, Vol. 3; Jiang Zhenghua 1995

of age-specific prevalence. However, the table discloses that understanding of the reasons for non-use is less than perfect, since high percentages of respondents give a catch-all 'other' reason for not practising contraception. Besides imperfections in questionnaire design, this may have to do with hidden resistance to birth control. The uneven distribution of 'other' reasons, if they are controlled for the sex of children born, hints in that direction.[61] But 'other' reasons can also cover a host of further factors such as separation of couples, voluntary abstention, inaccessibility of birth-control services, etc.

Most attempts to specify further reasons in the 1988 survey did not yield any significant results. Only breast-feeding, where figures for different age groups correlate closely with age-specific fertility, emerged as an important additional cause for non-use. This reflects the belief of women that lactation prevents conception in a natural way – an idea not backed up by medical research, which attributes insufficient reliability to the method. Accurate information on the link between breast-feeding and birth prevention in China is rare. One of the few studies investigating this topic has been an in-depth survey in Shanghai and Guizhou during 1985. While it showed the substantial impact of modern contraception, the figures for the reduction in birth numbers due to lactation remained low. In Shanghai they amounted to between 5 and 6 per cent of natural fertility, in Guizhou they rose to around 11 per cent.[62] As these regions mark the lower and upper end of the fertility spectrum in China and evince clearly different childrearing and weaning practices, this probably indicates the range to be expected within the country.

6.6 Abortions

The long road from the almost total ban on abortions in the early 1950s to their successive liberalization during later years has already been covered in the summary of birth-planning policies prior to the one-child campaign. The watershed was reached in 1963, when abortions were completely liberalized and the principle of cost-free availability with ten to fourteen days of rest was introduced. Already in 1958, Shanghai's hospitals had pioneered the use of new and easy-to-use vacuum techniques; after 1964 they became widely accessible in the rest of the country. Still, for a number of years a number of internal documents continued to lament that inadequate facilities failed to meet demand.[63] In the majority of cases, bottle-necks seem to have been created by the massive propaganda drive for birth control. However, although no precise information on the balance of voluntary versus 'recommended' applications is available, random references also hint at unfulfilled demand among parts of the population. Presumably, such instances were largely found in urban areas.

The character of things began to change in the 1970s, when abortion rates rose dramatically. Paralleling the call for contraceptive use in the course of the one-child campaign, abortions meanwhile have frequently turned into an obligatory measure not left to individual choice. Apart from married women whose childbearing would exceed the number of authorized births, they also involve all unmarried women who fall pregnant. Some recent birth-planning regulations contain the inconspicuous and seemingly self-evident sentence 'a couple is permitted to give birth to one child'. In the juridical literature this is interpreted as clearly prohibiting illegitimate childbearing, whether it results from premarital cohabitation, rape or artificial insemination.[64] Other provincial birth-planning regulations also explicitly spell out the ban on extra-marital births. Supplementary rules at local level stipulate penalty fines for premarital cohabitation, even if it has not resulted in pregnancy. If such instances are found among the student population, they can furnish sufficient ground for immediate expulsion.

Since 1979 birth-planning norms have usually treated abortions under the term 'remedial measures (*bujiu cuoshi*)'. This signals an awareness of the accompanying health hazards. Such awareness contributed to the earlier scepticism towards abortion in the 1950s, and it underlies the following supplementary rule decreed by the Birth Planning Leading Group of Tibet Autonomous Region in 1987:

> It must be pointed out that induced abortion is a remedial measure adopted for making up contraceptive failure. If induced abortions are performed many times in a row, they may impair women's health. Induced abortions therefore cannot be used as a contraceptive method. Women having two or more induced abortions within one year should be persuaded to undergo tubal ligation. Otherwise, they will pay the surgery expenses themselves and cease to receive wages during the period of rest.[65]

It is nevertheless remarkable that the relevant regulations contain many more stipulations on 'remedial measures' than rules on IUD use and sterilization. In some cases, they include the recommendation that women 'should take timely remedial measures (*yao jizao caiqu bujiu cuoshi*)' or should be 'persuaded and educated (*shuofu jiaoyu*)' to do so after becoming pregnant out of plan. Much more frequent is the severe admonition that 'remedial measures shall (*ying*) be practised'; most recent regulations also do not hesitate to use the unequivocal 'must (*bixu*)'.

This legal hair-splitting cannot hide the fact that pressures for termination of unauthorized pregnancies are extremely strong. Regional regulations vary from province to province and may contain the rule that those undergoing unauthorized pregnancies are immediately penalized by deducting 15 per cent to 30 per cent from their monthly wages. In March 1982, Gansu province ordered an immediate and complete freeze of all wage payments for offenders, and in the same year Shaanxi made the refusal of abortion a subject of criminal law. In January 1983, Jiangxi province decreed without much ado:

> All women with second or higher-order pregnancies outside plan must take remedial measures as soon as possible. Those who do not heed good advice will be punished with economic sanctions according to circumstances, and their pregnancy will be terminated within a fixed period. After termination of the pregnancy, no further sanctions will be administered, and all fines will be refunded.[66]

Regulations passed two years later in Inner Mongolia have been similarly unambiguous. Since then, they simply state: 'Getting information on pregnancies must be strengthened. As soon as a pregnancy outside plan is detected, timely remedial measures should be taken.'[67]

In 1984 Anhui ordered an immediate 15 per cent wage reduction per month for offenders after discovery of above-quota pregnancies. The regulations of the province valid at that time stated that 'whoever takes remedial measures within a specified time will receive a complete refund of the penalty sum'. Later, this formulation was still deemed to be insufficient. As of October 1988 revised regulations contain the additional sentence: 'If the specified time period is exceeded, the remedial measure will be ordered, and the penalty sum will not be reimbursed.' Other provinces emulated these procedures in later years, raising the threatened wage reduction to ever higher levels. In the Hainan regulations of 1989, this amounted to a monthly 60 per cent for cadres, workers and staff, and was raised to a flat 500 yuan in 1995.[68]

The Liaoning regulations of May 1988 have been equally stern. They simply proclaim: 'Those getting pregnant outside plan must terminate the pregnancy in time.' In 1997 an amendment clause was added: '... within the period prescribed by the township (town) people's governments or the street-committee offices.' Earlier, the provincial Party Committee circulated 'Some Opinions on Further Perfecting Birth Planning Policies' which contained a proposal that was also introduced in other provinces:

> If there are pregnancies outside plan, the granting of second-child quotas for the village shall be stopped, as long as no remedial measures are taken. If there are births outside plan, the granting of second-child quotas for the village shall cease for one year, starting with the month of birth. New second-child quotas can be only granted after thorough rectification.[69]

Pressures are particularly great if pregnancies result from cohabitation of unmarried persons. The designed system of contraceptive measures and abortions has been laid down most cogently in the birth-planning regulations of Henan province decreed in April 1990. Because of its high population numbers, its strong peasant traditionalism and repeated instances of fraudulent birth planning, this region has always been a problem case:

> All couples of reproductive age who have not obtained a birth quota shall practice contraception. Women shall get an IUD insertion after their first childbirth; in case of couples with two or more births, one spouse shall get sterilized. Women for whom IUD use is not appropriate according to medical review, as well as men or women for whom sterilization is not appropriate according to medical review, shall practice other effective contraceptive measures. Whoever gets pregnant out of plan, must take remedial measures and terminate the pregnancy.[70]

Although recent years have seen a renewed stress on contraceptive choice and some birth-planning norms have phrased the call for abortions more moderately, there is no doubt that in practice many unauthorized pregnancies are terminated by command.[71] The consequences of ignoring this command have varied widely from period to period and place to place. Extremes have ranged from turning a blind eye to immediate arrest, and in most cases they involve progressively steeper penalty sums and disciplinary sanctions. Since the mid-1990s, however, Chinese birth planning has also produced the opposite case of sanctions for having an abortion without proving 'valid reasons', such as eugenic indications, health hazards for the mother or an unauthorized pregnancy. Relevant stipulations have been written into a number of newly revised birth-planning regulations in order to check the increasing prevalence of prenatal sex determination with the consequent abortion of a female foetus.[72]

Table 7 presents the available figures on abortions. Fragmentary numbers begin with the second birth-planning campaign in 1963. There are no representative nationwide figures before that year; the few isolated regional reports for the 1950s all indicate abortion rates of well under 1 per cent. The data indicate a steep increase of abortion cases in the following two years. In Shanghai it assumed campaign proportions and produced a record figure of 100 abortions per 100 live births in 1964. No numbers are available for the second half of the decade, when book-keeping broke down during the Cultural Revolution. Records resume with the third birth-planning campaign in 1971, when the abortion rate already seems to have been twice as high as in 1965. After 1971 the figures rise consistently, and with the advent of the one-child policy they jump to hitherto unknown heights. Similar to the situation for sterilizations and IUD insertions, the years 1979 to 1980, 1983 and 1990 to 1991 have been peak periods. It is certainly no coincidence that these periods have witnessed the toughest political pronouncements on the one-child policy to date.

The abortion rate reflects the number of artificially terminated pregnancies per 100 live births. While it does not include spontaneous expulsions or miscarriages, it covers any removal or deliberately induced expulsion, no matter during which period of time. The rate therefore comprises both early terminations up to the end of the third month (*liuchan*) and later ones (*yinchan*). In the 1960s and 1970s late abortions were usually limited to surgery until the end of the fifth month. Revised Rules on Contraceptive Operations issued by the Ministry of Health and the Birth-Planning Commission in February 1984 extended this period to the end of the twenty-seventh week.[73] Under the high pressure of the one-child campaign, some places practise them even until the very last stages of pregnancy, if necessary. Apart from surgery, RU–486 abortion pills have been available in Chinese cities since the late 1990s. While regulations treat them as a prescription drug, they are also available on the black market for women eschewing official attention to their pregnancy.

All over the world, the abortion rate is notoriously dubious and highly vulnerable to distortions both in the birth numbers and the abortion figures *per*

Table 7 Contraceptive prevalence, operations, and abortions 1963–99 (contraceptive prevalence as % married women in reproductive age practicing various forms of contraception including sterilization; operations in millions; abortion rate per 100 live births)

	Contracept. prevalence	Male sterilization	Female sterilization	IUD insertion	Abortions	Abortion rate A	B
1963[1]		0.06	0.13	0.16	0.40	1.4	
1964[1]		0.20	0.61	1.63	1.80	6.4	
1965[1]	10.0	0.20	0.61	1.63	1.80	6.5	
1970	13.5						
	17.3	1.22	1.74	6.17	3.91	13.3	
	22.5	1.72	2.09	9.22	4.81	17.2	
	28.6	1.93	2.96	13.95	5.11	19.4	
	34.4	1.45	2.28	12.58	4.98	19.7	
1975	40.6	2.65	3.28	16.74	5.08	22.3	
	45.2	1.50	2.71	11.63	4.74	22.1	13.8
	48.4	2.62	2.78	12.97	5.23	26.3	13.0
	50.2	0.77	2.51	10.96	5.39	27.1	15.0
	53.7	1.67	5.29	13.47	7.86	37.8	17.5
1980	54.6	1.36	3.84	11.49	9.53	55.0	23.3
	54.7	0.65	1.56	10.34	8.70	41.5	20.4
	58.2	1.23	3.93	14.07	12.42	55.5	25.0
	64.2	4.36	16.40	17.76	14.37	69.8	31.0
	66.3	1.29	5.42	11.75	8.89	43.3	27.8
1985	66.2	0.58	2.28	9.58	10.93	49.6	27.7
	65.7	1.03	2.91	10.64	11.58	48.6	29.7
	69.4	1.75	4.41	13.45	10.49	41.6	27.5
	73.2	1.06	3.59	12.23	12.68	51.6	
		1.51	4.22	10.85	10.38	43.1	
1990		1.47	5.31	12.35	13.49	56.4	
		2.38	6.75	12.29	14.09	62.4	
	83.4	0.86	4.50	10.09	10.42	46.9	
		0.97	5.17	13.46	9.50	44.7	
	90.7	0.95	4.58	13.21	9.47	45.0	
1995	90.4	0.78	4.10	13.03	7.48	36.2	
	91.1	0.78	3.87	12.88	8.83	42.7	
	83.8	0.67	3.34	12.11	6.59	32.3	
	83.8	0.64	2.99	11.39	7.39	38.7	
	83.0	0.57	2.96	10.74	6.76	35.4	

Notes and Sources:
1 Own estimate on the basis of data for January to November 1963 and January 1963 to June 1965
Rates of contraceptive prevalence from survey data in: ZRN 1991, 529; Yuan Yongxi 1996, 296; ZJSN 1998, 122; www.sfpc.gov; rival data from the reporting system for 1981 and 1999 in table 3. Contraceptive operations 1963–92 and abortions 1963–99 according to data from the Ministry of Health in: ZJSQ 1997, 9, 898; ZWN 1993–. Contraceptive operations 1993–99 according to data from the State Birth Planning Commission in: ZRTN 1994–. Abortion rate A according to own calculations on the basis of registered birth numbers for 1963–65, adjusted birth numbers for 1971–81 from Judith Banister (Banister 1978, 180), retrospective calculations from 1990 census figures in ZRTN 1997 and birth numbers from the annual sample survey for 1991–99. Abortion rate B according to 1988 fertility survey of the Birth-Planning Commission in: Chang Chongxuan 1991, 170

se. Another weakness of the indicator is that it is heavily influenced by age structure and marriage patterns. In China's case, the abortion rates rise dramatically to between sixty-two and seventy-nine abortions per 100 live births, if the underestimated figures of the 1980s instead of the adjusted birth numbers from the 1990 population count are to be believed. Conversely, data from the 1988 national fertility survey convey yet another picture: they show a drastic decline in the abortion rate. The discrepancy is immense, and once again points to data problems and the possibility that abortion numbers were massively inflated due to corruption or political pressures. In later years, when illegitimate pregnancies increased and abortions came to be treated as indicators of birth-planning failure instead of success, over-reporting may have given way to a tendency to under-report.

Numbers in Table 7 hail from the Ministry of Health. Here, the abortion figures for the period 1992 to 1999 are considerably higher than those provided by the Birth-Planning Commission. The gap has been continuously widening, with the Ministry's figures for 1999 more than three times as high than those from the rival Commission.[74] Besides the all-pervading corruption of birth-planning statistics, such inconsistencies also point to major problems of inter-agency coordination. In part, they may be magnified by different systems of record-taking and tabulation by either place of surgery or place of residence. While the former method has been used for contraceptive operations and abortions in clinics of the public health system, the latter is used by the birth-planning stations subordinate to the birth-planning commissions. Generally, the abortion rate evinces the same ups and downs as contraceptive operations, but it differs in displaying a long-term rising trend. It is only since 1994 that it seems to have dropped continuously. Meanwhile, it seems to have levelled out at the beginning of the one-child campaign. However, in view of the many data problems, it remains to be seen whether this development is confirmed.

Estimates of annual pregnancies on the basis of reported birth and abortion numbers would indicate that nearly one-third of all pregnancies were terminated by induced abortions.[75] This percentage would drop to an average 21 per cent for the 1980s if data from the 1988 national fertility survey are used. This survey showed that about 33 per cent of urban and 18 per cent of rural pregnancies were artificially aborted during that decade. Such percentages are approximately double the figures for the 1970s (averages of 18 per cent and 8 per cent, respectively) and four to seven times larger than in the 1960s (averages of 9 per cent and 2 per cent, respectively). They dwarf the retrospective data for the 1950s (averages of 1 per cent and 0.2 per cent, respectively), when abortions were largely prohibited. The rural–urban differential has been a constant feature of the abortion rate. Rates for occupational groups and educational levels show a parallel tendency to rise with progression to urban characteristics.[76]

Once again, these numbers demonstrate the makeshift character of many birth-control measures, the lack of contraceptive effectiveness and stability in the campaign. Therefore, the high abortion numbers are symptoms of 'consistency' and negligence in birth control at the same time. It should be pointed out, however, that from an international perspective Chinese abortion figures do not appear to excessively high. Japan, Korea and Taiwan have known equally high or even higher abortion rates; ever since the mid-1980s abortion has been rising in many East and South Asian countries. East European abortion figures generally surpass the Chinese ones, while the West European and American figures approach them.[77] In this sense, state promotion of abortion as a last-resort birth-control measure rather than the prevalence of abortion as such is a Chinese peculiarity.

Table 8 lists the available regional abortion rate figures. Although figures for 1965 are approximate, they suffice to demonstrate the rural–urban gap prevailing at that time. Abortion levels in the three centrally administered municipalities were already approaching later levels, and Shanghai occupied its customary position as the region with the highest prevalence of abortion in China. Numbers in Jiangsu were also quite high. The other provinces, however, had only just begun to use this crash instrument of birth planning. Data from the 1988 national fertility survey are not strictly comparable either, as they are not computed for one year of reference but rather relate all past abortions of women respondents to all their past births. In most cases this raises the denominator of the abortion rate to a disproportionately large figure and thereby effects a drastic decline in the rate. It is only in urbanized regions like Beijing, Tianjin and Liaoning that data are roughly comparable to later annual figures. Figures for the period 1990 to 1996 are definitionally compatible. Their temporal trend confirms the existence of a new abortion campaign waged in 1991/92 after the census results of 1990 became known. With few exceptions, most regions report markedly increased abortion rates during these years.[78] The provinces singled out for a massive new abortion campaign can be readily identified: Anhui, Fujian, Shandong, Henan, Hunan and Guangxi. All these areas are problem cases of Chinese birth planning.

Apart from their definitional difficulties, abortion rates also pose other problems of interpretation. In the greater part of the 1980s most high fertility provinces were marked by low abortion figures and low contraceptive rates. This situation has changed since 1990, as most regions with traditionally high fertility levels now display above-average abortion figures and largely levelled out contraceptive rates. But high abortion rates are not only evinced by provinces with lagging birth control in the past. They can also reflect strict enforcement, easy availability of medical services and changing sexual habits in urban areas. Shanghai seems to be a case in point, followed by Beijing and Tianjin. Conversely, low abortion rates may also be interpreted in more than one way. They can either indicate successful birth planning with effective contraceptive measures or a lax population policy with high birth numbers. While the first interpretation would apply for the three Northeastern provinces and for Sichuan, the latter would hold true for the whole of the Northwest. Abortion rates for the national minorities settling there and in the Southwest have been only half those of the Han-Chinese population.

In 1988, almost 17 per cent of all married women in China had experienced one induced abortion, and a further 8 per cent had already had two or more.

Table 8 Abortion rate by provinces 1965–96 (abortions per 100 live births)

	1965	1988	1990	1991	1992	1994	1996
Beijing	35	35	35	55	30	18	13
Tianjin	38	27	35	36	25	20	21
Hebei	8	12	57	69	40	26	10
Shanxi		8	21	24	27	35	26
Inner Mongolia		9	25	23	27	16	12
Liaoning		16	15	21	16	9	7
Jilin	5	13	20	22	40	20	10
Heilongjiang		12	23	25	21	11	6
Shanghai	44	41	205	256	247	287	280
Jiangsu	15	21	48	57	47	27	25
Zhejiang		18	58	54	42	32	27
Anhui		12	29	45	55	48	25
Fujian		7	51	82	70	52	29
Jiangxi		10	33	41	51	30	34
Shandong		19	63	83	49	14	6
Henan		7	47	77	83	14	11
Hubei		16	42	48	46	37	24
Hunan	3	12	52	68	80	36	24
Guangdong	8	10	60	69	69	65	55
Guangxi		13	68	45	80	65	46
Hainan		10	47	50	41	40	31
Sichuan		28	45	48	33	26	24
Guizhou	2	6	38	41	41	39	36
Yunnan		12	55	57	51	30	19
Tibet							11
Shaanxi		8	41	47	39	39	25
Gansu		5	37	24	18	13	20
Qinghai		7	27	24	17	16	8
Ningxia		8	22	22	22	15	9
Xinjiang		9	33	21	23	16	8
China		13	45	50	47	30	22
			56	62	49		

Notes: Data for 1965 are own calculations based on population data for 1965 and approximations for all contraceptive operations 1962–65 in Peng Xizhe 1991. On the basis of data in table 5 it was assumed, that abortions made up 45 % of the total for abortions, sterilization's and IUD insertions. Abortion rates in 1988 are given as accumulated rates for all past abortions and births of respondent women according to the 1988 national fertility survey. Abortion rates for 1990–96 are period rates according to own calculations on the basis of census birth numbers for 1990, birth rates from sample surveys for 1991–96 plus provincial and national abortion numbers of the Birth Planning Commission; alternative rates for all China that result from use of the abortion numbers of the Ministry of Health are added.

Sources: contraceptive operations in 1965 calculated from Peng Xizhe 1991, 33; population numbers and vitality rates for 1965 from LTZH 1990; abortion rates for 1988 in: Chang Chongxuan 1991, 170; absolute numbers for abortions in later years: ZJSN 1990–; ZRTN 1991–; ZWN 1993.

Calculation of abortion rates for different age groups demonstrates the expected tendency of low figures for the cohorts of women between 15 and 24 years of age, who are either unmarried or expecting a child. Abortion rates mount thereafter, peaking with levels of 50 per cent to 75 per cent in the age group 35–44. They decline again in later years after the menopause sets in. In the same manner, they are very low for childless women, increase sharply for mothers with one child, and increase still further for those with two children or more. Between 1982 and 1987, the largest increases of abortion rates were recorded for women aged 15–24 and 35–39. In particular, the abortion rate for very young women aged 15–19 more than tripled during that period from 1.8 to 5.9 per cent. Today, it is probably still beyond that figure. This testifies to the problems created by a rising incidence of premarital sex combined with conservative attitudes towards sexual education and contraceptive use among the unmarried. Above all, it is the big cities that are affected by this development. Shanghai is a particularly serious case, for which some documentation is available. In 1990 the percentage of young, unmarried women in the city's abortion total had risen to nearly a quarter.[79]

While abortion due to non-use of contraceptives thus remains a critical issue with new problems, abortion despite contraceptive use is more significant in quantitative terms. The 1982 fertility survey yielded a figure of 48 per cent for abortions due to contraceptive failure; by 1990 this percentage is supposed to have risen to 70 per cent. Because of the low prevalence of short-term contraceptives, ineffective IUD insertions are chiefly responsible for this situation.[80]

6.7 Material incentives

Material incentives for birth control were slow in coming. In the few instances where they were introduced during the 1960s and early 1970s, they were limited to rather imprecise pledges of granting preference to two-child families as far as jobs or housing allocations were concerned. Under the Chinese system, such promises could apply only to the urban areas, where the state controlled all forms of employment and housing. For the villages they were largely meaningless.

The one-child policy with its massive violation of family interests led to a new approach. Already in 1979 the first provisional birth-planning rules started to list a number of material incentives for one-child families. Monthly bonuses, usually paid until a single child reaches the age of 14, have always counted among them. Some regulations left it to the discretion of local authorities to pay additional one-time rewards. In most cases, these have been abolished in later years due to problems of financing. In other more recent regulations, they have mutated into special bonuses for persons entitled to a second child, but who voluntarily forgo further pregnancy. All birth-planning norms have stipulated preferential treatment of one-child families in public services such as education, health and housing. Some of the early regulations contained a global list of incentives, while others laid down specific rules differentiated by urban and rural residence.

Although the basic idea of incentives and preferential treatment seems inherently plausible, it has once again entailed complicated problems of implementation. These problems begin with the one-child certificate that has to be produced in order to obtain the preferences mentioned above. In principle, only families committed to a long-term, preferably lifelong adherence to the one-child norm may obtain this certificate. Such prolonged commitment will only be guaranteed if one spouse gets sterilized after the first birth. However, many families wish to retain an option for a second child either because they hope for a later change of policy or because they are eligible for second-child permits.

In practice, this has posed the question: How long should the one-child norm be respected before a one-child certificate is issued? Procedures seem to have varied. A Hubei report from 1984 indicates that in this province one-child certificates were handed out only once couples had signed a written commitment for respecting the one-child norm for at least five years.[81] Today, the big cities insist on a yearly validation of the certificate by the street committee at the wife's place of residence. Street committees are also the organs responsible for receiving applications for one-child certificates from the self-employed or unemployed in urban areas. In contrast, workers and staff have to file an application with their work unit, and peasants have to visit the birth-planning bureau of their township or town.[82] One-child certificates have to be handed back after the birth of a second child. All regulations require that in such cases the one-child bonuses accumulated thus far have to be reimbursed.

Statistical data in Table 9 on the percentage of one-child certificates are confused due to definitional changes. Because the value of the rate could alter without indicating concomitant changes in programme performance, the definitions employed until 1983 were unsatisfactory. Examples were new cohorts of first children lowering the rate or women progressing to a second child who raised the percentage of one-child certificates by effecting changes in the denominator instead of the numerator. The rate was therefore only valid if its rise surpassed the rise in single children. A better and compatible time series starts in 1984. Nevertheless, in a broad sense the data for the years 1979 to 1982 indicate which provinces saw a speedy enforcement of the one-child appeals. Besides the heavily urbanized regions, these seem to have been the provinces of Jiangsu, Shandong and Sichuan, vanguards of rural birth control in earlier years. Precise numbers, however, are once again rather dubious and suffer from additional problems of falsification. The first national fertility survey of 1982, for instance, resulted in a national figure of more than 53 percentage points lower than the rival figure from the birth-planning reports. Differences in agrarian hinterland provinces could cause an increase of up to 70 percentage points.[83] This demonstrates the prevalence of massive falsification and fraudulent reporting of the rate of one-child certificates at an early date.

Nor is the compatible time series immune from problems of data quality, although at least it reflects the wide gap between lagging provinces and advanced birth-planning areas such as the three municipal regions of Beijing,

Table 9 Rate of one-child certificates by provinces 1979–99 (A = couples holding certificate/couples with 1 child; B = persons holding certificate/married women in reproductive age)

	A 1979	A 1980	A 1982	B 1985	B 1990	B 1999
Beijing	52.8	83.5	75.5	47.2	55.2	42.3
Tianjin	56.4	83.3	82.6	45.3	50.2	47.7
Hebei	72.8	78.7	34.1	18.2	14.1	13.9
Shanxi	7.3	76.8	16.1	11.8	13.0	12.6
Inner Mongolia	11.0	35.1	36.7	12.4	12.6	16.3
Liaoning	68.2	91.8	70.8	36.3	37.1	45.9
Jilin	15.3	50.6	40.9	27.7	26.6	36.1
Heilongjiang	54.3	82.4	35.2	25.1	25.8	32.3
Shanghai	87.2	74.8	78.1	54.0	67.5	49.8
Jiangsu	65.3	76.1	59.0	31.4	36.4	42.3
Zhejiang	18.5	39.0	26.5	18.8	22.0	20.4
Anhui	8.2	17.1	18.3	9.4	9.5	14.4
Fujian	5.5	15.5	15.5	7.7	9.5	20.3
Jiangxi		21.3	7.0	4.7	6.6	10.0
Shandong	58.9	88.3	54.2	26.6	21.5	29.1
Henan	2.8	25.8	20.6	17.6	10.0	14.8
Hubei	14.2	42.6	40.5	13.6	13.4	18.5
Hunan	34.8	40.2	17.3	8.3	9.0	11.6
Guangdong	3.2	21.9	12.8	7.6	8.8	13.5
Guangxi	1.9	6.5	10.3	4.6	6.0	6.8
Hainan					8.3	6.6
Sichuan	79.5	81.1	50.9	24.7	27.8	37.2
Guizhou	3.5	10.5	11.7	4.6	5.6	6.0
Yunnan	14.0	16.7	16.2	5.4	6.7	8.6
Tibet						8.1
Shaanxi	12.9	79.7	34.4	13.5	12.1	11.6
Gansu	22.3	25.0	16.7	8.2	10.2	10.8
Qinghai		13.3	9.7	5.8	10.0	12.1
Ningxia		6.9	29.3	5.4	9.3	12.7
Xinjiang	29.2	39.1	11.3	7.5	9.8	14.0
China	39.7	57.1	37.5	18.1	18.4	21.9

Sources: Calculations for 1979–80, 1985–98 from birth-planning report data in ZJSN 1986–; ZRTN 1994–; 1982 fertility survey results for 1982 in: Arnold and Liu Zhaoxiang 1986, 228

Tianjin and Shanghai, as well as the Northeastern region and the provinces of Jiangsu, Zhejiang and Sichuan. Problem areas with a long-range decline or stagnation of the one-child certificate rate such as Hebei, Shanxi, Shandong, Henan and Shaanxi provinces also show up in the yearly tabulations of the Birth-Planning Commission. According to the national fertility survey of 1982, acceptance of the certificate among couples with one boy was clearly higher than among those with one girl. Nine per cent of holders had handed back their certificates and gone on to have a second child. In the next fertility survey of

1988 the percentage of persons who had obtained a certificate between 1979 and 1988 and had returned it had risen to 15 per cent for the national total and 22 per cent for the rural areas. For individual years such as 1980 the figures increased to 27 per cent and 39 per cent, respectively. In agrarian hinterland provinces they were particularly high, where approximately half of second births were unauthorized.[84] No comparable data are available from the 1992 fertility survey.

If low numbers of one-child certificates are treated as a measure of non-compliance and an announcement of things to come, current figures from most provinces of the North, Center-South, Southwest and Northwest indicate that 80 to 90 per cent of women of reproductive age have already had either more than one birth or are serving notice that they are looking forward to another. The rates therefore correlate positively with provincial percentages for the non-agricultural population enjoying no second-child privileges. While at the outset this was only a moderate correlation (r=0.48 for 1979), the relationship became successively stronger over the years (r=0.79 and 0.82 for 1985 and 1997, respectively). This demonstrates the influence of the second-child concession, which, despite later attempts at back-pedalling, continues to play a major role. Today, few provinces deviate from the rule of a strong association between both indicators. These are minority areas and a few special cases such as Shanxi, Guangdong and Guangxi, where figures for one-child certificates are conspicuously below the non-agricultural population. With champions of strict birth control such as Jiangsu and Sichuan it is the other way round.

Apart from its function as an indicator of birth-control performance, the rate of one-child certificates signals financial liabilities, too.[85] This is why state organs may also have an interest in limiting the number of certificates issued. In the majority of cases, the one-child bonus conferred by the certificates is jointly paid by the work units of both spouses, each shouldering half of the expenses. However, some past regulations made the work unit of either the wife or the husband responsible for paying the total sum. In the urban areas there are clear rules about how to handle payments. Industrial and commercial enterprises pay the bonus out of their operating funds, and institutions use their budget appropriations. Of course, these are unwelcome burdens, aggravating once again the long-term problem of highly uneven social security expenses borne by work units. Another problem is the growing number of unemployed or self-employed persons. In these cases, the local birth-planning bureaux, the street committee offices or the administrations for industry and commerce have to foot the bill.

As shown in Table 10, there is a standard value of the one-child bonus which some provinces fall short of paying and which is only rarely exceeded. Starting in 1979, an annual total of 60 yuan became established as the standard sum. Although this level was reached by only a small number of provinces in 1979, subsequent years saw a growing number of regions implementing payments of that amount. For many years, provinces with a weak financial basis such as Jiangxi, Hunan and Guangxi have not been able to shoulder the burden. In a similar vein, densely settled provinces, which grant only a few second-child permissions and therefore have to finance a high number of one-child bonuses, also emerge as cases of low-level payments. Examples of such cases are Jiangsu and Zhejiang provinces.

Conversely, particularly high bonuses have been paid by Guangdong and Hainan provinces, which, by virtue of their special economic zones and high foreign investments, have developed into favoured regions. Shanghai also offers above-average conditions, since it was the only provincial-level unit to pay one-child bonuses for a period of sixteen years. This was surpassed in the 1990s by Heilongjiang, Jilin and Hebei provinces, which stipulate payments for eighteen years.

The stagnation of the one-child bonus has been quite serious. In 1990, Jiangsu province continued to pay the annual sum of approximately 40 yuan that it had already appropriated for one-child families in 1979. Table 10 also documents many years of stagnation in Shanxi, Liaoning and Shaanxi. In provinces where bonuses have been raised since the mid-1980s, increases have been modest and have rarely reached more than 100 yuan per year. This has brought about a continuous depreciation of the one-child bonus, which has not kept up with the increase in wages, prices and inflation rates. Although it still is a significant item in the balance of enterprises, it has lost its value as a material incentive for individual families.

It remains to be seen how experiments with special types of insurance will develop in the future. In the past, some places converted the one-child bonus into insurance premiums. Several types of insurance policy exist: a complete coverage of risks for single children, coverage of educational costs and dowries, an old-age insurance policy for the parents of single children, health insurance for mother and child, as well as insurance against health hazards of sterilization. The most favoured type is full coverage for single children, which in 1992 was used for two thirds of the then 15.68 million insurance policies.[86] For a long time the scheme has suffered from the problem that interest earned by insurance funds trailed behind inflation levels. Moreover, these types of insurances are not optimal, since it is not primarily children but elderly people without offspring who need assistance in the first place. Such old-age insurance policies are far more costly however, and depend on prolonged periods of contributions – the main reason why most rural areas are unable to finance them in the foreseeable future. They are only feasible, if villages earn enough from small-scale industries or obtain sufficient subsidies from the Ministry of Civil Administration. The Ministry has vowed to establish a rural system for guaranteeing a minimal standard of living in the future, but in contrast to the nearly 75 million rural contributors to the Ministry-sponsored old-age insurance scheme, only 0.61 million peasants were drawing old-age insurance payments in 1997. Only rich Guangdong province in the South has deemed it feasible to introduce the incentive of a township-run, mandatory old-age insurance scheme for one-child peasants into the newly revised provincial birth-planning regulations of September 1998. This is a step that even Shanghai municipality has shied away from, and where current regulations prescribe only 'a certain monthly reward' and 'favourable consideration in economic matters and living arrangements' for elderly peasants with a single child or no child at all.[87]

Table 10 Provincial birth-planning rules: one-child incentives 1979–99

	Date	Urban	Rural
Beijing	6-12-82	1 (60 ¥),2-5,7	1 (60 ¥) or 12 or 14;9
	15-1-91	1 or 2;3-6	1,3,7,15
Tianjin	14-10-82		
	2-11-88	1,3-5	1 or 7,15;3
	9-3-93		
	15-4-94		
	30-1-97	1,3-5	1 or 7;15;13
Hebei	5-4-82	1 (24-30 ¥),2-5,7	1 (15-20 ¥) or 12,14;3-5
	28-2-86		
	14-3-89	1 (60 ¥),2-5	1 (60 ¥),3-5,7,13
	2-9-94	1 (60 ¥),2-5	1 (60 ¥),3-5,7,13
	3-9-97	1 (60 ¥),2-5	1 (60 ¥),3-5,7,13
Shanxi	29-6-82	1 (60 ¥),3-5,7	1 (60 ¥),3-5,7,11
	28-12-86	1 (60 ¥)	1
	22-9-89	1,3-5	1 or 13,14
Inner Mongolia	15-6-82	1 (60 ¥) or 2-5,7	3-5,12 or 14
	15-1-85		
	1-12-88		
	12-10-90	1-4	7,12,13
	7-11-95	1-4	7,12,13,15
Liaoning	16-6-79	1 (60 ¥),2-5,7-9	1-5,7-9,11,12
	3-4-80		
	24-6-82	1 (60 ¥),2-5,7-9	1-5,7-9,11,12
	9-84		
	1-10-85		
	28-5-88	1 (60 ¥),3-5,9	1,3,7,9,12
	25-9-92	1 (60 ¥),3-5,9	1,3,7,9,12
	27-9-97	1 (120 ¥),3-5,9	1 (60-120 ¥),3,7,9,12
Jilin	21-7-88	1 (48-96 ¥),3-5,7	1 (48-96 ¥),3,7,13
	11-9-93	1 (48-96 ¥),3-5,7	1 (48-96 ¥),3,7,12
	14-11-97	1 (48-96 ¥),3-5,7	1 (48-96 ¥),3,7,12
Heilongjiang	9-79	1 (30-40 ¥),3,4,7	1 (30-40 ¥),3,7
	31-1-83	1 (60 ¥),3-5,7,9	1 (60 ¥),4,5,7,9,11,12
	13-12-89	1 (60 ¥),3,4,7,9	1 (60 ¥),3,7,12,13
	21-5-94	1 (60 ¥),3,4,7,9	1 (60 ¥),3,7,9,13
	18-12-99	1 (120 ¥),3,4,7,9	1 (120 ¥),3,7,9,12,13
Shanghai	28-7-81	1 (60 ¥),3,4,9	1 (60 ¥),3,4,9,12
	3-6-82		
	16-10-84		
	30-5-87	1 (60 ¥)	
	17-10-92	1,3,4,9	1,3,4,7,9
	16-6-95	1,3,4,9	1,3,4,7,9,12
	10-12-97	1,3,4,9	1,3,4,7,9,12
Jiangsu	31-7-79	1 (40 ¥),4,7	1 (40 ¥),3,4,7,11,12
	24-6-82	1 (50 ¥)	1 (50 ¥) or 14
	2-85		
	28-10-90	1 (40 ¥),3-5,7,9,16	1 (40 ¥),3-5,7,16
	16-6-95	1 (40 ¥),3-5,7,9,16	1 (40 ¥),3-5,7,16
	31-7-97	1 (40 ¥),3-5,7,9,16	1 (40 ¥),3-5,7,16
Zhejiang	4-3-82	1 (30-50 ¥) or 2-5,7	1 (> 30 ¥) or 14;4,5,7,12
	4-2-85	1 (50 ¥) or 2,3-5	5,7,9,13

	Date	Urban	Rural
	29-12-89	1 (60 ¥) or 2,3	1,3,7
	28-9-95	1 (100 ¥) or 2,3	1,3,7
Anhui	1-4-79	1 (30-60 ¥),3,4,7,11,12	
	9-5-81		
	17-8-84	1 (60-72 ¥),2-5,7,9	3-5,7,11
	31-10-88	1 (60-72 ¥),3-5,7,9,11,	1 (60-72 ¥),3-5,7,11
	30-8-92	1 (60-72 ¥),2-5,7,9,11	1 (60-72 ¥),3-5,7,9,11
	24-4-95	1 (60-72 ¥),2-5,7,9,11	1 (60-72 ¥),3-5,7,9,11
Fujian	28-5-82	1 (36-60 ¥),2-5,7	3-5,7,12,14,15
	29-4-88	1 (48-60 ¥),3-5,7	1 or 3,7,15;4,5,9
	28-6-91	1 (48-60 ¥),3-5,7	1 or 3,7,15;4,5,9
	25-10-97	1 (48-60 ¥),3-5,7	1 or 3,7,15;4,5,9
Jiangxi	18-1-83	1 (36-60 ¥),3-5,7	1 (36-60 ¥) or 14;3-5,7,12
	4-1-85	1 (36-60 ¥),3-5,7	1 (36-60 ¥) or 14;3-5,7,12
	16-6-90	1,3-5,7	1,3-5,7,13
	30-6-95		
	20-6-97	1,3-5,7	1,3-5,7,13
Shandong	29-7-82		
	20-7-88	1 (60 ¥),3-5,7,9	1 (60 ¥),3-5,7
	14-10-96	1 (60 ¥),3-5,7,9	1 (60 ¥),3-5,7,12
Henan	15-6-82	1 (60 ¥),3-5,7	1 (60 ¥)or 14;3-5,7
	11-12-85	1 (60 ¥),3-5,7	1 (60 ¥)or 14;3-5,7
	23-8-87		
	12-4-90	1 (60 ¥),3-5,7	1 (60 ¥),3-5,7,13
Hubei	27-9-79	1 (30-40 ¥),3-5,9	1 (30-40 ¥),3-5,9
	19-12-87	1 (48 ¥),3-5,7,9	1 (50 ¥),3-5,7,12
	1-12-91	1 (48 ¥),3-5,7,9	1 (50 ¥),3-5,7,12
	28-3-97	1 (96 ¥),3-5,7,9	1 (96 ¥),3-5,7,12
Hunan	6-79	1 (30-60 ¥),3,4,7,9,11,12	
	10-5-82	1 (40 ¥),4,5,9	1,3,12,14,15
	3-12-89	1 (60 ¥),3-5,7,9	1 (60 ¥),3-5,7,12,13
Guangdong	2-2-80	1 (60 ¥) or 4+5;3,9	1,3,7,9,12
	81		
	17-5-86	1 (84 ¥),2-5,7,9,10,16	3,7,9
	28-11-92	1 (120 ¥),2,3,5,9,16	3,7,9,13
	1-12-97		
	18-9-98	1 (120 ¥),2-5,9,16	3,7,9,13,17
Guangxi	25-11-82	1 (40 ¥),3-5,7,9	1,3-5,7,12,14
	4-85		
	17-9-88	1,3-5,7,9	1,4,5,7,13
	26-11-94	1,3-5,7,9	1,4,5,7,13,17
Hainan	12-6-84		
	85		
	11-3-89	1 (120 ¥),2-5,7,9,10,16	9,13
	27-10-95	1 (240-360 ¥),2-5,7,9	9,13
Chongqing	13-9-97	1(60-120 ¥),3-5,7,9,16	1(60-120 ¥),3-5,7,9,16
Sichuan	29-4-82	3-5,7,9	3-5,7,9
	5-84		
	2-7-87	1 (60 ¥),5	1 (60 ¥),5,7
	15-12-93		
	17-10-97	1(60-120 ¥),5,7,16	1(60-120 ¥)3,5,7,13,16
Guizhou	6-79		
	15-3-82		

	Date	Urban	Rural
	27-7-84		
	16-7-87	1,3,7,	1,3,7
	24-7-98	1 (>60 ¥),4,(5),7	1(>60 ¥),3,4,(5),7,(13),(17)
Yunnan	86	1 (60 ¥)	
	22-12-90	1 (60-120 ¥),3,4,9	1 (60-120 ¥),3,4,7,13
	3-12-97	1 (60-120 ¥),3,4,9	1 (60-120 ¥),3,4,7,13
Tibet	28-3-85		
	1-5-86	1 (60 ¥),2,4,5,7-9	
	8-5-92	1 (60 ¥),2,4,5,7,8	13
Shaanxi	6-79	1 (60 ¥),3-5,11	1 (36 ¥),4,5,7,11
	30-4-81	1 (60 ¥),3-5,7,9,11	1 (36 ¥),3-5,7,11
	1-10-82	1 (60 ¥),3,5,7,9	1 (36 ¥),3,5,7,11,12,14
	1-85		
	25-7-86	1 (60 ¥),3-5,7,11	1 (60 ¥),5
	5-11-88		
	3-3-91	1 (60 ¥),3-5,7,11	1 (60 ¥),3-5,7,12,13,17
	2-8-97	1 (60 ¥)	1 (60 ¥), 17
Gansu	16-3-82	1 (30 ¥),3-5	12 or 14;3-5
	15-6-85	1 (30 ¥),3-5	12 or 14;3-5
	28-11-89	1 (60 ¥),2-5,7	1 (60 ¥),3,15
	29-9-97	1 (60 ¥),2-5,7	1 (60 ¥),3,15
Qinghai	5-6-82	1 (60 ¥),3-5,7	1 (60 ¥),3-5,7
	9-85		
	17-4-86	1 (84-166 ¥),2-5,7	1 (84-166 ¥),3-5,7
	28-2-92	1 (84-166 ¥),2-5,7,16	1 (84-166 ¥),3-5,7,12,15
Ningxia	2-9-82	1 (72 ¥),2-5	1 (60 ¥),3-5,7,12
	28-8-86	1 (96 ¥),2-5,7	1 (96 ¥),3-5,7,12
	28-12-90	1 (96 ¥),2-7	1 (96 ¥),3,5,7,12,13,15
Xinjiang	4-4-81		
	30-4-88	1 (60 ¥),6,9	
	15-8-91	1 (120 ¥),2,4-7,9	1 (120 ¥),5,7,9

Incentives for one-child families (in Xinjiang partly for two children):

1 one-child bonus or health insurance fee up to age 14–18
2 extension of maternity leave or better financial conditions for paid maternity leave
3 preference in the allocation of housing or the allotment of building plots
4 preference in placement for nurseries and kindergartens and in school enrolment
5 preference in medical care and hospitalization
6 paid nursing or caretaking leave
7 preference in recruitment for non-agricultural jobs
8 preference in army recruitment
9 extra pension for employees or assistance for old peasants
10 pensioners with only one daughter covered by medical insurance of daughter or son-in-law
11 higher subsidized food ration
12 more allotment of farm land
13 preference in credit, relief and economic assistance
14 reduced procurement quotas of low-priced grain and other products, less collective fees
15 exemption from or reduction of compulsory labour
16 reward for areas or work units with commendation for birth planning
17 old-age insurance for peasants

Numbers in brackets show bonuses in yuan per year; in some cases these are minimum sums. Additional incentives for late marriages and late births, for childless persons, for persons undergoing sterilization after the first child, or or for those conforming to two-child conditions but not claiming a second-child permit are not listed. Some of the listed incentives are optional.

Sources and other notes: Compare table 1.

Financial problems also arise in urban areas if companies with accumulated deficits and facing imminent bankruptcy are required to shoulder one-child bonuses for their employees. This is also an issue for extended maternity leave and the periods of rest after contraceptive surgery granted to women who commit themselves to respecting the one-child norm. There are uniform national regulations specifying ordinary maternity leave for workers and staff, as well as post-operative care for any woman undergoing birth-control surgery.[88] However, stipulations as to the precise duration of an extended maternity leave differ, as they are contained in the provincial birth-planning regulations.

In 1988, nine provinces granted from twenty days to three months' extended maternity leave, and ten provinces increased this to four and up to twelve months.[89] The situation has not changed much since. As may be gleaned from Table 10, Zhejiang province is giving one-child families a choice between one year of maternity leave or fourteen years of monthly bonus payments, provided they obtain the consent of their unit and the superior department. Out of financial considerations, most other provinces do not grant such an option and limit the extended maternity leave to a period of between three and four months. Still others revoke it for couples not complying with the late-birth recommendation. In principle, a prolonged maternity leave should imply continuing wage payments, but only a few regions such as Shanghai, Zhejiang and Inner Mongolia have clearly stipulated that 70 to 100 per cent of the last wage will be paid. Since many urban families rely on the double income of both spouses, an extended maternity leave with partial wage deductions will not be regarded as an incentive.

Financing the one-child bonus in rural areas is an even greater problem. Table 10 documents that quite a number of provinces have not been able to enforce an equal level of payments for rural and urban areas. In many instances, bonus levels in rural areas have been lower than in urban areas by between one-third and half, and the discretionary powers given to lower echelons are often wide. Sometimes, one-child bonuses for the peasant population are not mentioned at all or carry no specification of the amounts paid.

The rural deficits have been caused by the decline in collective income. Already in 1980, many people's communes could no longer afford the high one-time bonuses paid for sterilizations one year earlier. An example is the commune studied by Mosher, which cut the bonus for sterilizations after the first birth from 500 to 100 yuan with an ensuing loss of real incentive.[90] Since 1982, the depletion of collective welfare funds after the abolishment of people's communes has further aggravated the situation. Many villages and townships do not have sufficient income to pay higher bonuses, so that the element of material incentives for rural one-child policies has diminished even more. In her field research in three villages of Shaanxi province during 1987, Greenhalgh concluded that bonuses and small incentives given to peasants amounted to only 3 per cent of average household incomes.[91] It is due to such circumstances that many birth-planning norms contain formulations that render the amount as well as the nature of material incentives dependent on local conditions.

Furthermore, most amended regulations of the 1990s have tried to forestall constant squabbling by laying down very detailed stipulations as to the sources of rural one-child bonuses. Their high degree of diversity documents the extremely different economic circumstances prevailing. In the early 1990s nine provinces prescribed payments out of collective fees or village-industry profits, two called upon the local birth-planning bureaux, one looked to the township or town budget, and another seized on state subsidies. Seven provincial regulations delegated the problem to local administration, three did not define financial sources, and two simply abolished one-child bonuses for peasants. Six others recommended alternatives that have since been implemented for more than a decade, namely one-time payments, preferential treatment of credit applications, lower community fees, a reduction of fixed procurement quotas, or exemption from unpaid corvee labour. Precise arrangements were left to the grass-roots units. The implementation of such measures leaves much to be desired. Furthermore, reliance on lower levels introduces an element of arbitrariness and leads to preferences along local affiliations and clan lines.[92]

There is no doubt that additional allotments of land would be one of the most potent incentives in rural areas. However, since the prolongation of contracts for responsibility land to periods of fifteen, thirty years or more, little disposable land is available. Recent birth-planning regulations therefore do not contain the former incentive of additional land allotments. At most, it survives with reference to the private plots (*ziliu di*) that are much smaller than responsibility land (*zeren tian*).

Preferential work allocation and retirement rules have met with similar problems of implementation. In principle, these are powerful economic levers for the authorities. In practice, however, cooperation between the departments of labour and personnel and the birth-planning authorities is often unsatisfactory, and there are no clear rules of implementation with regard to stipulated preferential treatment. With some exceptions, old-age insurance for rural areas is non-existent and cannot be realized due to financial problems. Often, peasants without families are impoverished and live in dire circumstances. With the dissolution of people's communes, the weak network of social support that had been woven for them has frequently been torn apart.[93] If they get social support at all, welfare payments generally amount to one-fifth of incomes officially considered as matching the poverty line.[94] Under such conditions, single old people all too often serve as living counter-propaganda against official birth-planning policy. Widows who continue to till the fields at the age of 80 are an example.

Implementation of preferential retirement rules contained in the birth-planning regulations should be easier for urban units. Such preferential rules stipulate increasing pensions by 5 or 10 per cent, and in some cases even to 100 per cent of former wage levels. The latter provision tends to be confined to childless pensioners; the latest birth-planning regulations from Liaoning, Shanghai and Anhui are examples. However, as documented in Table 10, pension-related instruments are listed in a small number of regulations only. Again, financial difficulties are the main reason for this lack of incentive.

Comprehensive improvements may be only realized in the course of urgent reform of the social security system. The same proviso applies to better health insurance for pensioners, which is only mentioned only in the Guangdong regulations.[95]

Since 1979 all birth-planning norms include a global promise of preferential treatment for single children in kindergarten and school enrolment, housing allocation or medical care. As these areas fall within the competence of other departments, the norms do not contain clear-cut rules of implementation. In practice, preferential treatment involves priority in registration and waiting lists, and sometimes it signifies the total or partial waiving of fees. Hospitals, in particular, can often muster good reasons for not recognizing priority in hospitalization of single children. Priority in the allocation of housing usually implies a better placement on the long waiting lists for the few larger flats available. Calculation of per capita space to which one-child families are entitled is handled inconsistantly. The housing reforms of the 1990s have blunted this instrument even more. In 1997, such difficulties prompted Liaoning province to remove housing allocation and medical care from its list of preferences. In the educational area, only Shanghai has enacted unambiguous rules prescribing exemption from all school fees for single children and the duty of employers to pay for kindergarten places. Because such rules have been largely non-existent in other provinces, preferential treatment for single children is frequently hampered or explicitly left to the 'discretion of local units'.[96] Moreover, urban areas, with their high degree of compliance with one-child norms, have a hard time offering preferential treatment, since almost all children are entitled to it.

All preferences mentioned so far are material incentives for individual practitioners of birth control. Provinces such as Fujian, Guangdong and Guizhou have also experimented with collective incentives. They have set a precedent that has been followed in recent regulations by Beijing, Tianjin and Shanxi. Most other provincial regulations also contain passages referring to 'advanced units with commendation for birth planning'. In most cases, collective incentives involve higher bonus payments for all employees of an enterprise. Even if this instrument for generating social pressures is not specified in provincial birth-planning norms, further details may be spelled out by additional rules at local level. There are many indications that this has been widely practised in recent years, and it is augmented by bonuses awarded to informants who truthfully report illicit births to the authorities. This latest unsavoury addition to the long list of control measures appears in newly amended regulations from Anhui, Liaoning and Shaanxi.

Another recent development has been the linkage of relief and subsidies for poverty regions with demonstrated adherence to birth-planning targets. National rules to that effect were promulgated in 1989 and have been broadened ever since. They involve various individual or collective incentives such as lifting certain fees and taxes or granting and withholding special benefits. The sums disbursed under such schemes have remained very modest however, and many villages complain that promised benefits have never materialized. Overall, a glaring gap between ever-increasing sanctions and highly deficient incentives remains.[97]

6.8 Economic and disciplinary sanctions

In its initial stages, Chinese birth control was conceived as a concession to couples overtaxed by too many children. After the emphasis shifted from family to state interests, the newly emerging campaign continued to rely largely on education and persuasion. Aware of the immense social resistance to intervention in fertility decisions of the family, leading politicians made it a point to emphasize flexible policies without applying coercion. The first punitive elements emerged in September 1963, when a central work conference on urban problems resolved that married youth would be excluded from university enrolment or apprenticeship training in non-agricultural work units. Grain rations for children were henceforth to be calculated by age rather than on a per-capita basis. Further regulations for urban workers and staff beefed up the late-marriage recommendation by decreeing that public housing would only be available for couples where the husband was over 28 and the wife over 25 years of age. Extra cotton coupons for marriage and birth or subsidies for employees in hardship were made contingent on compliance with birth-planning advice.[98] Furthermore, cost-free medical care for pregnant women with two children and paid maternity leave after third or higher-order deliveries were abolished in the cities.

While tight state control of the urban economy made enforcement of these measures relatively easy, their applicability to the countryside was limited to the new grain rationing rule for children. Its implementation depended on the support of the rural grass-roots organization and seems to have lagged behind. However, pressures built up with the third birth-planning campaign during the 1970s, at which time they were reinforced by ideological education and political campaigns, the intense social control and the unbridled state control of the economy prevalent during the Cultural Revolution. Yet few codified rules existed, and most of the few existing ones were decreed at grass-roots level. Lower-echelon cadres thus wielded almost unrestricted power to use deductions of income and rations, withholding of registration, threats of sacking, or organized group pressure for enforcing compliance with the gradually intensifying birth-control propaganda. Conversely, their great powers of discretion and their relative lack of accountability also gave these cadres ample opportunities to tacitly condon violations of policy.[99]

With the advent of the one-child campaign and the return to rule by regulations, sanctions developed into the main instrument of enforcement. Even so, Chinese policy has preferred the application of economic, administrative and disciplinary measures to resorting to criminal law. In an attempt to bridge the conflict between the professed preference for educational approaches and the reality of a stiff punitive regime, most revised birth-planning regulations from the late 1990s have favoured the phrase 'legal responsibilities' over the unadorned 'penalties' and substituted the neutral 'levying of fees' for the plain 'fining'. But while semantics have become lighter, penalties have become heavier.

Most present sanctions relate to the most blatant violation of birth-planning regulations, namely unauthorized childbirth. Moreover, recent years have seen a gradual extension of sanctions for other offences such as early marriage, non-compliance with formalities or breach of deadlines. While most regulations only stipulate mandatory contraception with sanctions for unauthorized births, some have begun to fine non-contraception, even if this has not yet led to pregnancy or the birth of an extra child.[100] For brevity's sake, discussion here will be limited to penalties for unauthorized births. In many recent birth-planning regulations these have come to specifically include illegitimate births out of wedlock, births before having reached 24 years of age, or rash births in disregard of spacing rules for second children.

With regard to urban workers and staff, wage deductions by specified percentages have always been the main sanction for violation of birth plans. This has been paralleled by equivalent income deductions for the peasant population. The relevant rules and other types of sanctions contained in the birth-planning regulations are listed in Table 11 which shows that sanctions have varied widely from province to province.

Until the late 1980s, the great majority of provinces decreed monthly wage deductions of 10 per cent; in a few instances, the deductions ranged from 5 per cent to 15 per cent. However, over recent years sanctions have become increasingly tougher, with nearly all provinces raising regular wage deductions to between 20 and 50 per cent of regular income. In recent years, one-time penalties have increased to sums equalling per-capita averages for one (Hebei) or one-and-a-half to three annual incomes (Shanghai, Jiangsu, Fujian, Hunan, Guangdong). Penalties for an unauthorized third child can surpass even these levels to six annual incomes. In former years, the time period specified for wage deductions ranged between seven and fourteen years; in some cases it amounted to three, five or sixteen years. In the 1990s, a trend of markedly higher deductions coupled with shorter periods of payment has become visible. If they are not replaced by a one-time payment of accumulated sums, wage deductions nowadays are enforced for a duration of seven years and always apply to both spouses.

Whereas these rules may be easily enforced for state or collective employees in urban areas, they have once again met major problems of implementation in the countryside. In the former system of people's communes, peasants could be fined by withholding work points (later converted into cash) or goods in kind. But with the abolishment of collective production units, peasants are now running their economic activities independently, and income is no longer distributed by rural cadres. Instead, cadres have to assess penalty payments on the basis of estimates of increasingly diversified peasant incomes. Moreover, they have to collect the specified fines regularly. Such collections are unpopular and hard to enforce over a prolonged period of time. Most rural birth-planning bureaux therefore prefer one-time penalty sums equalling the accumulated total of monthly payments. This can thwart the intended effect of penalties by creating the feeling that short-term deficit is traded for lifelong benefits. Furthermore, the method is prone to misuse and can lead to either insufficiently

Table 11 Provincial birth-planning rules: economic and disciplinary sanctions 1979–99

	Date	Urban	Rural
Beijing	6-12-82	2(7 y 10%),4-6,12,21	2,4,13,15,21
	16-5-91	1,3(5-50,000 ¥),4-7,9,11,12, 21,24	1,3(5-50,000 ¥),4,9,11,14,15,19,20,24
Tianjin	14-10-82		
	2-11-88	2(5 y 20%),4-6,12,22,24	2,4,6
	9-3-93		
	15-4-94		
	30-1-97	2(5 y 20%),4-6,12,22,24	2,4,6
Hebei	5-4-82	2 (14 y 10%),5,14	2 (14 y 10%) or 16-18;14
	28-2-86		
	14-3-89	1,2(1 a.i.),4-6,14,21,23,24	1,2(2.5 per-capita a.i.),4,14, 23,24
	2-9-94		
	3-9-97	1,2(1 a.i.),3-6,8,14,21,23,24	1,2(2.5 per-capita a.i.),3,4,14, 23,24
Shanxi	29-6-82	2(7 y 15%),4,5,21	2 (7 y 10%),4 or 7,17,18
	28-12-86	2(7 y 25%), 4	2 (7 y 25%),4
	22-9-89	1,2(7 y 20%),4-7,14,21,23,24	1,2 (7 y 20%),4,14,15,19, 20,24
Inner Mongolia	15-6-82	2(14 y 10%),5,6,21	15,16,21
	15-1-85		
	1-12-88	2,21	2
	12-10-90	1,2,4-7,9,19,21	1,2,4,15
	7-11-95	1,2(2-20,000 ¥),4-7,9,19,21	1,2(2-20,000 ¥),4,15
Liaoning	16-6-79	2(14 y 10%),5-7,14,21	2 (14 y 10%),13-15,21
	3-4-80	2(14 y 10%),5-7,14,21	2 (14 y 10%),13-15,21
	24-6-82		
	9-84		
	1-10-85		
	28-5-88	1,2(14 y 10%),4,6,7,14,23,24	1,2 (14 y 10%),4
	25-9-92	1,2(5-50,000 ¥),4,6,7,14,23,24	1,2(5-50,000 ¥),4,24
	27-9-97	1,2(5-50,000 ¥),3,4,6,7,14,23,24	1,2(5-50,000 ¥),3,4,24
Jilin	21-7-88	2(10-30%),4-6,8,9,13-15,21,24	2(10-30%),4,9
	11-9-93	1-3,21,24	1-3
	14-11-97	1-3,21,24	1-3
Heilongjiang	9-79	2(14 y 10%),5	2 (14 y 10%)
	31-1-83	2(> 1200 ¥),4,5,7,21	2 (>1200 ¥),4,21
	13-12-89	1,2(14 y 10%),4-7,21,23,24	1,2 (14 y 10%),4,24
	21-5-94	1-3,21	1-3
	18-12-99	1-3,21	1-3
Shanghai	28-7-81	2(16 y 10%),5	2 (16 y 10%)
	3-6-82	2(3 y 10%)	2 (3 y 10%)
	16-10-84		
	30-5-87		
	17-10-92	2(3 a.i.),4,5,12,14,21,24	2 (3 a.i.),4,14,24
	16-6-95	2(3 a.i.),4,5,12,14,21,24	2 (3 a.i.),4,14,24
	10-12-97	2(3 a.i.),4,5,12,14,21,24	2 (3 a.i.),4,14,24

	Date	Urban	Rural
Jiangsu	31-7-79	4,14	4,14,15
	24-6-82	2(7-10 y 10%),4-7	2 (7 y 10%),4 or 15-17
	2-85		
	28-10-90	1,2(3 a.i.),4,5,12,14,21,24,25	1,2(3 a.i.),4,5,14,21,24
	16-6-95	1,2(3 a.i.),4,5,14,21,24,25	1,2(3 a.i.),4,5,14,21,24
	31-7-97	1,2(3 a.i.),4,5,14,21,24,25	1,2(3 a.i.),4,5,14,21,24
Zhejiang	4-3-82	2(7 y 5%),4,5,12,21	2 (7 y 5%),4 or 16,17; 21
	4-2-85	2(5 y 15%),4-6,21	2 (5 y 15%),4,6
	29-12-89	1,2(5 y 20-50%),3-5,9,21,23,24	1,2 (5 y 20-50%),3,4,9,24
	28-9-95	1,2(5 y 20-50%),3-5,9,21,23,24	1,2 (5 y 20-50%),3,4,9,24
Anhui	1-4-79	4(14 y 5%),5,13,14,15	
	9-5-81		
	17-8-84		
	31-10-88	1,2(7 y 10%),4-8,21	1,2 (7 y 10%),4
	30-8-92	1,2(7 y 10%),4-8,19-21	1,2 (7 y 10%),4,15,20
	24-4-95	1,2(7 y 10%),4-8,19-21	1,2 (7 y 10%),4,15,20
Fujian	28-5-82	2(10-14 y 5% or 500-800 ¥)	15,17
	29-4-88	1,2(7 y 20%),4-8,13,24	1,2(7 y 20%),4,19,20
	28-6-91	1,2(<3a.i.),4-8,13,24	1,2(<3a.i.),4,16,19,20,24
	25-10-97	1,2(<3a.i.),4-8,13,24	1,2(<3a.i.),4,16,19,20,24
Jiangxi	18-1-83	2,4 or 11;5-8,21	2,4,15,17,18,21
	4-1-85	2,4 or 11;5-8,21	2,4,15,17,18,21
	16-6-90	1,2,4-9,14,19,21,24	2,4,14,19,20,24
	30-6-95		
	20-6-97	1,2(<30,000 ¥) ,4-8,14,19,21,24	2(<30,000 ¥),4,14,19,20,24
Shandong	29-7-82		
	20-7-88	1,2,4-8,12,21,23	1,2,4,23
	14-10-96	1,2(3-10,000 ¥),4-8,12,21,23	1,2(3-10,000 ¥),4,23
Henan	15-6-82	2(7 y 15%),4-7	2 (7 y 15%),4 or 16; 5,15
	11-12-85	2(7 y 15%),5-7	2 (7 y 15%) or 16;5,15
	23-8-87		
	12-4-90	1,2(7 y 20-30%),4,6-8,10,21	1,2 (7 y 20-30%),4,10,14,15
Hubei	27-9-79	2(14 y 10%)	2 (14 y 10%)
	19-12-87	1,2(5 y 20%),5,7,21,24	2 (5 y 20%)
	1-12-91	1,2(5 y 20-60%),5,7,21,24	2 (5 y 20-60%)
	28-3-97	1,2(5 y 20-60%),5,7,21,24	2 (5 y 20-60%)
Hunan	6-79	4(14 y 5%),5,13-15	
	10-5-82	2(5 y 10%),4,5,13,21	5,13;15 or 17 or 18
	3-12-89	1,2(1.5 a.i.),4,21	1,2(2 a.i.),4
Guangdong	2-2-80	4(14 y 10%),5-7	5
	81		
	17-5-86	1,2(7 y 20%),4-7,12,14,24	1,2,4,5,12,14,19,20
	28-11-92	1,2(2.1-3.5 a.i.),4-7,12,14,21,24	1,2 (2.1-3.5 a.i.),4-6,9,12,14,19,20
	1-12-97		
	18-9-98	1,2(2.1-3.5 a.i.),4-7,14,21,24	1,2(2.1-3.5 a.i.),4-6,9,14,19,20
Guangxi	25-11-82	2,4-7,13,21	5,13-15,21;16 or 17
	4-85		

	Date	Urban	Rural
	17-9-88	1,2,5,12,21	1,2
	26-11-94	1,2(2-50,000 ¥),5-7,21	1,2(2-50,000 ¥),19,20
Hainan	12-6-84		
	85		
	11-3-89	1,2(7 y 20%),4-7,12,14,21,24	1,2(500 ¥),4,12,14,19,20
	27-10-95	1,2(2-3 a.i.),4-8,14,21	1,2(2-3 a.i.),4,14,19,20
Chongqing	13-9-97	1,2(2-3 a.i.),5,21,23,24,25	1,2(2-3 a.i.),16
Sichuan	29-4-82		
	5-84	2(7 y 5%)	
	2-7-87	1,2(7 y 10-20%),4,21	1,2 (7 y 10-20%),4
	15-12-93		
	17-10-97	1,2(7 y 20-30%),4,21	1,2(7 y 20-30%),4,21
Guizhou	6-79		
	15-3-82		15
	27-7-84		
	16-7-87	2(7-14 y 10%),4-7,12,21	2,4
	24-7-98	1,2(2-5 a.i.),21,24	1,2(2-5 a.i.),24
Yunnan	86	2(10%)	
	22-12-90	1,2(7 y 30-40%),4-8,12,21	1,2,4,6,14
	3-12-97	1,2(7 y 30-40%),4-8,12,21	1,2,4,6,14
Tibet	28-3-85		
	1-5-86	Han:3(1000 ¥),Tib:3(300 ¥)	
	8-5-92	Han:1,3 (3000 ¥),4-7,12,13,21 Tib.:1,3 (500 ¥),4-7,12,13	
Shaanxi	6-79	5,12-14	13-15
	30-4-81	2(7 y 10%),4,14	2 (7 y 10%),4,14,15
	1-10-82	2(7 y 10%),4,14	2 (7 y 10%),4,14-18
	1-85		
	25-7-86	2(7 y 10%),4-7	2 (7 y 10%),4,5
	5-11-88		
	3-3-91	1,2(7 y 15-30%),4-8,19,21,24	1,2 (7 y 15-30%),4,10,14,15, 19,24
	2-8-97	1,2(7 y 20-30%),4-8,19,21,23	1,2(7 y 20-30%),4,14,15,19,23
Gansu	16-3-82	2(10 y 10%),4,5,7,11,19,21	2,4,5,11,14,15,19,21
	15-6-85	2(10 y 10%),4,5,7,11,19,21	2,4,5,11,14,15,19,21
	28-11-89	1,2(7 y 30%),4-7,19,21,22	1,2(7 y 30%),4,6,14,19-22
	29-9-97	1,2(7 y 30%),4-7,19,21,22	1,2(7 y 30%),4,6,14,19-22
Qinghai	5-6-82	2(7 y 10%),4,12,14,21	2,14-16,18
	9-85		
	17-4-86	1,2(7 y 10%),4-6,12,14,21	1,2(300-500 ¥),4,5,14
	28-2-92	1,2(7 y 25%),4-7,9,12,19,21	1,2(7 y 30-50%),4,6,12,14,15
Ningxia	2-9-82	2(14 y 10%),5-7,21	5,15,21
	28-8-86	1,2(14 y 10%),6,7,12,21,24	1,2 (14 y 10%),15
	28-12-90	1,2(14 y 10-30%),4-7,12,21,24	1,2 (14 y 10%),12,14-16,19,24
Xinjiang	4-4-81		
	30-4-88	2(7 y 10%),5,6	2 (7 y 10%),5
	15-8-91	1,2(14 y 10-30%),5-7,14,19,21, 22,24	1,2,14,15,19,22,24

Sanctions for unauthorized births:

1 fines for illegitimate or early births, neglect of spacing rules or disregard of formalities for permitted first, second or higher-order births
2 above-quota birth fines (regular or one-time income deductions for both parents of non-authorized child)
3 social-support fee for non-authorized birth, one-time or in installments
4 more severe wage and income deductions or fines for third and higher-order child
5 privately paid medical and maternity expenses, no paid maternity leave
6 no bonus payments, welfare items or commendation benefits (limited in time)
7 no job promotion (limited in time)
8 demotion
9 possible revocation of business license for persons self-employed or holding provisional registration
10 possible abrogation of leases of state or collective enterprises
11 possible discharge of non-tenured employees
12 no medical insurance and social welfare benefits for unauthorized children (limited in time), no relief
13 no subsidized grain rations
14 no higher allocation of housing or allotment of building tracts
15 no higher allotment of farm land, no social relief
16 reduction of land allotments
17 higher procurement quotas for low-priced grain and other produce
18 higher fees for the collective
19 no work allocation in state or collective enterprises for peasants or urban unemployed
20 no non-agricultural household registration or provisional registration in urban areas
21 disciplinary sanctions for cadres and state employees up to discharge from work
22 public criticism and account of cadres
23 fines for responsible cadres
24 economic sanctions and no commendation benefits for work unit or area
25 further sanctions according to birth-planning contract

Information in brackets signifies the amount of annual income (a.i.) fined, a total penalty sum in Yuan (¥), or the years (y) of wage deductions and the percentage deducted. Sanctions under points 5-24 mostly apply to unauthorized second or higher-order births only. The Heilongjiang regulations of 21 March 1994 leave further details of sanctions to special rules decreed by the provincial government.

Sources: Compare table 1.

high or grossly inflated sums. Another reason for widely fluctuating penalty sums is the discretionary power of city and county authorities, which are entitled to levy additional one-time fines in order to enforce birth plans.

There is a multitude of reports illustrating the highly divergent range of sanctions resulting from these procedures. Mosher, who witnessed the first peak of the one-child campaign in a people's commune of Guangdong province in 1979 and 1980, documented a 10 per cent deduction of work points. This deduction began in the fourth month of an unlicensed pregnancy and was intended to serve as an incentive for abortion. If the pregnancy resulted in an unauthorized birth, an additional one-off penalty of 300 yuan was levied, and the monthly health insurance premium was doubled. As coupons for rationed and subsidized daily necessities were withheld at the same time, couples who did not respect the policy were effectively driven to ruin. This situation, however, presented the birth-planning cadres with the embarrassing alternative to either refrain from enforcement or to take over responsibility for suicides.[101] In the investigation by Potter and Potter, exactly the opposite situation prevailed where, in this village of the same area, a one-time birth-control fine of 250 yuan was collected. This was sufficiently affordable to be regarded by many peasants as a small price to pay for an extra child. It was only in 1981 that the production brigade became tough. This time it overreacted and meted out lifelong penalty sums for third children.[102]

While the one-child bonus has stagnated for a long time, penalty payments have kept pace with quickly rising incomes and different standards of living in the various regions of China. The researches by White on a people's commune in the vicinity of Wuhan highlighted the fact that two production brigades there collected one-off payments of between 200 and 300 yuan for unauthorized births. However, four other brigades did not levy any fines at all.[103] Reports from Xiamen region in Fujian province and from the Kunming area in Yunnan document one-off penalty sums of between 800 and 1000 yuan in 1986.[104] In their 1987 survey of two rural counties in Fujian and Heilongjiang provinces respectively, Kaufman and Zhang Zhirong reported penalties of between 400 and 800 yuan for an unauthorized second child in Fujian and a minimum of 1200 yuan in Heilongjiang. This Northeastern province also accepted instalment payments over a period of fourteen years. Birth-control fines in the Shaanxi villages investigated by Greenhalgh in 1987 varied even more and ranged from a one-off fine of 420 yuan for unauthorized second children to double this amount for third births.[105]

Whereas many localities started to raise penalty sums in the mid-1980s, the effectiveness of fine collection declined noticeably at that time. Because of the tedious and unpopular nature of this work, many cadres dispensed with collection completely. In their 1987 survey of two rural counties in Fujian province, Kaufman and Zhang Zhirong counted some 30 per cent of women with more than one child born since 1980, only one of whom had paid a fine of 300 yuan. In the two rural counties of Heilongjiang, the percentage of unauthorized births being fined climbed to 50 per cent. Greenhalgh's study reported that in the three villages under investigation, fine collection had declined from 87 per cent of birth-control penalties in 1979 to only 37 per cent in 1985. In 1986 and 1987, fine collection there ceased altogether.[106] Survey results for penalty patterns in Hebei between 1980 and 1988 clearly established that risks of getting fined increased until 1984 and diminished thereafter.[107]

The problems of penalty assessment and collection may be divined by the following widespread complaint of birth-planning cadres: the rich pay high birth-control fines without wincing and are not deterred from having unauthorized births; poor people, however, continue with more childbirths, because no fines can be collected from them anyway.[108] A 1987 implementation report from impoverished Hunan illustrates the situation:

> Fines are always collected from well-to-do persons. Those who pay 100 to 150 yuan for a child born outside plan do not consider this to be a hard punishment. They therefore do not take contraceptive measures and cause repeated above-quota births. Those, however, who are not well-off cannot pay fines anyway. They do not care at all. You are just helpless in confronting them.[109]

At the same time, a classical field report from rich Guangdong noted:

> There's a fine of 1,200 yuan for having a third child, but people consider that as nothing serious. The pregnant women just run away into hiding with relatives in other villages. When they come back with the newborn, they just pay the fine and that's that.[110]

Similar problems arise in the cities when the income of self-employed artisans, private entrepreneurs, migrant workers or casual labourers comes up for assessment. This is one of the reasons why penalty sums can differ markedly. A report from a Beijing district, dated January 1987, mentions additional one-off payments of 2000 yuan for second children, rising to 4000 yuan for unauthorized fourth children.[111] Current birth-planning regulations for Beijing contain extremely wide discretionary powers for the local authorities. Instead of regular, long-term wage deductions, they stipulate high 'social support fees' for unauthorized births. These range from 5000 to 50,000 yuan for second children and between 20,000 and 100,000 yuan for third births.[112] In Liaoning province, normal fines are comparably high. For 'particularly serious cases of births outside plan', the province even permitted a fine of up to 150,000 yuan in 1997. Social support fees are also stipulated in the birth-planning regulations of Zhejiang province, promulgated in December 1989. In contrast to Beijing, the level of these one-off payments is set at lower amounts of 3000 to 5000 yuan for urban residents and 1000 to 3000 yuan for peasants. However, since Zhejiang continues to enforce additional wage deductions of 10 per cent to 25 per cent for a period of five years, the 'social support fee' here assumes the character of an additional charge for second children. In the province's revised birth-planning regulations of 1995, 'social support fees' are also demanded for authorized second births. The same procedure was introduced between 1992 and 1997 into the newly revised birth-planning regulations of Hebei, Guangxi, Shandong and the three Northeastern provinces.[113]

In recent years the general increase of penalties has accelerated. This has been the case for one-time payments as well as for regular wage deductions. The Henan birth-planning regulations from April 1990, which doubled the monthly wage deductions, are an example. Between 1989 and 1996, wage deductions in Southern Zhejiang also doubled and began to include new fines for first children born without authorization, for disregard of stipulated birth intervals, or for not attending regular pregnancy check-ups. Penalty sums reached 2000 to 5000 yuan for an unauthorized second child and 5000 to 10,000 yuan for an unauthorized third child in 1996. Similar penalties have been introduced in other provinces. Some areas have not hesitated to fine cohabitation outside wedlock, even it has not resulted in pregnancy. The most drastic penalty increases of the 1990s were implemented by Shanghai and Jiangsu. Regulations there stipulate birth-control fines of three times the annual income for both spouses in case of second births without proper permits; this amount is raised to from four to six times the annual income for non-authorized higher-order births. Interest for arrears and further penalty sums specified by individual 'birth-planning contracts' between employers and employees may be added.[114]

The discretionary powers of local authorities continue to be wide, so it is difficult to calculate individual fines in advance. The propaganda value of the cases concerned, the social status of individuals, personal connections, the situation of public finances and many other factors play a role. This is the reason why penalty sums for unauthorized births are often the subject of 'bargaining' and why no clear-cut standard of fines can be ascertained. The link between local levels of affluence and the amount of penalty sums remains tenuous. In reaction to such circumstances, some recently amended birth-planning regulations empower counties to decree penalties should local townships fail to do so.[115]

For many years, statistical figures for birth-control fines have been a well-guarded state secret. It was only in 1996/97 that some data became available for the first time. These data were revealed in an auditing report on the birth-control budget that contained the following information: birth-planning commissions at various levels had decreed 21.40 billion yuan in fines between 1985 and 1993; at the end of 1993 some 78 per cent of this sum had been settled. Altogether, 24.18 million persons had been penalized, of whom 91 per cent had already effected payment. Additional information for 1995 and 1996 indicated 3.7 billion and 2.5 billion yuan in fines for these two years, respectively.[116] Although no further details were given, the terminology employed suggests that all kinds of fines for unauthorized births, including illegitimate, early or rash births, were contained in these figures.

At first sight, the dimensions are shocking. By very rough calculations the numbers for 1985 to 1993 translate into approximately 20 per cent of all couples in the age groups 20–29 being penalized. On closer scrutiny, however, this share is moderate in relation to the average 40 per cent of unauthorized births during the period in question. The volume of fines implies an average of 885 yuan per capita. It conforms with information from a 1992 survey on fertility and household economics, which resulted in an average 870 yuan in fines for a second child born without a permit. These sums are high in view of the many reports on low penalty sums or lagging fine collection during the second half of the 1980s. Even so, they conform to regulations and statistical data on average earnings in the countryside, as they equal fourteen years of 10 per cent deductions from the average peasant per capita income in 1990.[117] This result could only have been realized by markedly stiffer fines during the early 1990s. Yet the reports also signify that an element of social consideration remains, as per capita income accounts for the different number of dependants in peasant families. It would therefore act as a more favourable yardstick than individual income of full labourers. Technically, most provincial birth-planning regulations used to stipulate that the gross annual income of both spoused serves as the basis of penalty assessment. As this is often hard to fathom, recent amendments have also prescribed calculations on the basis of standard sums or annual per capita averages for either total population or earners.

Birth-control penalties are not the only instruments in the arsenal of punitive actions. Other punishments widely used in recent years are sanctions such as denial of bonus payments or health and welfare benefits for specified time periods, no job promotions, or demotions by one, two or even three wage grades for persons employed in urban units. Self-employed businessmen are threatened with the revocation of business licences, and private entrepreneurs leasing state or collective enterprises may face cancellation of their terms of lease. Moreover, parents of unauthorized second children have always been obliged to pay the delivery costs themselves. They have been refused wage payments during maternity leave, have to pay for a subsequent sterilization themselves, and are not permitted to apply for more living space.

The allotment of housing tracts in the villages is the equivalent of housing allocation in urban areas. It has been typical of the marked egalitarianism and welfare considerations of the rural land system that the size of housing tracts has always been reckoned by family size. If peasants could not add new floors to their buildings, they were awarded new building plots for their offspring. Many grass-roots cadres have questioned this principle and refused additional housing tracts for unauthorized births. Table 11 documents that birth-planning norms have vacillated. In many cases, the denial of additional housing tracts has entered the regulations only recently. In 1990, Chinese authorities proposed allotting housing tracts on the basis of a standard family size of three to five persons only.[118] Such proposals carry a latent message with them. They were put forward eight years after decollectivization, namely eight years after such problems arose for the first time. In this sense, they once again testify to the stubborn resistance met by many birth-control policies at the grass-roots level.

Comparable problems arise with the allotment of 'responsibility lands', i.e. land handed over to private management of peasant households with specified production quotas. In practice, most plots have been allotted on a per capita basis. Grass-roots cadres are under constant pressure from peasants demanding consideration of growing family size due to marriages and births. Although the term of land-use rights has become extended to thirty years or more, a large number of villages effect periodical adjustments in consideration of household changes.

Many current birth-planning norms demand a termination of allotments according to family size, and some also urge a reduction of land holdings in case of unauthorized births. Inner Mongolia offers a compromise by denying additional plots to extra children for five years. But once again Table 11 points to cases in which none of these sanctions are applied. Directives of the Central Committee, the State Council and the Ministry of Agriculture from 1993/94 have urged an end to demographically based land adjustments.[119] New provincial legislation on land-use contracts from the late 1980s and early 1990s also contains the clause that contracts become invalid if a contractor violates state law, regulations or policies.[120] Such calls are clashing with the government's guarantee not to terminate long-term contracts for responsibility land. It remains to be seen which principle prevails in the protracted conflicts that can be expected at village level. Field reports indicate that demographic adjustments of land holdings persist. According to a 1997 survey by the Ministry of Agriculture, only 30 per cent of the villages investigated had concluded new land-use contracts for periods of thirty years or more without the possibility of demographic adjustments within that time. Thirteen per cent had concluded contracts for up to five years, 29 per cent for periods of between six and fourteen years and 28 per cent for durations of fifteen to twenty-nine years.[121] The abolition of land allotment on a per capita basis therefore continues to be on the political agenda, and a renewed call by the Central Committee in March 2000 for upholding a policy of 'No more land for more people, no less land for less people' is far from being fulfilled.[122]

Gaps in implementation are also likely for those sanctions that threaten peasants with the denial of work allocation for industrial enterprises or non-agricultural household registration. Such rules require a state monopoly in labour allocation and efficient migration controls. Both conditions have been given in former times, but they have become increasingly eroded by the growing freedom of movement, the privatization of the economy and the slow re-emergence of a labour market. The state retains the ability to complicate matters by requiring the presentation of birth-control documents before new workers can be engaged, but it cannot totally supervise private job-searching in collective, private or individual small-scale enterprises. Discharge from work, which was a dreadful threat in former times, has therefore lost some of its intimidation. It is telling that some new birth-planning norms do not list this sanction any more.

Another controversial sanction is the threat to withhold health insurance for children born outside plan until their fourteenth birthday. Some provinces continue to uphold individual responsibility for medical treatment of unauthorized children to this very day, but in most cases the recognition that these children cannot be held responsible for their own birth seems to have gained ground. This was bolstered by a ruling of the Supreme Court in August 1990 which confirmed the status of unauthorized children as surviving dependants entitled to receive death grants and support for orphans. The progressive decline of state influence in economic life has also affected other sanctions employed at the outset of the one-child campaign. In the early period, the refusal to register unauthorized births resulted in no additional coupons for grain rations, edible oil or cotton cloth. Contemporaneous measures for the cities included the denial of grain rations, a total wage freeze in case of resistance against abortions or immediate expulsion from the Party.[123]

In May 1980, the Central Disciplinary Commission of the Party criticized these measures as being excessively hard. In a similar vein, the Shanghai Birth-Planning Commission notified its compliance with the Central Committee's Document No. 7/1984 by abolishing further sanctions not covered by birth-planning regulations. These included: refusing marriage registration for couples not complying with the late-marriage recommendation; refusing to issue birth certificates; refusing household registration for unauthorized children; and raising penalty sums at will.[124] But indications are that these and similar measures continue to be practised in many regions as unwritten laws. Up until this very day, the birth-planning procedures of Tibet Autonomous Region contain a reference to withhold household registration of unauthorized children until all fines are paid and other sanctions have been meted out. Other reports leaking out of the country every once in a while have mentioned incarceration for unauthorized births without payment of fines.[125] And it is hardly a coincidence that an article published in a social science journal during 1989 opposed 'coercive measures in present population policy such as demolishing houses, felling trees, confiscating cattle, tractors, and other agricultural machinery, as well as refusing household registration'.[126]

Similar practices have been reported by a Chinese survey of 1995 on birth-control practices in the villages, which documented both signs of cadre resignation and frank admissions of violent conflicts. Among the latter, the following responses from cadres were recorded:

'We first resort to persuasion and education. If somebody still does not mend his ways, we mete out fines. In serious cases, we tear down the houses and take away land.'

'First, we employ reasoning and education. Then, we order a pregnancy fine and forced abortion. For persons with above-quota births, we mete out fines; for those with many births, we confiscate land and revoke household registration.'

'Legal restrictions, demolition of houses, confiscation of cattle, arrest.' [127]

In a criminal case leaked from Wuhan, birth-planning cadres were accused of drowning a newborn child, the fourth born to a local peasant family, in a paddy-field.[128] Such measures seem to express a double frustration. Although they document the brutality prevailing in some instances of birth-planning enforcement, they also testify to the helplessness of grass-roots cadres who meet popular resistance to one-child norms by resorting to violence.

Such violence is not condoned by upper-level organs. Periodically, the centre has tried to curb excesses by internal rectification measures. The last such attempt started in 1991 and led to the issuing of a Directive Against Seven Transgressions in July 1995. It condemned the following actions of birth-planning cadres against violators of the rules: illegal detentions and beatings; destruction of property and houses; mortgaging of personal possessions without court orders; unreasonable confiscations and fines; incriminations of relatives and neighbours or retaliations against persons filing complaints; prohibiting legal childbearing in order to meet the population plan; and pregnancy tests for unmarried women. The need to issue this directive speaks for itself, but equally telling is the fact that it has been circulating only internally without any public report on the subject. In the view of the government, maintaining face and respect for birth-planning cadres clearly continues to be of paramount importance.

Instead of self-administered justice, the authorities prefer to condone intimidation by law. Some birth-planning norms therefore introduce collective sanctions designed to employ social pressures for birth-control enforcement. The regulations amount to a system of twofold guarantees for compliance with birth quotas: work units vouch for their employees, employees vouch for their families.[129] Early model rules for collective sanctions were promulgated by Guangdong in February 1980. The province decreed that all enterprises and work units exceeding their birth quotas would be fined with a two per thousand deduction of profits. The modified regulations of 1986 upheld and specified this rule. In recent years other provinces such as Liaoning, Heilongjiang, Zhejiang and Hubei have followed suit. Liaoning has decreed a 5 per cent deduction of profits for the work unit concerned. The other provinces employ global collective penalties of 500 to 10,000 yuan per unauthorized birth. In rural areas, collective sanctions have included the threat to withhold all second-child permits for villages with unauthorized births. In 1993, Shandong and Guangxi provinces broadened this injunction with the announcement that counties with more than 30 per cent unauthorized births would suffer penalty payments and global deductions of bonuses. Moreover, the leadership threatened to put their birth-planning work under direct provincial supervision.[130] Other counties have included denials of promotions, wage increases and regular work contracts under their lists of collective intimidation.

As public models of birth planning, cadres have always been singled out for special treatment by the Party. At an early date, many birth-planning norms already included additional disciplinary sanctions for cadres with above-quota births. Such disciplinary punishment was explicitly endorsed by the Central Disciplinary Commission in July 1980. In 1989/90, violations of birth-control policies made up some 40 per cent of all cases of disciplinary punishment for Party members.[131] Most regulations do not specify the type of disciplinary measures applied. At times, they use the formulation of 'measures up to discharge from work'; in some instances, they list 'cancelling of appointments, demotions or expulsions'. Other options are entries in the personal file on admonitions or grave admonitions.

Disciplinary sanctions have not prevented cadres from becoming focal points in the criticism of unauthorized births. Unlicensed births in cadre families are dreaded, because they can develop a dynamic of their own. Subordinates begin to circumvent birth-planning regulations by citing precedences, and this may in turn provoke new fraud and data falsification. In recent years, higher-level Party organs have therefore taken exemplary action and convened public meetings for the criticism of non-complying cadres. The Henan birth-planning regulations of April 1990 explicitly mention public criticism as an integral part of disciplinary punishment.[132]

A report from Shaanxi illustrates the nature of such meetings and the standards employed in sanctions against cadres. A public meeting, convened in autumn 1993 before a public audience of more than 1000 spectators, resolved to punish fifty-three cadres as follows: all accused persons had to pay a one-time penalty of 1000 to 2500 yuan for fathering unauthorized children, and three of them were expelled from the Party. Eighteen cadres with two births outside plan were discharged on two years' probation with minimal monthly support; at the end of their probationary period a demotion by two wage grades was decreed; and even this was considered insufficient, as an additional social fee for above-quota births amounting to five years of 30 per cent wage deductions had to be paid. The meeting was adjourned after thirty-five other cadres who had more than three children outside plan were immediately dismissed.[133]

While such punishments apply to the unauthorized births of officials themselves, cadres have also been forced to take responsibility for enforcement of birth-planning regulations within their sphere of jurisdiction. The precise procedures for the newly introduced responsibility systems have differed from place to place. Therefore, only examples of prevailing practices and standards can be cited. One example is a rural township in Hebei province that has been granting a qualified second-child permit for peasants. In 1991, the birth-planning cadres of this township were threatened with the following wage deductions for non-compliance with birth plans: 30 per cent for each third or higher-order birth; 10 per cent for each case of non-compliance with birth-spacing rules; 2 per cent for each planned but non-enforced sterilization; 1 per cent for each planned but non-enforced IUD insertion, for errors in quarterly reports exceeding a 5 per cent margin and for each 1000 yuan of non-collected birth-control fines.[134] The amended Heilongjiang birth-planning regulations of May 1994 threaten lump sums of 300 to 500 yuan per under-reported or misreported birth to be paid by the leader of the work unit and the directly responsible cadre, respectively. Guangdong, which has to counter constant criticism for lax policies and high fertility numbers, is another example of stiff administrative punishments during recent years. In a widely publicized case, the province punished the Party secretaries and administrative heads of four towns in 1998 for failing to reach birth-control targets in their areas. They were demoted by one rank, dismissed from concurrent posts, and forced to repay rewards and subsidies. Two years later, the province cracked down on Jieyang municipality, publicly criticizing this area for being backward in birth planning, ordering direct rule of some counties and the dismissal of leadership personnel.[135]

Cadre remuneration and promotion have thus become linked to an increasingly sophisticated system of 'efficiency wages' and regular evaluations. Still tougher standards apply for the leading cadres of urban units with unauthorized births. Already in 1983, the birth-planning regulations of Heilongjiang were threatening them with a deduction of 10 to 20 per cent of their monthly wage; in 1989 this was increased to 10 per cent of the annual wage.[136] Although this sanction is not mentioned in other provincial regulations, it seems to have become the norm in supplementary rules at the lower level. In any case, the National Birth Planning Conference of April 1993 decided that managers of urban enterprises should be personally responsible for birth planning in their work unit.[137] Present birth-planning regulations have taken up the cause by stipulating personal responsibility of all 'legal representatives' of enterprises and institutions. This formulation is intended to cover the complicated issues created by the proliferation of private and foreign enterprises, joint ventures, stock companies and other new forms of ownership.

6.9 Special group rules

6.9.1 *National minorities*

Since the onset of Chinese birth-control efforts in 1955 and throughout the 1960s and 1970s China's national minorities were exempt from family planning. If they mattered at all in official pronouncements on population policy, they were mentioned as groups to which pro-natalist policies applied. However, apart from efforts to promote population growth by raising economic, educational and health standards for the minorities, no specific birth incentives were employed. In practice, the dispensation from birth planning was translated as a privilege for all autonomous areas at regional, district and county level. When in September 1980 the Open Letter of the Central Committee also addressed the ethnic groups of China, this was the first time they were mentioned in the context of birth control.[138] In May 1981, Ulanfu, the long-time Party secretary of Inner Mongolia and then director of the Party's United Front Department, was asked for instructions on birth planning among the national minorities. He carefully weighed his words, emphasizing the distinctions between urban and rural areas, border regions and hinterland, autonomous regions and normal provinces, Han-Chinese and minority nationals in the autonomous areas.[139]

Since birth planning for the national minorities is a highly emotional subject prone to provoke ethnic strife, later directives of the Central Committee dated February 1982 contained only the lapidary statement that 'birth planning should be promoted among the national minorities, too, but requirements can be a little more lenient in an adequate way. Specific rules should be passed by the autonomous areas, and the provinces or autonomous regions concerned, on the basis of the real situation prevailing there.'[140] A number of academic conferences have convened to discuss this topic since 1981 and have proceeded with the utmost caution. While they point out that the constraints prompting birth control increasingly applied to the minority regions too, they have refrained from any suggestion of a unified policy.[141]

At the end of 1982 the notion of birth control for densely settled minority areas entered the sixth five-year plan. It has been repeatedly confirmed ever since in a number of policy pronouncements, and increasingly without any further qualifications. Still, the Party is proceeding with the utmost caution. The currently valid points are contained in the Central Committee's Document No. 7 of April 1984. This grants a global second-child permit for all minorities with under 10 million members, concedes special third-child permits, and strictly opposes all higher-order births. Later experience shows that these rules have been applied with considerable latitude. Although in the great majority of cases they define the limits of minority privileges, some areas continue to grant permits for fourth children, absolve small nationalities from any type of birth control, or lift requirements in border areas. These modifications seem to enjoy the support of the centre. At a conference on birth planning for the national minorities convened in June 1992, Peng Peiyun delivered a very carefully worded speech and confirmed the principle of differentiated policies with regard to regional specifics.[142]

In contrast to their minority populations proper, autonomous regions started to implement birth control for Han-Chinese living there already between 1971 and 1975. Since then, new regulations have slowly come into being. In June 1982, Inner Mongolia Autonomous Region laid down formalized birth-planning rules for the region's majority population of Han-Chinese. Special rules and 'recommendations' applied for minority nationals. For the first time, the preliminary birth-planning regulations of December 1988 made these groups subject to a moderate form of birth control. They permitted two children for Mongol inhabitants of the region's cities and three children for Mongols settling in the countryside, since 1990 with the added proviso that one of the first two children be a girl. Two births were also conceded to Koreans and members of the Muslim Hui minority living in the Inner Mongolian cities. Members of the small Tungus minorities (Dagur, Evenki and Oroqon) were exempt from birth planning altogether. In the newly amended regulations of the 1990s, they are counselled to practise eugenics and 'lower childbirths suitably'.[143]

Birth-control regulations for the three Northeastern provinces were likewise introduced in 1982. They are stricter than in neighbouring Inner Mongolia. Significantly tight regulations have been decreed in Liaoning province, the homeland of China's numerous but highly assimilated Manchu minority. Because of the large numbers of Manchus living in the cities, in 1982 the province limited second-child permits to endogamous unions of minority nationals settling in the villages. Slight modifications were enacted in 1985 and 1988. Neighbouring Jilin first granted second-child permits to all urban and rural minority nationals in endogamous unions, restricting this concession in 1990 to minorities with a population of under 10 million. Nowadays, this caveat should also apply to Manchus, who in the last micro-census of 1995 are shown to have surpassed the 10 million mark. In Heilongjiang, Tungus tribesmen are allowed three children. Other, more populous minorities such as Manchus, Mongols, Xibe and Hui are conceded a second child only for endogamous marriages.[144]

The provinces of the Chinese core region in North, East and Central-South China with their small minority populations have adopted different rules. In some instances they have also extended second-child permits to minority nationals in urban areas (Fujian, Shandong, Guangdong).[145] In other cases they have limited such favours to the minority peasant population (Henan). Practices in the Southwestern provinces of Guizhou and Yunnan have varied. Starting in 1984, Sichuan implemented a policy that discriminated between plains, hill country and mountainous regions. In accord with the directives from Beijing, Guangxi Autonomous Region in the South of the country introduced birth planning for many areas of Han-Chinese settlement in 1974. In 1985 it subjected its titular Zhuang nationality with more than 10 million members to the same kind of modified one-child policies prevalent in Han-Chinese areas, but it does grant second-child permits to its smaller minorities.

Regulations for the national minorities of Tibet, Xinjiang, Ningxia and Qinghai are particularly sensitive, as these are the minority areas with the greatest political problems. For Tibetans settling in the herding districts of Qinghai province, 1982 rules replaced the former total exemption from birth control with a general permit of second and third births. In 1986 these permits were extended to minority nationals living in urban areas. Regulations in the Tibetan areas of Sichuan, Yunnan and Gansu provinces are tighter and have brought about a noticeably lower fertility level there. Tibet Autonomous Region set up tenuous birth-planning offices in 1975 that only five years later allowed the same formalized birth control for Han-Chinese cadres and employees as in the rest of the country. In 1985 this was extended to a cautious form of birth control for the urban population of the region. Tibetan cadres and state employees living in the urban areas of Tibet were restricted to two children. In special cases they were allowed three children. A Party directive of 1983 aimed at controlling fourth births of Tibetan peasants and herdsman in the central region around Lhasa and Shigatse, but in the region's provisional regulations of 1986 this objective was abandoned. According to the presently valid, stricter rules of 1992, Han-Chinese personnel in urban areas are to honour the one-child requirement, while all Tibetan city dwellers are allowed two children. Under special circumstances, both groups may also apply for an additional birth. The rural areas of Tibet are targeted for the gradual introduction of a three-child limit. Border areas and smaller ethnic groups continue to be exempt from any restrictions.[146] At the end of the 1990s some rural counties seem to have begun to enforce the three-child limit by requiring IUD insertions and sterilizations from peasants and herdsmen, too. Rates for contraceptive use and late marriage in the region have constantly increased.

The Tibetan government in exile paints a much more sombre picture of birth-control policies in the region. According to its White Paper of 1996, since the mid-1980s third births have been fined in rural areas too. This would indicate disregard for official regulations and is hard to substantiate. However, in view of the many reports on over-zealous cadre behaviour and breaches of law, it cannot be ruled out for individual cases or places. The White Paper also insinuates that a conscious policy of ethnic suppression is followed by bolstering Chinese migration to the region, while subjecting some 30 per cent of all married Tibetan women of reproductive age to IUD insertions or sterilizations. This allegation seems exaggerated as far as the period of reference (1987) is concerned.[147]

Nevertheless, the controversy vividly illustrates the dynamite buried in the issue of birth control for the minority areas. It can quickly explode into highly emotional rows and culminate in the reproach that problems of overpopulation are not home made, but rather created by the resettlement of Han-Chinese, who try to solve their problems to the detriment of the natives. Besides the political issue of Han-Chinese migration to minority areas, birth control also touches on religious attitudes there. Chinese policy-makers are therefore consciously wooing public opinion leaders from the clergy. In Tibet their efforts have produced lukewarm statements from lamas, who profess an understanding of the economic motives for birth control while pointing out the conflict with the Buddhist concept of karma. Among most minorities, popular acceptance and support for birth planning is therefore very low. Some hazard canvassing of cadres in Tibet and Xinjiang confirms this view.[148]

A less well-known but equally sensitive case is the small Ningxia Autonomous Region of the Chinese Muslim (Hui) community, which introduced a two-child limit for the cities and a limit of two to three children for the densely settled irrigation areas of the Huanghe river plain in 1975. In the traditional-minded mountainous South of the region three to four children were permitted. Tightening began in 1980. A series of new regulations in 1982, 1986 and 1990 finally established a 'one-two-three rule' (i.e. limits of one, two or three children) for the cities, the plains and the mountainous area, respectively. Since early marriages and higher-order births are extremely prevalent in Ningxia, the rules are particularly hard to enforce. Moreover, birth control in Muslim areas has to wrestle with the problem of forceful religious opposition to abortion and contraceptive measures interfering with godly life. Muslim clergy in the region are known to have closed mosques to believers who practise birth control. In Ningxia as in other Muslim regions of China, the resistance of conservative Islam to fertility control may be gauged from the notably lower rates of sterilization and IUD use in comparison to those prevalent in the areas of Han-Chinese settlement.

Finally, there is the strategically important Xinjiang Autonomous Region on the Western border of China, where separatist movements are active and similar complaints are raised as in the Tibetan case. After a number of adjacent Central-Asian republics gained their independence following the dissolution of the Soviet Union, Chinese policy is currently operating under even more constraints. As with Tibet, for many years Xinjiang did not lay down any fixed birth-planning requirement for the Muslim majority of its population and limited itself to propaganda only. Only in 1974 did it start to distribute contraceptives free of charge. A year later birth control was introduced for Han-Chinese in their typical areas of concentration such as the cities of Urumqi, Karamay, Ili and Hami and the various military settlements of the land reclamation zones. This was extended to all Han-Chinese in the region's first formalized birth-control rules of April 1981. New regulations of April 1988 introduced birth planning for the minorities. In comparison with rules for the core region of China, these were rather relaxed. Minority nationals living in the region's cities had to respect a limit of two children; in the countryside they were permitted three children; in special hardship cases, an additional child was allowed. Members of small ethnic groups with under 50,000 members could even give birth to five children. This lenient ruling applied to Tajiks, Uzbeks, Russians, Tatars, Xibe and Dagur. The amended Xinjiang birth-planning regulations of August 1991 have seen a tightening of the rules. Although the general permit for two children (in the cities), three children (in the villages), or even an additional child (in special hardship cases) for minority nationals stayed in force, special rules for the small minorities were scrapped and second-child permits for Han-Chinese peasants were restricted in a number of areas. In addition, fines and other penalties for violation of the rules were steeply increased.[149]

While Tibet and the Muslim regions of the Northwest are characterized by marked ethnic tensions and endogamous marriages within ethnic groups, mixed marriages between Han-Chinese and national minorities are more widespread in other parts of the country. In most cases these are unions between a Han-Chinese man and a woman belonging to a minority group. Minority women often see such a union as an avenue to social advancement, whereas male Han-Chinese appreciate the opportunity to save the sometimes abhorrent marriage expenses that come up in many rural areas of China. There is a general tendency of government promotion of such marriages, which are viewed as instrumental in alleviating ethnic tensions. Promotion is most marked in autonomous areas and in regions with strong national antagonism. Because of these differences in the social and political environment, rules for mixed marriages also vary. Whereas Tibet, Xinjiang, Ningxia, Qinghai, Hainan, Sichuan and Jilin extend second-child permits to mixed marriages, other provinces such as Liaoning, Shandong and Henan issue such permits only in cases where both spouses can prove minority status. Hunan, Guangdong and Yunnan mostly grant second- or even third-child permits for mixed marriages but limit such privileges to particular minority areas. Yet other provinces like Zhejiang and Guizhou operate with separate rules for urban and rural areas.

Fertility policies for the minorities are intimately tied to the question of how to declare nationality status. Change of ethnic affiliation has been a major problem. After the Cultural Revolution reclassification was permitted in order to compensate for persecution of minorities in the past. Rules finalized in a circular of November 1981 governed this major step. For mixed marriages they stipulated that parents should decide the nationality status of their children under age 18; adults should decide for themselves; and orphans could revert to the nationality of their grandparents. Since there was no age limit for those desiring a change of nationality status due to past discrimination, and since all wrong registrations were to be corrected, the rules permitted reclassification for millions of people. In some parts of the country this led to a complete reshaping of ethnic composition. Reclassification is furthered by the incentive structure for minority nationals, who are granted special preferences in schooling, employment and cadre promotion in addition to fertility privileges. It tends to involve mainly those descended from mixed couples or minority women married to Han-Chinese.

Liaoning province, in particular, has had to cope with massive numbers of people changing back from Han nationality to Manchu minority status. During the period 1982 to 1990, between the third and fourth population censuses, an estimated 85 per cent of its Manchu population growth has been due to reclassification. In October 1985, the province therefore modified the second-child privilege to include only endogamous couples having held minority status before that date. Mongols and smaller Tungus minorities of the Northeast, as well as equally assimilated minorities in Hubei, Hunan and Guizhou, offer further examples of strikingly high growth rates resulting from reclassification. In reaction to such problems, in 1990 the State Commission for Nationality Affairs limited the right to change nationality status. Those who desire such a change must now prove beyond doubt the minority status of at least one parent. Children from mixed marriages are only allowed to change their ethnic affiliation between 18 and 20 years of age.[150] Up until now, the new rules seem to have had only limited effect. The micro-census results of 1995 demonstrate that the tide of minority reclassification has not yet subsided. Comparing population numbers for Mongols, Manchu and Tujia in the micro-census with the 1990 census figures still results in abnormally high growth rates far beyond a natural increase.

6.9.2 Others

Besides the national minorities, other groups have also created particular problems for Chinese birth planning. Above all, this pertains to the migrant population, which has grown markedly since the mid-1980s.[151] These are predominantly peasants who migrate to urban areas in search of work and better income opportunities. Although a number of regulations on household registration and labour policies are designed to curb population movement, economic reforms make them ever harder to enforce. The same applies to birth-planning regulations, which are difficult to implement for persons with high mobility. Thus migrant workers are able to take advantage of problems of jurisdiction that arise in the division of labour between birth-planning authorities at places of origin and places of destination. They also profit from the lack of control as far as population movement and the labour market is concerned. In the late 1980s up to 70 per cent of migrants had not registered at their present place of residence; by 1995 this figure was still estimated at 45 per cent.[152]

Since 1985, a number of provinces have promulgated regional regulations on birth planning among the migrant population. Sometimes these regulations take the form of separate rules; at other times they are integrated into the general birth-planning norms. Special documents are available from eleven provinces.[153] The 'Administrative Procedures of Birth Planning for the Floating Population' issued by the central government in December 1991 were intended to serve as an instrument for unifying these local regulations. This aim has been accomplished in the newly amended birth-planning regulations from the 1990s, which show a high degree of standardization and a tendency of continuously tightened controls.[154]

The latest administrative measures make the official place of household registration responsible for the issuing of documents, while the implementation of birth planning and the necessary controls are entrusted to the place of residence. Migrants are required to respect the birth-planning rules of their permanent registration place. The regulations strive for a tight control of fertility, making employers, landlords and local authorities responsible for the checking or signing of proper documents and the reporting of unlicensed pregnancies. In particular, work permits, business licences, provisional house-hold registration, lease and rental documents will be refused if migrants cannot produce valid birth-planning documents. If migrants have unauthorized births away from home or fail to attend pregnancy check-ups, the departments concerned at the present place of residence are required to revoke licences and provisional registration, to set deadlines for returning home, and to notify the birth-planning office at the home residence.

But these rules are hard to put into practice. In particular, persons without a permanent residence and regular work are hard to classify by place of registration and place of residence. In these cases, the rules require the authorities at both places to approach the persons in question. But the authorities often pass on their responsibility to other organs so that in reality nobody takes action. Similar problems arise with regard to the necessary cooperation of various authorities at places of in-migration. This has resulted in the resignation of many urban administrations which do not ask for the required documents and openly declare themselves unable to control migrant fertility. A 1996 migrant survey in Beijing highlighted the fact that 46 per cent of married migrant women did not carry birth-planning documents of their places of household registration, while 52 per cent had not completed birth-planning formalities at their place of in-migration.[155]

Activities are further hampered by the lack of extra personnel, sufficiently clear registration rules and the difficulties of collecting fines from itinerant persons. A core problem has been the fact that the financial burden resulting from control measures in areas of in-migration had to be met out of budgets calculated for registered, long-term residents only. It is against this background that new amendments to the rules for birth planning among the migrant population in 1998 have further buttressed the responsibilities of host areas, charging them with the validation of birth-planning documents, the establish-ment of files and regular supervisory activities. An increasing number of host places oblige migrants to carry special birth-planning documents with them which contain information on number of births, contraceptive measures taken, the penalties meted out to them and the status of fine collection. Cities with a particularly high concentration of migrants have created special cadre positions and budget provisions for birth control among this part of their population. Host areas have also obtained the right to levy birth-control fees from the migrants themselves.[156]

Similar problems arise with those belonging to the private sector or who are self-employed. Because people in this sector are not salaried and not dependent on state employers, the usual controls and sanctions are hard to implement. If these who belong to the private sector are long-term urban inhabitants living on small incomes in crowded housing, they do not usually possess the means for raising a large number of children. Conditions are different, though, if private businessmen are registered elsewhere, if they realize large earnings or employ many people from the countryside. The authorities then confront similar problems as in the case of migrant workers. Because of such problems, a number of recent birth-planning regulations from the lower levels have required sharply increased deposits from migrants and those discharged from the state sector. Guarantee sums for respecting birth-control measures can range from 1000 to 5000 yuan. In addition, private employers have been made responsible for setting up birth-planning arrangements for their employees to parallel similar measures in state enterprises. Finally, the work of informants and militia squads working under the public security committees of urban neighbourhoods seems to be focused on law enforcement among the informal employment sector and the migrant population.

The 'Administrative Procedures for Birth Control Among the Self-Employed in Industry and Commerce' of 1987 stipulated that the Administrations for Industry and Commerce provide the birth-planning authorities with numbers and names from their registration records. Birth planning itself fell within the responsibility of authorities at the permanent registration places of women. Furthermore, the regulations made detailed prescriptions on the question of financial responsibilities for birth planning among this segment of the labouring population. However, just as in the case of the migrant population, the increasing population mobility and the growth of the private sector make enforcement of such rules exceedingly difficult. In recent years, local branches of the Administration for Industry and Commerce have been exhorted to revoke business licences in cases of unauthorized births and to follow the example of other grass-roots organizations by undertaking regular check-ups and filing regular birth-planning reports. Some newly revised regional birth-planning regulations also charge them with handling the one-child bonus for the self-employed or with levying administrative fees. These fees can be turned into an incentive mechanism by collecting them from all members of the private sector and then lowering them for persons respecting the one-child rule.

Similar to the private sector, implementation of birth-planning rules for foreign enterprises and joint ventures in the special economic zones has been less than perfect. In principle, Chinese employees of foreign companies have to respect the same rules as other citizens, but the awkward problem arises of how to manage enforcement in a different organizational and cultural environment. Birth control in these enterprises has therefore lagged behind. In recent years, it has tended to become vested in the semi-official Birth-Planning Association, which enables the state to intervene in a less obnoxious way. In addition, the Chinese parties to sino–foreign joint ventures have been made responsible for enforcing birth control among employees.[157]

The increased mobility of the population, the diversification of property relations, the empowerment of enterprises and the gradual extension of a labour market have also forced the authorities to devise special rules for employees dismissed from work, for the unemployed, or for the larger group of people suspended from work while still holding social security coverage from their old work unit. These people tend to be forgotten by the various administrations, which deny further responsibility for such cases. Recent birth-planning regulations from the late 1990s have reacted to the increasing prevalence of such problems by establishing clear-cut rules. They usually stipulate a continuing responsibility of the former work unit to care for contraceptive measures and compliance with birth control among employees suspended from work. It is only with the start of new employment that responsibility passes to the new employer. For registered unemployed persons in urban areas, the regulations specify birth-planning duties of either the local street committee or, in cases of existing insurance coverage, the authority handling unemployment insurance. Birth planning for employees dismissed from work is vested with the local street committee.

Chinese from Hongkong, Macao, Taiwan and overseas constitute another important group for which special rules apply. Ever since the opening up of the country, their numbers have multiplied in the coastal areas, where they are valued as a source of know-how and investment. Against this background, the leadership has granted birth-planning concessions for returned overseas Chinese. Special rules were first formulated by a work conference of August 1982, which discussed new rules for second children in rural areas. Spouses who both hailed from overseas were included in the types of cases eligible for second-child permits.[158] The rules were further relaxed in June 1983. Ever since, overseas Chinese living in urban areas are also entitled to second-child permits if they have returned to China within the last six years. Overseas Chinese women who have two or more children and who return to China while pregnant are not required to undergo an abortion.[159] Another directive of July 1992 ruled that marriages between Chinese citizens and ethnic Chinese from other territories who are residing in China are allowed a further birth, provided the other children are living abroad.[160]

7   Problems of organization

7.1 Institutions

7.1.1 The role of the Party

During the 1950s birth planning was entrusted to the health departments, with some token participation of other ministries and mass organizations. Handling it as a Party affair is an invention of the 1960s and the Cultural Revolution period, which replaced organization with indoctrination and left many decisions to the discretion of grass-roots units. With the beginning of the third birth-planning campaign in the early 1970s, the revolutionary committees, followed by Party committees, stepped in to fill the vacuum left by the weakening of central government institutions. Repeated admonitions to the local Party secretaries to take over coordinating tasks became standard fare at that time. Since 1978 they have intensified.

In February 1978 the State Council as the highest government organ endorsed the report of a national birth-planning conference, which had decided that 'Party committees on all levels should strengthen leadership over birth planning and put it on their agenda'. Echoing similar calls since 1963, the conference resolved to make one of the Party secretaries of each Party committee personally responsible for this new task.[1] Eight months later, another birth-planning conference and the Central Committee reconfirmed this ruling. They decreed that 'all Party committees from the county level upward are required to have quarterly deliberations on birth planning'.[2] The final steps for implementing the directive were taken in May 1979 at the work conference of the Central Committee meeting at that time.

After the close of this conference, the CC Secretariat took up the regular discussion of birth planning for the first time. As the Party organ responsible for daily operational work, and as a *de facto* second government of the country, this institution was chaired by General-Secretary Hu Yaobang. In the struggles between followers of Deng Xiaoping and leftists around former Party Chairman Hua Guofeng, it had acquired extra weight as a bastion of reformist forces. It seems that within the CC Secretariat the influential chief theoretician of the Party, former Secretary Hu Qiaomu, acted as the person responsible for birth planning. A number of top-level directives to the Birth-Planning Commission bear his signature. These directives called for new proposals on how to enforce rural birth planning after decollectivization, urged effective measures against the illegal removal of IUDs, and action against encroachments on infant girls and their mothers.[3]

In the period 1979 to 1987, all important changes of population policy were decided by either the CC Secretariat collectively or by its presiding officer, the General-Secretary of the Party. The CC Secretariat defined the subjects for the regular work conferences on birth planning, and discussed, endorsed, and circulated the minutes of these conferences, having the final say in all critical points. After the retirement of Hu Qiaomu and the dismissal of Hu Yaobang, his successor, General-Secretary Zhao Ziyang, assumed responsibility for all important decisions from January 1987 until his demise in June 1989.

In March 1988, the alarming reports on problems of birth planning led to a change of jurisdiction within the Party leadership. Ever since, it appears that the Standing Committee of the Politburo holds regular discussions on birth planning in February or March each year. Some more precise information on the sessions of March 1988 and February 1989 is available.[4] The change in the sphere of responsibility has underlined the extraordinary importance of birth planning in the eyes of the Party leaders. At the same time, it has also strengthened the influence of proponents of a hard-line one-child policy.

When all members of the Standing Committee of the Politburo participated in the National Birth Planning Conference held in April 1993, the personal involvement of the top leaders became visible to everyone. Party leader Jiang Zemin and Premier Li Peng insisted on using this occasion to personally present new provincial birth-planning targets to the First Party Secretaries of all provinces.[5] Their personal responsibility for birth-planning performance was thereby underlined once more. Despite recent emphasis on legal accountability and the joint birth-planning duties of leading cadres from both Party and state organs,[6] Party supremacy remains intact.

7.1.2   *Birth-planning commissions*

Until 1964, the first tentative birth-control measures remained under the jurisdiction of the Ministry of Health and its Department for Maternity and Child Care. In 1962, this department set up a special Section for Birth Planning. In most cases, the Ministry of Health was also the organization steering the few provincial birth-control committees founded between 1954 and 1958. In other instances these embryonic organizations were formally registered as committees subordinate to the Chinese People's Political Consultative Conference, the united front organ of the country. The birth-control committees were umbrella organizations bringing together representatives from the health establishment and other ministries, from intellectual circles, and the three large mass organizations active in mobilization and propaganda work: the Women's Federation, the Trade Union and the Communist Youth League. Typically, they existed in only a few provinces of the coastal belt such as Tianjin, Hebei, Liaoning, Shanghai, Jiangsu, Shandong and Guangdong. The major exception in the interior was Hunan, which in 1957 set up a particularly wide network of more than 1500 birth-control committees in all prefectures, cities and counties of the province. However, all these committees had ceased functioning by the second half of 1958. Some were revived in summer 1963 after the Great Leap Forward, either under their old name or under a new designation.

The establishment of a nationwide organization was completed only after a further year. In January 1964 the State Council charged its general-secretary Zhou Rongxin to head a special Birth-Planning Commission, which was responsible for coordinating respective policies and served as the model for similar organs at lower levels. The organizational arrangements for these hybrid institutions carried all the marks of improvisation, financial constraints and manifold compromises. Terminology at the lower levels wavered between birth-planning commissions and leading groups for birth planning, indicating that their exact status as executive or coordinating organs was left undecided. The commissions had very little personnel. A large part of their limited budget was disposed of by the Ministry of Health. In most cases their general offices were combined with the premises of the maternity and child care sections in the departments of health. Time was too short for the Commission to make much of an impression, as it soon ceased to function in the Cultural Revolution. It shared this fate with the majority of the other government ministries and commissions, which were similarly dissolved or stopped operating between 1966 and 1968. When in August 1968 at least the Ministry of Health was restored under the supervision of a Military Control Commission, birth planning completely reverted to the jurisdiction of the Ministry.

Things started to change in 1971, when some provinces re-established the leading groups or birth-planning commissions under the provincial ersatz governments, the revolutionary committees. In June 1973, this was followed by a Leading Group for Birth Planning operating under the State Council at national level. During the first two years of its existence it was chaired by later Party chairman Hua Guofeng. In 1975 he was replaced by Politburo candidate Wu Guixian, a female model worker from the Cultural Revolution. Such groups or commissions became the established norm for all provinces and cities, as well as for a growing number of counties; the last regions to establish them were Xinjiang and Tibet in 1975. Members of the leading groups were representatives of the state organs responsible for planning, civil administration, public security, health, education, production and distribution of contraceptives, as well as cadres from the Party's Propaganda Department and Disciplinary Commission, the Women's Federation, the Youth League and the Trade Union, the Army and a number of provincial Party committees. In 1978, these totalled thirty-four persons in the Leading Group at the central level.

During the last years of the Cultural Revolution, the groups were responsible for coordinating policies within the state administration, propagating birth planning, and drawing up plans for population development, the production of contraceptives and contraceptive research. They had a general office but no subordinate institutions or staff offices. Moreover, the weak and understaffed general office continued to be set up within the Ministry of Health and its provincial departments. At the central level, it was headed by Su Xiuzhen, a female cadre from the Ministry of Health who weathered the storms of the Cultural Revolution. Only a limited number of provinces made the general office independent from the health organs. The competencies of the national organ *vis-à-vis* the regional institutions were largely confined to convening an annual meeting of their directors.[7]

After the end of the Cultural Revolution the general intensification of birth control led to a large-scale expansion of the apparatus. In June 1978, Zhou Enlai's former protegée, Vice-Premier Chen Muhua, took over the chair of the Leading Group for Birth Planning. Four months later, the State Council acted on the recommendation of a national birth-planning conference convened by her and decreed a nationwide extension to all counties. In January 1979, this was followed by the decision to establish birth-planning offices with specialized personnel in rural people's communes and urban street committees, too. Large enterprises with more than 500 employees also appointed birth-planning personnel of their own.[8]

But the biggest change was yet to come. As the leading groups had to confine themselves to discussion and coordination without being able to effect implementation, this set-up was considered insufficient. In 1981 the State Council therefore took the decision to establish the State Birth-Planning Commission under the leadership of Chen Muhua and four deputies. The Commission comprised twenty-six ordinary members from the Standing Committee of the National People's Congress, the Chinese People's Political Consultative Conference, various ministries and commissions, the People's Liberation Army and a number of mass organizations. In later years this was regularized to *ex-officio* membership at the vice-ministerial level for presently eighteen government organs. This arrangement largely paralleled the former Leading Group for Birth Planning, but, unlike the former set-up, this time the Birth-Planning Commission acquired its own functional departments. It also established its own vertical structure of birth-planning commissions for all administrative units of the country. Instead of just convening coordinating conferences, between 1981 and 1983 an entirely new bureaucracy with regularized work started to develop. Only Tibet, with its chronically weak governmental apparatus, still largely relies on the former arrangement of working from within the health departments.[9]

This embryonic organization was constantly enlarged during later years. Today, the State Birth-Planning Commission has staff departments for policy and legislation, planning and statistics, propaganda and education, science and technology, finances and pharmaceuticals, liaison and personnel. Furthermore, it has its own auditing office and separate bureaux for investment, administration, petitions and archival work under a general office. The general office also handles an internal network for communicating information on current birth-control developments to the Central Committee and the State Council.[10]

At its first plenary session of May 1981, the duties of the Birth-Planning Commission were spelled out as follows: managing birth-planning measures, implementing relevant rules, formulating birth plans in cooperation with the Planning Commission, organizing propaganda and educational work, training birth-control cadres, conducting scientific studies on subjects of birth control, and planning the production and distribution of contraceptives. Two years later, it also acquired the right to independent planning in the areas of finances and investment, employment and wages. Ordinances of 1988 and 1989 basically restated these responsibilities and specified the tasks of the Commission's functional departments; revised statutes from 1993 contain the most recent rules for duties, powers and procedural matters. [11]

Following the model of other functional bureaucracies with vertical organization, the thirty provincial birth-planning commissions are placed under dual leadership. They are subject to operational guidance by the State Birth-Planning Commission in Beijing, which also receives quarterly and half-yearly reports from them. The national-level organ in Beijing has the right to decide on procedures and definitions in the reporting system, it coordinates training programmes, planning procedures, annual meetings of the directors of provincial birth-planning commissions, research activities, as well as the production and distribution of contraceptives. It can also demand information and offer advice on regional birth-planning norms.

The division of powers in the normative process has always been a crucial issue. The statutes of the Commission testify to its gradual empowerment *vis-à-vis* the provinces and other government organs. Although the earliest government documents of 1981 only granted it the right to 'implement' regulations, a later version of 1988 added the privilege to 'draft' such rules. In May 1989, a circular issued by the Commission on the instruction of the Politburo's Standing Committee and the State Council went even further and 'asked' all regions to 'contact' the State Birth-Planning Commission before promulgating new regional birth-planning regulations. Although the delicately worded circular stopped short of requiring the provinces to obtain prior consent and thus preserved their formal right of final decisions, it indicated the growing stature of the centre in birth-planning legislation.[12] The presently valid statutes of 1993 give the Commission the right to 'determine' birth-planning regulations either alone or in 'coordination' with other bureaucracies. It is reinforced by the newly acquired prerogative to exert 'overall management, inspection and guidance' in relation to local birth-planning stations. Provincial birth-planning regulations, however, continue to be promulgated by provincial legislatures and governments, which also establish grass-roots level institutions, appoint personnel, and exercise political leadership over the provincial birth-planning commissions. If the centre wants to rule decisive issues of birth planning, for instance, second-child permits, vertical chains of command within the birth-planning bureaucracy are insufficient. Instead, it must invoke State Council directives or, even better, directives of the CC Secretariat, the Politburo or its Standing Committee.

The regular duties of the provincial birth-planning commissions consist of formulating regional population plans, staging annual propaganda campaigns before the Chinese New Year Festival, organizing an annual work conference for the evaluation of past performance and the planning of future measures, and performing annual inspections of grass-roots organs in different localities. In addition, the provincial birth-planning commissions receive statements of local demand for contraceptives as well as monthly work reports from the cities and quarterly reports from the rural areas. These regular reports are then used for compiling the quarterly and half-yearly reports to the centre in Beijing.

The tasks of the approximately 360 municipal or prefectural birth-planning commissions more or less correspond to this pattern of duties. Hierarchical arrangements at this and the lower levels vary, however. A multitude of different methods for combining vertical leadership by upper echelons with horizontal leadership through Party and government organs at the same level coexist. Vertical leadership tends to be stronger than in relations between the centre and the provinces. The municipal or prefectural commissions exercise leadership over the nearly 2800 birth-planning commissions of counties or urban districts, which in turn give guidance to the more than 60,000 birth-planning bureaux established in townships or towns. In urban areas, this level is equivalent to the street committee. At the lowest level of towns and townships, birth-planning bureaux have been established only since 1991. Financial difficulties and lack of personnel have retarded the nationwide extension of such grass-roots bureaux for many years.[13]

Completely outside this vertical organization are special offices responsible for birth planning among the military, the armed police, as well as among cadres and employees of organs directly under the Central Committee or the State Council. Sometimes, the history of these special offices reaches back to a period prior to the start of nationwide birth planning. Their separate existence once again shows the complicated nature of organizational setups in China. It pinpoints the organs that claim special prerogatives and which do not accept guidance from a government commission at the same hierarchical level.[14]

Similar to other ministries and state commissions, the Birth-Planning Commission is at the apex of a large number of subordinate institutions. At the national level, these include a medical and pharmacological research institute, a centre for population information and research, a publishing house and the editorial offices of a newspaper dedicated to population issues. A national centre for birth-planning propaganda and education produces films and television programmes, educational pamphlets, slides and poster series; it also organizes exhibitions and symposia. Furthermore, the Birth-Planning Commission is in charge of a training centre for higher cadres in Nanjing, a similar school for middle-level personnel in Taian (Shandong), as well as thirty provincial distribution centres for contraceptives. Since 1992, Chinese economic reforms have made inroads and led to the establishment of five additional institutions offering services and contracting on a commercial basis. They consist of a publishing house for audio-visual media, a supply centre for birth-planning offices, a management training and exchange centre, a centre selling new health products and technology, and a consulting company offering information, exhibition, conference and patent transfer services. At the provincial level, there are twenty-nine further cadre training institutions, as well as seventeen regional research institutes, seven technological service centres, twenty-three newspapers, and thirty-six institutions for information, propaganda and educational work. Whereas in the beginning these institutions were confined to the big macro-regional centres of Shenyang, Shanghai, Wuhan, Beijing, Chengdu and Xi'an, they have now extended to almost all Chinese provinces.[15]

A glance at this organizational framework shows that since 1981 China has created another huge, nationwide bureaucracy. This demonstrates the organizational capacity of the Chinese state with its tight, centralized hierarchy. However, there is also another constant element. Just as in the imperial period, direct state control ends at county level. Extending the reach of the state to the rural township or village level has been tried ever since the Guomindang era in the 1930s, but even today it remains far from being totally accomplished. From a Chinese perspective this can be a grave deficiency, as rural counties can contain up to 1.5 million inhabitants.

7.1.3 Coordination with other government organs

Quite early on, China discovered the truth of a basic rule applying to family planning everywhere in the world: since birth control is interwoven with all aspects of economic and social life, it requires integration with other departmental policies. Without such coordination, birth-planning norms will not be in tune with other regulations embodying unintended incentives for childbearing. Earlier examples from the Chinese case include uniform grain rations both to adults and children, housing and land allotment on a per capita basis, cost-free medical provisions for all births, or other social services increasing with family size.

Mechanisms for coordination have already been discussed in connection with the Birth-Planning Commission and its various predecessors. It is an organizational weakness of the Commission, though, that it ranks at the same level as other ministries and state commissions without enjoying global planning competencies. Empowering the Birth-Planning Commission with such rights, however, could easily turn it into a higher-level organ claiming rights of interference in other policy arenas. This would put the Birth-Planning Commission on a par with the State Planning Commission – an organizational arrangement that leading politicians found unacceptable. Failure to raise the status of the Birth-Planning Commission has resulted in the unsatisfactory situation that at least twenty other central ministries, bureaux, and institutions are directly or indirectly involved in birth planning. In the early 1980s, these included the following organs:

- *The State Planning Commission* has to approve, decree and supervise the population plans of all provinces, integrating them with economic planning; the Planning Commission has its own research institute with a population section.
- *The State Commission for Science and Technology* is responsible for defining, organizing and approving central research projects.

- *The State Commission for Agriculture*; before its duties were taken over by the Ministry of Agriculture, it was charged with devising and implementing rural responsibility systems, linking agricultural production with a birth-planning component.
- *The State Commission for Nationality Affairs* is responsible for population policies among the national minorities.
- *The Ministry of Health* is responsible for disseminating information on medical aspects of birth planning, training medical personnel for contra-ceptive operations, promoting relevant research, issuing medical certifi-cates, investigating malpractices, and performing IUD insertions, sterilizations and abortions in its subordinate hospitals.
- *The Ministry of Chemical Industry* is charged with the production and development of condoms.
- *The State Pharmaceutical Administration* supervises the State Corporation for Pharmaceutical Production, which produces oral contraceptives, and the State Pharmacy Corporation, which stores, administrates, and distributes all contraceptives.
- *The Ministry of Culture*, which publishes and subsidizes popular literature and posters for the birth-planning campaign.
- *The State Commission for Education* is responsible for coordinating birth-control teaching and research in the country's institutions of higher learning.
- *The Ministry of Civil Administration* is entrusted with marriage registration, late-marriage propaganda and the organization of relief.
- *The Ministry of Finance* appropriates and controls the birth-planning budget.
- *The Ministry of Public Security*; besides commanding the police forces, it is also charged with household registration and the promulgation of relevant rules.
- *The Ministry of Labour*, which has to implement preferential treatment in work allocation for single children.
- *The Trade Union, the Communist Youth League and the Women's Federation* are responsible for effecting propaganda work and mobilization among their constituencies, and they provide unpaid part-time cadres at the grass-roots level.
- *The Army's General Political Department and General Department of Logistics*, which promote birth planning within the military.
- A *Scientific Advisory Committee* attached to the Birth-Planning Commission.

This is a conservative and limited roster of institutions listed in a State Council ordinance of July 1981 on the division of competencies for birth planning.[16] The list could easily be continued. It would thus have to include the Ministry of Machine Building and its subordinate National Corporation for Medical Appliance Industries charged with the production of IUDs. In the 1990s, a complete list would also include the Ministry of Personnel responsible for the appointment of cadres and specialists, the Central Disciplinary Commission of the Party, the Ministry of Supervision and the People's Courts, meting out administrative punishment and sanctions, the Ministry of Urban Construction and the Administration for Industry and Commerce, controlling migrant workers in construction projects, industry and the tertiary sector, the Ministry of Foreign Economic Relations and Trade, licensing joint ventures and foreign enterprises, the Ministry of Education, the Ministry of Radio, Film and Television, the Party's Propaganda Department, the State Statistical Bureau and the People's Bank, the Administrations for Housing and Real Estate, Land Management and Resources, the Departments of Traffic and Transportation, and at least ten other authorities disbursing various economic incentives.[17] The majority of these organizations have their own vertical bureaucracy with subordinate offices at the provincial, city and sometimes even county level. Many delegate *ex-officio* members to the Birth-Planning Commission.

It is revealing that the State Council ordinance of 1981 did not mention the inclusion of birth-planning propaganda in the school curricula. It was only after 1981 that such a project was initiated with support from the United Nations Fund for Population Activities. A number of senior high schools experimented with either half-year birth-planning courses or with the inclusion of relevant elements in geography and biology lessons. This was also the first time that a textbook on birth planning was produced for the school system. However, the project was limited to China's major cities, demonstrating the tenacity of a social environment not conducive to birth planning. Rather than organizational problems, it is the strong resistance to sex education in schools that is responsible for this state of affairs. In China's prudish society, this has long continued to be a taboo subject. Even in the nation's capital, implementing such measures encounters enormous problems. It was only in 1988 that the State Commission for Education ordered all schools to introduce population courses in elementary and junior high schools and sex education at the senior-high school level, but execution of this directive has lagged behind.[18]

Other examples of problems of coordination are the contradictions between the Ministry of Health and the Birth-Planning Commission in the spheres of medical education and research, gynaecological check-ups and contraceptive surgery. Because the birth-planning commissions were only set up in the early 1980s, they have had to cope without medical cadres of their own for some time, which is why they tried to effect a transfer of doctors and medical assistants from hospitals and health offices. Their efforts aroused the strong resistance of the Ministry of Health, which insisted on other sources of recruitment for the birth-planning commissions. Frictions increased in the 1990s with the large-scale extension of a separate medical network under the jurisdiction of the birth-planning commissions. A joint circular from both authorities from January 1995 on the division and overlapping of competencies bears witness to the manifold problems involved.[19] Similar tension exists between the birth-planning commissions and the departments of public security, urban construction, labour and business administration, all of which have to cooperate in controlling migrant fertility.[20]

These are merely glimpses of the numerous problems of coordination between the birth-planning commissions and other departments. Reading the long list of bureaucracies involved can cause dizziness! Coordinating this huge bureaucracy which jealously defends its prerogatives requires Herculean efforts. Frequently, there is little horizontal cooperation and much vertical rivalry between the different administrations. Recent provincial birth-planning regulations have tried to tackle these perennial problems by conferring to staff of birth-planning offices a right of leadership, control and inspection *vis-à-vis* enterprise birth-planning personnel, by turning interdepartmental cooperation into a legal requirement, and by vesting local birth-planning commissions with the right and duty to report other departmental measures not in accord with birth-planning policies to superior authorities. However, this still calls into question the institution in charge.

It is the declared will of the central leadership that coordination should be shouldered by the Party committees and local governments at all levels. These bodies are required to guarantee the provision of the necessary finances, personnel and equipment, so that the birth-planning commissions are able to meet the population targets decreed by the five-year plan. Because existing mechanisms for coordination are unwieldy, it has been repeatedly suggested that the State Council's Leading Group for Birth Planning parallel to the Birth-Planning Commission be revived, or to empower the latter institution with the right to instruct other state organs. In February 1989, Premier Li Peng turned down this proposal, using the arguments mentioned above. Rather than establishing an all-powerful organ, he appointed State Councilor Li Tieying as the person in charge of mediating conflicts between the various bureaucracies. Moreover, he ordered that the State Council should organize interdepartmental meetings on birth planning twice a year. The government reorganization introduced by the new premier Zhu Rongji in March 1998 also failed to take up the more far-reaching ideas that continue to be voiced by influential population specialists.[21]

While the State Council's interdepartmental meetings are restricted to the discussion of problems within the administration, national birth-planning conferences involve the participation of a much larger audience. Initial conferences with national representation were staged in 1958 and 1965, and after 1971 they became a regular event with a changing format. Since 1992 they have been convened on an annual basis, partly replacing the usual meetings of directors of provincial birth-planning commissions. National birth-planning conferences last from between one to four days. In addition to the national and provincial leadership of the birth-planning commissions, they also bring together representatives from the Army, the National People's Congress and the Political Consultative Conference, as well as from all relevant departments, commissions and ministries under the Central Committee or the State Council. In some instances, vice-governors from problem regions have been cited to join the meetings and deliver self-critical reports. Altogether, attendance has ranged from between 100 to 200 delegates. The conferences have been twinned with national symposia on birth planning jointly organized by the Party's Central

Committee and the State Council. During these one-day events, the participants of the national birth-planning conferences are joined by the top leadership of the Party and government, as well as the First Party Secretaries and Governors of all provinces and cities with independent planning status.[22]

The national birth-planning conferences and symposia thus function as a coordinating mechanism at the national level. Developments in the regions have shown some deviation from this pattern. Here, some provinces have retained the leading groups for birth planning from the 1970s, while others established or revived them in the 1980s and 1990s. A new wave of founding such coordinating organs started in 1991.[23] Essentially duplicating the functions of the national conferences at a lower level, they are meant to effect even closer coordination on a more regular basis. It remains to be seen, however, whether these new organizational devices will succeed in reducing friction. Increasing bureaucracy remains a distinct possibility.

7.1.4 Grass-roots organization

In its initial stages birth control was an elite subject, discussed among intellectuals and leadership circles, largely limited to the urban population and executed by a small health administration with few rural extensions. During the later period of the Cultural Revolution its focus shifted as it came to engulf the countryside's semi-autonomous villages. This meant it had to rely on the efforts of millions of poorly trained grass-roots cadres, whose ranks were augmented by a host of unpaid or inadequately rewarded propagandists. In contrast, the birth-planning administrative structure of regular, budgeted posts was extremely tenuous. This was indicative of the general situation of the Mao period, when ideological mobilization substituted for organizational and financial resources. The 1980s saw events turn full circle. They witnessed the construction of an elaborate administrative superstructure rising from the county or township level. However, as with other Chinese bureaucracies, the birth-planning apparatus has long been top-heavy. It struggled with the problem of extension to the grass-roots level and was further enfeebled by decollectivization and the retreat of the state in the reform era.

This has again exacerbated the cleavage between cities and villages. Today, the organizational set-up in urban areas is still superior to that in the countryside. Large- and medium-sized urban enterprises and institutions have appointed their own birth-planning cadres. Newly established private enterprises have been obliged to follow the lead of the state and collective sector and to set up their own birth-planning offices with specialized personnel. Cadres at the grass-roots level are commissioned to maintain a list of women of reproductive age in order to supervise contraceptive measures and distribute contraceptive devices. Neighbourhood committees, as the lowest urban units of self-administration, are trusted with implementing birth control for non-employed persons. They are accountable to birth-planning offices of street committees and urban districts, creating a tight vertical hierarchy in the process.[24]

The main problem, however, arises at the rural grass-roots level. In the 1960s and 1970s most people's communes appointed special cadres for birth-control work. These tasks usually rested with female vice-leaders of the units concerned, who were also assigned many other duties. Their efforts were supported by barefoot doctors and political activists. Just as during the first birth-planning campaign of the 1950s, these were mostly unpaid activists from the Women's Federation or the Youth League. Production brigades or villages under the township level did not have any specialized personnel at all, but restricted themselves to sending women cadres to birth-control meetings organized by the people's commune. Production teams, equivalent to current village groups, charged one cadre with the whole range of women's work. Sometimes, she was assisted by other female activists who joined in the activities for birth-control propaganda and the arduous house visits required. However, these forces have been inadequate to shoulder the increasingly heavy duties entailed by the continuous tightening of birth-control policy. For people's communes or townships, these involve regular inspections, the distribution of contraceptives, the collection and tabulation of report figures from the lower levels, and the fixing of annual birth quotas and their breakdown by villages.[25]

Starting in 1977 the government urged the creation of regular, specialized positions on a full-time basis. However, it typically could not offer financial support and had to pass the problem on to the provinces. Recruitment, payment and accommodation for grass-roots cadres and offices continued to be an unsolved problem. The dissolution of people's communes in the early 1980s exacerbated the problem, as it frequently resulted in a reduction of personnel and finances. Often, the re-established township administrations were unable to help. Even today, many township offices are understaffed and cannot handle the work efficiently.

Part-time cadres for birth control in rural villages or urban neighbourhood committees are said to have totalled 0.5 million in 1981. This seems to have been the zenith of mobilization during the early one-child campaign. Only in urban areas did the figure increase further to 2 million by 1994. However, even the figures for 1981 are low in comparison with the Cultural Revolution period, when fragmentary reports indicated levels of up to 0.5 million people for just one province. These numbers were certainly inflated by including all paramedics and propagandists in the count. With the advent of economic reforms, mass mobilization ceased to be a viable strategy. Since many part-time cadres are mobilized for unpaid work, they do not enjoy any special training and have suffered a loss of authority in the wake of rural decollectivization. Motivational problems and low work effectiveness are widespread.[26]

Most provincial birth-planning regulations of the 1990s prescribe the establishment of township (town) birth-planning offices and the appointment of personnel at village level. Ten years before, this was anything but a self-evident arrangement. In cases where the dismantling of people's communes left a vacuum at township level, coordinating groups had to substitute for non-existing permanent birth-planning bureaus. They comprised responsible cadres from organs that even today remain the cornerstones of birth planning at the grass-roots level: the township administration, the Women's Federation, the Youth League, the militia and the civil administration. Since the late 1980s they have acted as a committee of mandators and supervisors *vis-à-vis* the village committees elected by the peasantry. Just as at central government level, committees are also required to handle the manifold problems of coordination between various bureaucracies. In the townships and towns, these are mainly the following offices and institutions: the Party committee and township government exercising overall leadership; the finance department effecting and auditing the necessary appropriations; the local hospital and/or birth-planning station performing contraceptive surgery, abortions and relevant education; the education department, the Youth League and the Women's Federation, the culture and the radio stations all carrying out propaganda work; the civil administration and the police station responsible for marriage and household registration; and the credit cooperative or the local branch of the People's Insurance Company managing one-child insurances.[27]

Yet the weakest link in the long chain of delegation is the village unit. In the 1980s, there were neither full-time cadres nor offices in the villages, so that birth planning at this level largely depended on the cooperation of all parties involved. In the 1990s, a number of newly revised birth-planning regulations stipulated that a vice-head of the village committee assume responsibility for birth-planning duties. Some have also explicitly stated that in birth-planning affairs the village committee is under the leadership of the township or town government. The most time-consuming and difficult work is at village level, namely the control of contraceptive measures and the supervision of women of reproductive age, the constant visits to women with unauthorized pregnancies and the concomitant efforts to persuade and pressure them to have an abortion, the hearing of medical complaints and appropriate counselling, the proclaiming of village birth quotas and the handing out of licences to applicants, the collection of fines from violators of policy, and the gathering and filing of raw data on births, deaths and marriages. Current relevant handbooks propagate that all women of reproductive age should be visited monthly or at least once every three months.

The large-scale expansion of Birth-Planning Associations to the villages in the early 1990s must be seen as an attempt to meet these exigencies. As of June 1994, more than 55,000 township and more than 780,000 village chapters of the Birth-Planning Association had become involved in a new membership drive. This is more than the total number of townships, towns and administrative villages throughout China. Until 1999 the total for affiliated chapters in both urban and rural areas had further grown to more than a million. Just as awesome is the recent growth of Association membership to a 1994 total of more than 83 million in both rural and urban areas. The implications of this figure may be fully understood only when it is contrasted with a contemporary total of more than 160 million young women between 20 and 34 years of age. It signifies that half of all women in the critical age groups have been forced to join. Moreover, the Association has started to pay grass-roots personnel. In 1994 these included nearly 1.5 million people. Wherever possible, village heads and

Party secretaries, who used to shoulder the tiring and unpopular duties of birth-control work, have delegated these tasks to the local Birth-Planning Association. Its office then effectively assumes responsibilities that at higher levels are handled by state organs.[28]

A further measure of the last decade has been the large-scale promotion of birth-planning contracts that specify a maximum birth number, regular contraception with required guarantee sums, rewards for respecting the one-child rule and penalties in case of contract violations. Although in principle all couples of reproductive age are urged to sign relevant statements, certain segments of the population have been targeted as the main objective of such additional efforts to enforce compliance: peasants with second children, staff on prolonged leave from duty, floating population leaving for other places, unemployed or laid-off labourers, those working in the private sector – in short, anyone not under easy supervision at the workplace. While some provincial regulations give lower-level units an option to introduce such a system, others make it mandatory. The latest birth-planning regulations from Guangdong even stipulate that birth-planning obligations have to be integrated into all work contracts, lease and rental agreements covering more than one year.

A number of provincial and local regulations also prescribe birth-planning contracts between village committees and township authorities. Relevant procedures include a written list of prescribed birth-control indicators, powers and duties for lower-level cadres. All parties involved have to sign two different contracts. One is drawn up between the township government and the local birth-planning bureau. It obliges the township Party committee and government to guarantee specified financial resources and material allocations. Another contract is laid down between township governments and Party committees on the one hand and village committees on the other. While the former embody the lowest level of state organization, the latter act in their capacity as non-state, autonomous peasant representations. Village committees and their birth-planning cadres pledge the fulfilment of detailed targets, non-adherence of which is sanctioned by progressive wage deductions. Such arrangements place the elected village committees into perennial conflict with their rural constituencies and their government mandators.[29]

Wages of birth-planning personnel are calculated by a system of work points; they are linked to regular cadre evaluations with a threat of sizeable income losses. Table 12 reproduces an evaluation form dating from 1992 and recommended by the Birth-Planning Commission for use at town and township level. Although the selection, definition and weighting of specific items differs throughout the country, the basic system of cadre wages and collective benefits linked to ratings for birth-planning performance remains the same. The form reproduced in Table 12 reveals that overriding birth-planning goals clearly precede local interests and concerns in the evaluation process. While penalty enforcement is stressed, individual benefits are not even mentioned, and only sketchily outlined collective benefits are taken into consideration. The document also contains other hazily defined items. As with all similar schemes, it suffers from the difficulties of finding objective indicators for individual

Table 12 Birth-planning evaluation form for townships and towns 1992

Name of township/town: Evaluation date:

	Maximum credit points
A. Birth-planning targets	35
1. Target formulation	12
according to upper-level mandate, by scientific reasoning	12
self-decreed, without sufficient basis	6
transmitted by upper level	4
no targets existing	0
2. Target fulfillment	23
fulfilled, birth rate < 15‰	23
not fulfilled, birth rate 15–16‰	16
not fulfilled, birth rate 16–18‰	10
not fulfilled, birth rate > 18‰	4
B. Birth-planning work	35
1. Propaganda work	12
> 80% of couples of reproductive age grasp present birth policy	12
70–80% of couples of reproductive age grasp present birth policy	9
60–70% of couples of reproductive age grasp present birth policy	6
< 60% of couples of reproductive age grasp present birth policy	3
2. Technical services	12
contraceptive prevalence (married women of reproductive age) > 80%	12
contraceptive prevalence (married women of reproductive age) 70–80%	9
contraceptive prevalence (married women of reproductive age) 60–70%	6
contraceptive prevalence (married women of reproductive age) < 60%	3
3. Policy implementation	11
penalty rate for above-quota births > 95%	11
penalty rate for above-quota births 80–95%	8
penalty rate for above-quota births 65–80%	5
penalty rate for above-quota births < 65%	2
C. Economic benefits of birth planning	15
good economic benefits	15
satisfactory economic benefits	10
medium economic benefits	6
poor economic benefits	2
D. Social benefits of birth planning and image of birth-planning personnel	15
> 90% of canvassed population have good opinion of birth-planning dept.	15
80–90% of canvassed population have good opinion of birth-planning dept.	10
70–80% of canvassed population have good opinion of birth-planning dept.	6
< 70% of canvassed population have good opinion of birth-planning dept.	2

Total credit points: Head of evaluation team (signature):

Source: Li Jinfeng 1992, 128–129

performance that are not influenced by outside factors and do not lend themselves to manipulation.[30]

In its incessant drive for the perfection of regulations and procedures, the centre introduced standardized Evaluation Rules for Birth Planning in 1993. These fix four basic indicators: birth rate, birth-planning rate, a percentage of grass-roots units conforming to birth-control standards, and a maximum error for birth statistics. Further optional indicators include the early- and late-marriage rates, the rate of contraceptive prevalence, figures for the popularization of birth-control knowledge, work attendance of birth-planning cadres and so on. Different weighting procedures are explicitly permitted, but errors in birth statistics exceeding a prescribed level cannot be compensated and will lead to immediate economic sanctions. Many provincial implementation rules for birth-planning regulations from the 1990s explicitly prescribe annual evaluations of lower-level birth-planning offices by the superior organ at the next highest level.[31]

It is telling that in addition to regular check-ups by superiors in the normal chain of command, special provincial investigation teams have started to clamp down on the villages. Their unannounced visits have created an increasingly tense atmosphere in the countryside. Investigation manuals of 1996 urge personal visits to local households and patrolling of villages in order to prevent the hiding of women or the passing of illicit information; they counsel watching for nappies, toys and baby food in order to detect unregistered births, or examining children's teeth and physical coordination movements for conformity with declared age. All persons checked are required to produce documents for proving correct household, marriage and birth registration. Furthermore, they have to sign all sensitive items in a protocol. The records are then cross-checked with neighbours and compared with the vaccination records, birth-control filing cards, household registers and report forms of the village cadres.[32] A discussion of practices in the annual sample survey includes these revealing passages:

> For discovering the correct birth numbers, the areas have to use infinite ruses in conducting surveys, like the Eight Immortals, who all used their personal piece of magic for crossing the sea. Some ask about the next household, while investigating and recording circumstances in the one before; and they cross-check the results of the earlier household, while entering the numbers in the next one. Some visit hospitals, vaccination stations and midwives in order to find out about births. Some provinces send statistical cadres back to a sampled village for discreet inquiries, so that public surveys and inside knowledge are combined. In still other cases, the personnel pretends to be salesmen for children's clothes and thus collects household information. Some provinces decree that the grass roots select experienced statistical cadres with a strong sense of responsibility as interviewers for direct questioning in the households, to be accompanied by a person familiar with the local situation. And, finally, there are not a few provinces confronting low-fertility places with several investigation groups

that enter the villages without prior notification of the county, the township and the village and that conduct both open and covert investigations for finding non-reported births.[33]

Mutual surveillance of villages is another measure from the arsenal of the authorities. How investigations may be conducted in practice can be gleaned from the following report on poor areas, where high fertility leads to tight control measures:

> These areas need annually three to four months of stress on birth planning. For each surprise attack, a great number of people are drawn from various county and township departments in order to go down to the villages. There can be dozens of them, who weigh upon a place for some days. In addition to this, there are the mutual checkups in birth planning. Often there are up to twenty or even dozens of people from the opposite township, who come to a number of villages in the township under investigation. After entering a village, they check one family after another, have talks, examine the records, and even count how many children's clothes are around. It goes without saying that in relation to the backward economic circumstances the expenses created by such activities are huge. The anger of peasants about these excessive burdens and their fury about the feasting connected with it is like adding oil to the fire.[34]

This is not the way authorities would like it to be. In recent years, their preferred procedures have been propagated under the heading of the 'Three-One-One Method'. This catchword designates a fixed schedule for propaganda and control measures that was first introduced in rural areas of Shandong province. It involves the following sequence of activities. Every month on a given date all peasant women are required to attend compulsory birth-planning classes, where contraceptive knowledge and fertility policies of the state are taught. On the same day, contraceptives are distributed and village cadres visit women who have recently had a delivery or an abortion. There are also monthly medical consultations for those suffering from sterility or gynaecological ailments. Every two months medical personnel visit the villages in order to examine pregnant women, check for eugenic problems and hold maternity courses. Every three months there is a random check of advanced, average and backward villages that serves to control plan compliance. It involves investigation of prescribed propaganda efforts, book-keeping and fine collection, as well as ultrasound examinations of all women who are required to practise contraception. Results of this investigation are then compared with the written pledges and birth-control targets, and credit points are awarded according to an evaluation scheme. They are made public in an open meeting co-chaired by the township Party secretary and the head of the township administration. Attendance of the village Party secretary, the village head and the person in charge of local birth planning is compulsory. Irregularities have to be explained on the spot, and there must be proven enforcement of penalty regulations together with proposals for remedial action.[35]

Similarly tight controls have been reported from Jiangsu, where village women have been forced to line up for bimonthly pregnancy tests, including supervised urinalysis, with abortions following if necessary. Liaoning and Jiangxi have written the pregnancy test into their newly revised provincial birth-planning regulations of 1997. It is only in recent years that recognition of the humiliating nature of such exercises shows up. Some local birth-planning commissions have therefore begun to replace the unembellished 'check-up' with friendly worded 'services'; dependent on the degree of compliance with birth control, they have also substituted the compulsory administering of pregnancy tests with gynaecological self-reports during regular meetings of all women of reproductive age.[36]

Such arm-twisting methods together with the large-scale expansion of the Birth-Planning Association signal a renewed attempt to submit all women in the critical age groups to constant mandatory birth-planning propaganda and fertility control. Birth planning has been promoted to such a degree that in many county administrations it may take up a quarter to one-third of all work capacity. But the reports cited above hail from villages in more affluent regions. Although central authorities have eagerly recommended them as models for the rest of the country, organizational and financial deficiencies hardly allow for their wholesale adoption. Deviant field reports and random surveys in different parts of the country confirm the continued existence of large variations, with the percentages of childbearing women not receiving any 'fertility services' ranging from 10 to 100 per cent.[37]

7.1.5 Medical network

The establishment of a medical network for maternity and child care that is also charged with birth-planning services has met with similar problems as those encountered by grass-roots administration. From modest, predominantly privately organized beginnings in 1949, a government-run system has slowly progressed along a bumpy road. Steady growth during the early 1950s was followed by spectacular expansion in the Great Leap of 1958, retrenchment and stagnation between 1959 and 1965, accelerated decline during the Cultural Revolution 1966 to 1972, and new growth since 1973. It was revealing for the situation in the villages that until 1984 three-quarters of all urban births, but barely one-third of all rural births, were delivered in hospitals. By 1995 the percentage of hospital deliveries had fallen to 71 per cent in the cities, while it had risen to 50 per cent in the countryside, again with noticeable regional differences. In 1999 these percentages had increased up to 83 per cent and 62 per cent, respectively.[38] Comparing the institutional figures in Table 13 with the corresponding totals for administrative units points to the fact that even in 1998 only 19 per cent of all cities and counties, 6 per cent of all towns and townships and an even smaller percentage of villages were covered by the system of maternity and child care.

Public health policy has vacillated between distinctly different approaches to closing these glaring gaps. The ups and downs shown in Table 13 indicate the

Table 13 Institutions and personnel for maternity and child care 1949–99

| | Institutions for maternity and childcare | | | | | | Part-time personnel with child delivery skills | |
| | Hospitals | | | Health stations | | | | |
	Institutions	Beds	Personnel	Institutions	Beds	Personnel	Barefoot doctors	Midwives
1949	80	1,762		9				...
1950	77	3,000		349				...
1953	98	5,000		4,046				...
1957	96	6,794		4,599				...
1958	230	9,000		4,315			...	...
1963	104	9,000	10,400	2,863			...	...
1965	115	9,223	11,500	2,795			...	686,000
1967	103	8,000	10,900	1,536			...	...
1970	66	7,000	6,600	1,058			...	...
1973	90	7,000	9,000	1,446			190,000	...
1977	106	9,000	10,600	2,353	3,000		468,000	755,000
1980	135	11,013	14,000	2,610	5,000	24,000	356,000	635,000
1985	272	24,000	31,000	2,724	10,000	39,000	294,000	514,000
1988	310	30,000	38,000	2,793	13,000	49,000	291,000	467,000
1998	467	36,000	69,000	2,724	27,000	88,000	...	359,000[1]
1999	550	37,000	75,000	2,630	28,000		...	290,000

1 figure for 1995

Note: Institutions for maternity and child care are predominantly run by the health departments but include a small number of establishments run by other government departments and collective units. Hospitals designate better endowed institutions on the city and county level or above, health stations are organized on the town, township or village level. Personnel of all these institutions includes full-time doctors, nurses, pharmacists, technicians and paramedics.

Sources: health statistics in ZTN 1981–; ZWN 1986–; ZFTZ 1991, 478–483

changing fortunes of the Ministry of Health and its subordinate departments which manage the vast majority of maternity institutions. Although the share of institutions run by the Ministry rose sharply during the heyday of Soviet-style socialism between 1953 and 1957, 1958 saw a two-pronged strategy that increased the number of state hospitals at the higher levels while turning over health stations at the lower levels to collective management. After the Great Leap, policy was again reversed, but a return to the former strategy was hampered by severe budget constraints for the Ministry, which forced it to close down lower-level health stations. During the Cultural Revolution it came under attack as a bourgeois institution favouring an urban constituency. These years therefore saw a high increase of health stations run by the people's communes, the creation of mobile medical teams touring the countryside and the proliferation of barefoot doctors, namely rural paramedics paid from collective funds and working on a part-time basis. From 0.094 million in 1965 their total numbers grew dramatically to a peak of 1.802 million in 1976, one-third of them women. More than half a million part-time midwives had to be added to this number.

Besides performing regular healthcare, this large-scale grass-roots organization was charged with the dissemination of birth-planning knowledge. To some extent, it was also trained for performing contraceptive surgery and abortions. Table 13 gives some approximate numbers of part-time midwives and barefoot doctors possessing child-delivery skills, who were the primary agents for propagandizing, counselling and administering birth control in the countryside. Other barefoot doctors who administered abortions and vasectomies would have to be added to the list. There can be no doubt that this large army of paramedics must be credited for low-cost extension work and positive contributions to the lowering of the fertility rate in the 1970s. By paying them out of the welfare budget of people's communes the state was able to pass on the burden to lower units. Sending the paramedics to the vast number of villages spread birth control to an extent that would have been impossible through exclusive reliance on a small body of professionals.

But the lack of sufficient medical qualification and equipment was the Achilles heel of the scheme. It led to a renewed shift in favour of a centralized medical network after the Cultural Revolution. The number of part-time paramedics and midwives in the countryside has greatly diminished ever since, while figures for fully employed medical-technical personnel in the government-run maternity institutions has grown.[39] Although balancing of losses and gains remains a complex issue, both strategies failed to satisfy the requirements of a continuously tightening birth-planning campaign.

Precise information on the birth-planning efforts of the medical network is hard to come by. The first details are contained in an internal report of a vice-minister of health, outlining the situation of subordinate institutions as of January 1964. At that time, more than 4900 medics at the senior and middle levels had received special birth-control training, 3000 to 3300 clinics were capable of rendering tubal ligations and vasectomies, while 4000 to 4100 were considered capable of performing IUD insertions and abortions. This number exceeded the 1963 total of specialized hospitals and health stations for maternity and child care. It therefore must have included a number of gynaecological or urological wards in ordinary clinics, too. Representative figures for the birth-planning efforts of part-time paramedics during the Cultural Revolution period are lacking, and further information on their role is largely limited to heavily politicized case reports. As propagators of birth-control knowledge and distributors of the necessary devices, the barefoot doctors seem to have been a success. Their training for performing IUD insertions, sterilizations and abortions has been likewise hailed as a major achievement. However, it probably also resulted in innumerable tragedies and ordeals for women, who were submitted to surgery under the most awkward and primitive circumstances.

Permanent injuries or fatal accidents due to malpractices are one of the sensitive spots of Chinese birth planning. Time and again, such malpratices have poisoned the relationship between population and leadership or even provoked mass violence. Although muted reference to the issue shows up regularly in medical reports, it took a long time for the state to react with more than just exhortations. It is certainly no coincidence that rules for diagnosis, certification and restitution for malpractices and concomitant ailments were finally promulgated after the massive campaigns for contraceptive surgery in 1982/83 and 1988/89. A number of recent birth-planning regulations lay down a requirement that medical personnel performing contraceptive surgery have to carry the relevant licences with them. Some specify special bonuses for performing a large number of flawless surgeries in a row.[40]

Professionalization and extension of the medical network for birth planning has therefore remained an urgent problem. There was a long time lapse after 1964 before the next set of precise figures was issued. In 1983 the institutions for maternity and child care under the Ministry of Health employed 27,000 gynaecologists and 71,000 midwives to perform an annual total of some 20 to 30 million IUD insertions and to meet the gynaecological needs of approximately 20 million women. Starting in 1983, the rapidly growing incidence of contraceptive surgery caused these hospitals and health stations to establish special birth-planning wards. The facilities have never been sufficient, however, and many interim solutions have had to be adopted.[41]

Because regular hospitals have been overtaxed and the collectively run institutions began to break down after the Cultural Revolution, big gaps in the medical network showed up in the 1980s. Yet, despite the relicensing of private physicians in other sectors, the state has shunned turning to privatization as the way out for birth planning. Of course, this reflects the sensitive nature of birth control and the large-scale evasion of regulations. Typically enough, invectives against private physicians interfering with birth-control measures have increased over the years, and a number of recent birth-planning regulations expressly bar private physicians from performing contraceptive surgery.

Instead of privatization, the state has opted for the extension of state-run medical services. A new network of birth-planning stations was thus started in 1979. Originally, the birth-planning stations were designed to hand out contraceptives and condoms or to perform IUD insertions and regular check-ups. Later on, their duties were enlarged to perform sterilizations, to offer prenatal examinations and to give genetic advise. Until they went into operation, these services had to be rendered by the county hospitals. In 1992, some 38 per cent of all contraceptive surgery was rendered by birth-planning stations. In addition to their medical duties, they also assumed responsibility for propaganda, education and training in birth-planning work. In this way, a new medical network has been created that functions parallel with the county hospitals.[42] However, due to financial bottle-necks and the lack of qualified manpower, it is not up to the standards of regular hospitals.

County birth-planning stations were first established in areas of Henan and Sichuan at the start of the one-child campaign. After 1985 they increasingly extended to the rest of the country, reaching more than 90 per cent of all counties by 1991. They usually employ a staff of fifteen to thirty specialists who conduct propaganda work and hold training courses, organize the distribution of contraceptive devices within the county, supervise the quantity and quality of contraceptive operations, issue various medical certificates required for birth-

Table 14 Birth-planning stations in townships/towns and villages 1991–95 (in % of administrative units)

	1991		1993		1995	
	Townships & towns	Villages	Townships & towns	Villages	Townships & towns	Villages
Tianjin	68.0	47.4	92.0	80.0		
Shanxi			64.5	5.0		
Jilin			88.0	90.0		
Heilongjiang			92.6	88.7	96.3	88.0
Jiangsu						90.0
Zhejiang			42.8		76.5	
Anhui			73.0	30.0	95.0	90.0
Fujian			53.7		97.0	
Jiangxi	60.0	10.9				
Shandong	40.0	30.0		95.0	99.3	70.0
Henan			98.2	80.0	97.0	39.0
Hubei	60.0		90.0			
Hunan						
Guangdong	88.0		96.3	66.7	98.0	
Guizhou	72.5	38.6	97.7	43.8	98.4	90.0
Yunnan					53.8	
Shaanxi	65.0	65.0				
Gansu	72.3		98.5			
Qinghai			87.0	80.0		
Xinjiang					51.0	
China	47.2				70.0	

Sources: ZJSN 1992–; ZJSQ 1997, 973

planning formalities, as well as perform gynaecological check-ups, contraceptive surgery and abortions.

The situation below the county level is much tighter. Until 1985, little more than 10 per cent of townships or towns had established birth-planning stations, and massive increases occurred only in the 1990s. Birth-planning stations in towns and townships used to employ two to ten medical assistants, who concentrated on medical check-ups, contraceptive surgery and abortions besides various administrative, educational and propagandist duties. A 1997 survey of birth-planning stations in seven predominantly backward provinces showed that this number had increased to an average seven persons. Because of the size of many counties, the medical network ideally also extends to the villages, where the work of one full-time birth-planning cadre largely comprises organizing marriage and contraceptive guidance courses, visiting married women of reproductive age and regularly checking their IUDs. In most cases no medical appliances are available in the villages,[43] but in recent years wealthy areas and a centrally funded crash programme has started to send mobile clinics on regular tours through the countryside. These are equipped with facilities for pregnancy tests, gynaecological and contraceptive surgery, deliveries or abortions.

Table 14 summarizes the incomplete data from the provinces. It documents the great weaknesses at grass-roots level that existed at the beginning of the last decade. Lack of data usually signifies very small numbers of birth-planning stations. If there are no birth-planning stations in villages or townships, the women concerned only have the choice of either visiting the neighbouring county town or accepting the services of paramedics with even lower levels of specialized training. As in administrative matters, the extension of medical services to the villages remains the core problem of organization. As demonstrated by Table 14, recent years have seen considerable efforts to tackle this problem. Yet even today, the network is anything but complete. Although recent reports treat rural extension as an almost accomplished fact, many newly formed birth-planning stations remain empty shells without sufficient resources. Many women continue to complain about physical side-effects of contraceptive measures, and special investigations show that sterilizations or IUD insertions in township clinics or birth-planning stations clearly cause more abdominal pain than contraceptive operations in county or city hospitals.[44] Village extension therefore remains not merely an organizational problem of quantity but involves medical standards of quality, too. Closing this gap will need many years of continuing efforts.

7.1.6 Production and supply of contraceptives

The selling of contraceptives pre-dates their mass production in China. It began in July 1954, directly after the Ministry of Health had finally scrapped its former ban of imports. At that time, the State Pharmacy Corporation started to retail small and obviously insufficient quantities of imported contraceptives over the counter of some of its sales outlets in the major cities. Initial regulations on supply and production of contraceptives, together with relevant device specifications, were promulgated by the Ministry of Health in November 1954 and February 1955. The devices included condoms (targeted for 55 per cent of all contraceptives produced), diaphragms (10 per cent), contraceptive suppositories (30 per cent) and creams (5 per cent). Moreover, the directives ordered the establishment of a state monopoly for the production and import of contraceptives and the licensing of all sales outlets. Responsibilities for production, import, wholesaling and retailing were divided between subordinate corporations of the Ministry of Light Industry and the Ministry of Health.[45] These ministries were also responsible for diversifying the contraceptive mix, which in the 1960s came to rely more and more on upgraded, modern devices.

The first plants for the production of contraceptives were established in 1955 and 1956. In some cases they could build on extremely small numbers of handmade devices that were produced on medical demand in previous years. Trial production of the first IUDs started in 1957. For many years demand exceeded supply. Some sources claim that in early 1958 all domestically produced devices were sufficient to meet the needs of only 2 per cent of all couples of reproductive age. Condoms continued to be the most widespread form of contraception in the early 1960s. Although their supply was still insufficient, it was considered large enough to earmark one-third of the production for export in 1964. The situation for the increasingly popular IUDs was tighter. In 1965, a leading official of the Birth-Planning Commission judged their supply to meet just 8 per cent of demand. Although production seems to have caught up with demand by the late 1970s, the devices employed were long plagued by problems of reliability and compatibility. Change to more modern forms of IUDs with lower failure and expulsion rates was only achieved a decade later.

Research on oral contraceptives and clinical testing began in 1963. It received a tremendous boost, when Mao Zedong pledged his support for 'anti-baby pills' in an interview with Edgar Snow two years later. In reaction to Mao's remarks, a small Japanese plant for the production of the pill was imported during that same year. Mass production was taken up in 1967 and expanded in 1969, when pills were included in the national economic plan. But ever since the mid-1970s their use has declined as they have become largely superseded by the more reliable and less costly IUDs. Long-term injections and implants have also since been added to the list. The production of modern contraceptives has been a success. It now numbers about sixty certified products and has accelerated to such a degree that the minutes of a 1992 work conference on contraceptives contain references to the problem of oversupplies and costly stocks.[46]

In contrast, projects for developing contraceptives on the basis of traditional native recipes proved to be more or less futile. They were first taken up in 1956 and revived in 1963, when research on the 'Five Flavours Abortion Pill' and various teas, powders and herbs was pursued. Efforts to improve the low effectiveness of such traditional recipes, to rid them of unwanted side-effects and to develop drugs for mass production on their basis continued well into the 1980s. Most important among them was a project for the production of a pill for men that experimented with phenol from cotton oil for preventing sperm production. But despite decades of research, no real breakthrough was achieved.[47]

Over the years, the production and supply system underwent a number of changes. Its broad outlines in the 1980s and 1990s may be outlined as follows.

Responsibilities for the production of contraceptives are widespread. They conform to the system of industrial organization in accordance with raw material use. Production of IUDs is delegated to the National Corporation for Medical Appliance Industries, which is functioning as a monopoly enterprise under the Ministry of Machine Building. The Ministry of Chemical Industry with its subordinate China United Rubber (Group) Corporation is charged in turn with producing condoms in production plants appointed by the government. Other contraceptives fall within the jurisdiction of the State Pharmaceutical Administration, a separate organization under the State Council with two subordinate corporations: the State Corporation for Pharmaceutical Production, responsible for the production of pills, injections and implants, and the State Pharmacy Corporation, with responsibilities for storing, administering and distributing these products. Further bureaucracies involved in the production, specification and distribution of contraceptives are the Ministry of Health, the State Pricing Bureau, the Ministry of Finance and the transportation departments.[48]

These various administrations have traditionally stood at the apex of a complicated hierarchical system linking the thirty-four Chinese production units for contraceptive devices with their final users. Among them have been twelve enterprises manufacturing IUDs, seven charged with producing condoms, and approximately twelve producing various oral contraceptives and implants.[49] Since the mid-1980s the list has grown to include some six sino–foreign joint ventures for the production of contraceptive pharmaceuticals and devices. Up until 1985, products were first given to twelve interregional and twenty-five regional procurement centres, which then passed them on to the provincial birth-planning commissions. The latter dispatched the products to birth-planning bureaux at city, county or street committee level, which in turn handed them over to persons responsible for contraceptive use in rural townships, urban neighbourhood committees, industrial enterprises, state institutions and army units. Only a limited number of contraceptives could be bought in pharmacies and hospitals.

Since 1985, this clumsy system has been streamlined in order to combat its high internal costs, the ineffectiveness of distribution channels and problems of quality control and retailing. The number of intermediate links has become reduced to thirty provincial distribution centres, thirteen distribution centres for municipalities with independent planning status, 249 centres for ordinary municipalities or provincial prefectures, and 1900 centres for rural counties. Townships usually employ a special cadre for the administration of contraceptives. As in other spheres of economic life, responsibility systems have been introduced in order to suppress unnecessary expense. At present, lower administrative units receive given sums for independent management and distribution. While expenses are not allowed to exceed fixed limits, savings may be kept.[50] Such regulations result in high pressure to lower costs. They can make it unaffordable to practise expensive types of contraception, and they can seriously limit the free choice of methods.

State enterprises and institutions report a list of their female employees of reproductive age to the proper birth-planning bureau. After proving their right for allocations free of charge, they receive the necessary contraceptives to be handed out to all married women of reproductive age among their employees. Married housewives, self-employed persons and people out of work obtain their contraceptives directly from the neighbourhood committee. Non-residents and those avoiding the distribution office may also buy condoms and contraceptives in pharmacies. This new distributional channel was opened in the mid-1980s. Whereas in 1988 only 10 per cent of all contraceptives were retailed, four years later already up to 10 per cent of ordinary pills, 20 per cent of one-month pills, 41 per cent of all condoms and 54 per cent of pills for short-term effectiveness were sold via pharmacy counters. Typically, these are all more expensive pharmaceuticals that place a burden on the state budget. Initial results of the national survey on population and reproductive health in 1997 indicate that the share of retailed contraceptives has risen further. Less than 63 per cent of the married women interviewed had obtained their contraceptives via cost-free allocation; nearly 29 per cent (36 per cent in the cities, 16 per cent in the villages) had bought them over the counter; 9 per cent had received them through other channels.[51]

Paying for contraceptives is a welcome measure for lowering state expenses, but it creates dilemmas for the moral guardians of the nation, because unmarried persons can now have intercourse without the fear of unwanted pregnancies. This is why many localities continue to restrict the sale of contraceptives to unmarried persons.[52]

7.1.7 Academic bodies and mass organizations

Until the late 1970s, no specialized institutes for population research existed in China. There were only two exceptions to the rule. One was the Institute of Population Geography at East China Normal University. Established in 1957 as a product of the political thaw and the first birth-planning campaign, its brief existence was terminated a year later by the Great Leap Forward. The other exception was the Institute of Population Studies of People's University in Beijing, whose beginnings date back to initial provisional arrangements in late 1973. Strictly avoiding the public eye during the first years of its existence, it functioned as a service institution for the State Council's Leading Group for Birth Planning. It was only after the end of the Cultural Revolution in late 1977 that a decision was reached to establish more institutes for demographic research in Beijing, Shanghai and other major cities. By 1987 the number of these institutes had already multiplied to the present figure of more than sixty. Including university and academy institutes, as well as institutes under various state authorities and regional party schools, their ranks are characterized by a great diversity of organization.[53]

Extension in the academic sphere was accompanied by the establishment of a national umbrella organization, the Chinese Association for Population Studies. This association was founded in February 1981; ever since, it has established branches in all provinces of the country and grown to more than 2000 individuals with over 200 corporate members on its membership rolls. Activities have included a number of national conferences for the discussion of current problems of birth planning. Guiding the association from behind the scenes is the Birth-Planning Commission, which also appoints cadres for the leading bodies. In 1988 it appointed twenty-five demographers to serve on a scientific advisory board for birth planning that is paralleled by expert committees for contraceptive technology and birth-planning education. The Ministry of Health has a similar arrangement with advisory committees for contraceptive technology, established under the Chinese Medical Association and five of its regional chapters.

In May 1980, the State Council resolved to found another nationwide organization, the Birth-Planning Association, functioning as a transmission belt in the classic Leninist sense. Its mission is to engage in propaganda, educational and supervisory work at the grass-roots level, where it conducts presentations, study sessions and personal counselling. It also hands out production credits and implements for one-child peasant families, and it has established its own kindergartens, old-people's homes and insurance fund. These activities are designed to augment the ranks of birth-planning cadres and the weak material incentives available for birth planning via other channels. In particular, the Association is trusted with enforcing birth control among groups such as peasants and migrant workers, private and foreign-sector employees, where the state finds it hard to penetrate with its own organization. In practice, membership for demographers and sociologists, responsible persons from the trade unions, the Youth League and the Women's Federation, as well as birth-planning personnel and grass-roots cadres, has become compulsory.

Although the Association could claim a membership of only about 1 million in 1987, it had already grown to 1.7 million members by 1989. Under Chinese conditions this was still a small number, but since then, the advocates of hard-line one-child policies have succeeded in whipping up a large-scale recruitment drive, creating full-time personnel and establishing local chapters in almost every village and urban area. Within the short span of three years, the Association enlarged its membership to 50 million by late 1992. In mid-1994 it stood at 83 million. Although regional extension continues to be uneven, these members, plus the nearly 1.5 million personnel of the Association and the large-scale network at grass-roots level, have turned it into one of the biggest mass organizations of the country.[54]

A third organization, formally established as an independent body but in reality answering to the Birth-Planning Commission, is the Foundation for Population and Welfare Activities, set up in 1987 to assist poor areas, to facilitate international contacts, and to receive aid from international donors. In the same vein, a National Study Association for Politico-Ideological Work Among Birth-Planning Personnel, a China Council for the Promotion of Population Culture, and a Population Branch of the National Association of Journalism Workers were set up in 1992/93 to cater for birth-planning education among different constituencies.[55] The existence of these various organizations documents the thoroughness of the concerted propaganda drive accompanying the tightened birth-control policy of the 1990s.

7.2 Personnel and remuneration

Since its establishment in March 1981, the State Birth-Planning Commission and its subordinate regional organs have struggled with huge problems of staffing. New personnel had either to be recruited independently or transferred from other administrations. As documented by Table 15, until the mid-1980s the number of full-time cadres at the levels of townships, towns and street committees was extremely limited for a country the size of China. An initial increase in numbers occurred in 1985 in reaction to the Central Committee's Document No. 7/1984. A second marked acceleration of recruitment may be discerned after 1990, testifying to the renewed emphasis on strict enforcement of birth-planning rules. Today, the apparatus of the birth-planning commissions and their subordinate institutions constitutes one of the largest bureaucracies in the country. This is mainly due to the recent extension in townships and towns. More than 70 per cent of all cadres listed in Table 15 are working at this level, which also includes urban street committees.

The figures do not contain part-time cadres in rural villages or urban neighbourhood committees; nor do they cover full-time employees of state institutions and enterprises, who are responsible for birth-planning efforts of their own. Large-scale state enterprises have their own specialized birth-control cadres, who cooperate with personnel from the Party, the Women's League, and the management. Data on this type of cadres are very fragmentary. Their number totalled more than 33,000 in 1985, rising to 38,000 by 1989. In 1991, the total equalled an average six to seven birth-control cadres in large and medium-sized enterprises. A further 2000 birth-control cadres work in the Army and in the armed police forces.[56]

Some information about the breakdown of the number of cadres by administrative echelons is available. At national level, the State Birth-Planning Commission budgeted for 110 permanent posts in 1981. Between 1988 and 1993 this number expanded to 150 to 190. This contrasted with just one person in the Ministry of Health responsible for contraception in 1954, and two persons looking after birth control in the 'streamlined' Ministry from 1968 to the beginning of the 1970s. Two persons was also the average size of re-established provincial birth-planning sections in 1971.[57] During more normal years, provincial birth-planning commissions or their equivalents in the departments of health grew from under ten in 1964 and around forty-two in 1981 to an average of fifty budgeted posts eleven years later. At municipal or prefectural level, the figures amounted to two, twelve and sixteen, respectively.

During the 1960s there was just one birth-planning cadre for each county. In the early 1980s this number increased to approximately twelve. However, these were largely provisional positions. At the end of the decade some 70 per cent of the county commissions still did not have a fully budgeted permanent post. Due

Table 15 Personnel of birth-planning commissions 1979–95 (full-time personnel down to the level of townships, towns and street committees)

1979	44,878
1980	59,250
1982	67,968
1985	134,671
1986	142,157
1987	146,884
1989	180,000
1991	292,363
1995	405,999

Sources: ZJSN 1986–; Chang Chongxuan 1992, 295; Sun Muhan 1987, 228

to this highly unsatisfactory situation, 1989 saw a dramatic increase of appropriations for the specific purpose of financing 8000 new permanent county posts. Even in 1992, though, approximately 17 per cent of the county cadres continued to be commissioned from other administrations. Over the years all echelons have shown a tendency of increasing regional differences at recruitment levels, with numbers varying according to population size. One county cadre per 30,000 to 50,000 inhabitants is considered appropriate.[58] This ratio is approximately three times lower than in the cities.

All positions mentioned so far are directly attached to the birth-planning commissions. To these must be added 5000 further posts for various subordinate institutions in research, documentation, publication and educational work, among which some 1000 are in central institutions. The numbers also do not include approximately 20,000 employees of county birth-planning stations, which on average have ten positions for medical and technical services each.[59]

It has been mentioned repeatedly that the greatest problems of personnel reside at grass-roots level. Until recently, birth-planning bureaux of townships and towns had only one full-time employee. Calculated by population data from 1995, this equals one cadre handling birth-planning work for more than 3000 married women of reproductive age. Only a few rich areas like Shanghai could afford to establish two positions. But even this is still far below the desirable level that has been defined as two to four cadres for townships with under 10,000 inhabitants and four to six cadres for those with more – figures amounting to roughly one cadre per 600 married women of reproductive age. In recent years, the strong pressures for enforcing compliance with birth plans has pushed even these standards continuously upwards. Counties complain that a quarter to one-third of their work is devoted to birth planning, without sufficient resources for other tasks. Nowadays some of them urge townships to establish eight to ten birth-planning cadre positions and to install a total of ten to twenty village cadres as well.[60]

The educational standard of many birth-planning cadres tends to be low. In 1983, only 13 per cent of cadres at county level and above had academic qualifications, and 51 per cent had twelve years' education. Targets for future recruitment and training of personnel aimed to raise these percentages by the year 1990 to 30 per cent and 70 per cent respectively, but they have not been fully met.[61] Formerly, medical and technical specialists constituted only 15 per cent of cadres. At county level, where the better birth-planning stations are established, this percentage has risen to 39 per cent in recent years. Other frequently met occupations are teachers, statisticians, accountants or legal experts, who altogether make up 8 per cent of personnel. The great mass of all birth-planning cadres, however, are ordinary civil servants or activists from the mass organizations, and there are few training courses available to them. This is due both to the high workload and the lack of additional capacities in colleges and schools. In 1985, institutions of higher learning enrolled only 820 birth-planning cadres. Another 500 received instruction in middle-level technical schools, where they were trained as medical assistants, technicians and clerks. Before the Nanjing Academy for Birth Planning, established in 1984 as the highest training centre subordinate to the Birth-Planning Commission, started to enrol students, there existed only two-month courses for birth-planning work. Training capacity increased to approximately 4000 persons graduating from special birth-planning programmes in 1989. Crash courses in 1993 enrolled approximately 36,000 persons. Two years later, the number of cadres enrolled in various college extension programmes amounted to around 30,000.[62]

Just as unsatisfactory is the situation with regard to wages and social security benefits for employees of the birth-planning commissions. More than once, their cadres have complained about the low wage level. In 1990, birth-planning cadres in townships and towns earned 70 yuan per month, and the wages of county-level specialists for medical and technical work rose to an average 85 to 100 yuan. Part-time activists in the villages and urban neighbourhood committees, who shoulder the main burden of unpopular control, persuasion and intimidation work, received a monthly bonus of just 3 to 5 yuan. These were minuscule amounts that in no way sufficed to meet the rising expectations of the reform period. Recent years have seen substantial wage rises. Some provincial regulations have specified that subsidies for birth-planning personnel should equal 70 to 80 per cent that of leading cadres at the same administrative level. Figures from a 1997 survey of birth-planning stations in townships and towns of seven provinces showed monthly wage averages for medical personnel of 287, 532 and 597 yuan in the years 1994 to 1996, respectively. In remote areas with special allowances for high price levels, wages have risen even further; for example, counties of Linzhi prefecture in Tibet pay more than 900 yuan per month. The dramatic increases in the numbers have resulted partly from subsidies paid by higher echelons, partly from extra income earned via additional medical services, partly from raised local payments.[63] It may be surmised that the improved bargaining position of doctors, who can threaten to leave their work, also plays a role.

There is no way one can judge the representativeness of these figures, which must also be evaluated against a background of annual inflation that has eaten away more than half of the increase between 1990 and 1996. Yet there is still substantial improvement. If the data prove to be reliable, they would indicate that in recent years remuneration of medical personnel in local birth-planning stations has equalled or even surpassed the average wage for the health sector as a whole.[64]

Because birth-planning commissions are a newly established bureaucracy without assets accumulated over the years, they have long suffered from lack of office and housing space. Their cadres frequently do not receive social security benefits and encounter problems of obtaining the coveted non-agricultural household registration. This registration is indispensable for enjoying subsidized housing, health insurance and better schooling opportunities. In the period of the eigth five-year plan for the period 1991 to 1995, great efforts have been made to improve this situation. An important initiative was the decision of April 1993 to recruit one to two full-time birth-planning cadres for each township and town, and to grant them the social and economic privileges connected with a transfer from agricultural to non-agricultural status. However, it is revealing that all persons benefiting from this measure have been required to pledge a work commitment of at least ten years.[65] Other, regionally varying incentives such as pension supplements have also been made contingent on long-term service.

It remains to be seen whether these material improvements have effected the desired fundamental changes in the outlook of birth-planning cadres. In the late 1980s many were demoralized and had to be subjected to increased ideological schooling. Facing frequent antagonism from their friends and acquaintances, they continue to be burdened with one of the most unpopular jobs in China. In early 1988, the Party organ quoted their comments on their work conditions as follows: 'We frequently have to act against our own wishes, we need strong nerves and have to do a lot of talking. We must run around the whole day long, and we are always hungry.'[66]

A number of surveys on work attitudes among birth-planning cadres have therefore produced alarming results. In 1988, 57 per cent of the cadres who were questioned in six provinces wanted to quit their jobs. A smaller hazard survey in 1995 produced similar results. And even a more docile investigation in 1992 still yielded a figure of only 48 per cent of county birth-planning personnel who professed 'a relative interest' in the future continuation of their work.[67]

Under these circumstances the doubling of the birth-planning budget in 1991 was more than necessary, but the additional funds can be used only partly for remuneration, and constant wrangling between the different echelons about responsibilities for the wage bill continues. Although in recent years the number of employees under work contracts specifying subsidies, floating wages and special bonuses has grown, and the few wage figures available indicate marked improvement, the material and motivational problems are far from being solved.

7.3 Budget and financing

In 1964, birth planning became an independently budgeted item dispensed by the Ministry of Health and the Birth-Planning Commission. This is why first figures are available for 1965. Directives jointly issued with the Ministry of Finance ruled that the item covered all expenses for contraceptive surgery of peasants. The expenses for city residents on state payroll were to be borne by enterprise funds or institutional budgets. For the individuals concerned, the services were provided free of charge. The birth-planning item in the national budget was further used for financing wages and running costs, as well as expenses for the training of personnel and the equipment of birth-planning institutions. There was no clear ruling on short-term contraceptives, and all further details were referred to the discretion of provincial authorities. A clear directive for state coverage of all contraceptives was issued only in 1970. It seems that together with the Birth-Planning Commission, the independently budgeted item was abolished during the Cultural Revolution. In 1978 it was re-established within the account for culture, education, science and health in the table of state expenditures. Although birth control at that time still stayed within the jurisdiction of the Ministry of Health, the new procedures again secured a dependable flow of resources.[68]

Table 16 shows the increases in birth-planning expenditure since 1963. It highlights the fact that the costs for birth-planning efforts have largely been borne by state and collective enterprises in the cities or by people's communes, rural enterprises, and town and township administrations in the countryside. In

Table 16 Birth-planning expenditures 1963–98 (million yuan, budget allocations and social expenditures)

	Grand total	Budget allocations			Social expenditure
		Subtotal	Central share	Regional share	
1963		16.61			
1965		27.63		27.63	
1971	202.65	59.52		59.52	143.13
	256.44	75.47		75.47	180.97
	419.52	123.48	15.00	108.48	296.04
	476.30	140.31	20.00	120.31	335.99
1975	574.34	169.20	26.00	143.20	405.14
	567.83	167.81	29.00	138.81	400.02
	593.28	175.27	25.00	150.27	418.01
	670.44	197.64	25.12	172.52	472.80
	859.18	251.30	22.46	228.84	607.88
1980	1038.13	331.52	33.79	297.73	706.61
	1147.82	344.07	50.08	293.99	803.75
	1557.22				
	2494.97				
	2537.78				
1985	2582.42	745.00			1837.42
	2837.84	778.00			
	3101.76	852.00			2249.76
	3512.45	977.00		841.41	2535.45
	4218.87	1100.00			3188.87
1990	4858.96	1340.00	200.00	1017.20	3518.96
		1560.00			
		1936.00			
		2262.00			
		2699.00			
1995		3190.00			
	5676.00	3700.00			1976.00
		4293.00	488.00	3805.00	
		4820.00	470.00	4350.00	

Note: The grand total and the social expenditures for 1996 do not include birth-planning expenses of urban enterprises.

Sources: Sun Muhan 1987, 164, 273; Chang Chongxuan 1992, 277; ZJSN 1991–; ZRN 1994, 544; ZJSQ 1997, 128. Slightly different figures for both the grand total and the sub-items are given in Gao Erling et al. 1997, 23.

these latter cases, they are raised collectively via fees and indirect contributions from the peasantry. With the weakening of the state sector in the 1990s, private enterprises have been required to shoulder a part of the burden, too. All these areas of total expenditure are bracketed under the heading 'social expenditure'. For most of the period covered in Table 16, they have comprised approximately 70 per cent of the grand total. It is only in the 1990s that this share has declined slightly. Within it, rural enterprises have always been the major contributors of funds, followed by urban state enterprises and – with a noticeable gap – by collective or private units.[69]

In the past, budget allocations covered the smaller part of the costs incurred. However, in most years their growth far outpaced the average increase of all government expenditure. Spectacularly high growth rates were registered at the outset of the third birth-planning campaign between 1971 and 1973, at the start of the one-child campaign in 1979 to 1980, with its intensification in 1983 to 1985, and again with the large-scale expansion of rural birth-control work in 1990 to 1992. But for many years, increases in birth-planning appropriations have trailed behind budgetary growth in other categories. Furthermore, over the years inflation has eaten into the budget. During the last two plan periods, the average rates of increase for birth-planning appropriations of 13 per cent (1986–90) and 19 per cent (1991–95) have to be balanced with average annual inflation rates of 10 per cent and 12 per cent for both periods, respectively.[70]

In 1963 birth-planning allocations amounted to just 0.05 per cent of all state expenditure. In the seventies this level quadrupled, in the late 1980s it increased to 0.39 per cent – still an extremely tight budget for this wide and complicated policy arena. Even the substantial budget increases ever since raised this share to just 0.45 per cent in 1998.[71] Complaints about the lack of financial support have been a consistent element in all discussions on how to improve birth planning. As the allocations of central government are obviously insufficient, the main responsibilities have been shifted to the lower levels. In this way, central government contributes only 10 per cent to 15 per cent of all birth-planning appropriations. Until 1973 the central government did not accept any financial obligations at all. Although specialized personnel at national level are currently paid by central contributions, administrative cadres in birth-planning work are paid out of the ordinary budget. The contributions of central government are further used for subsidizing provincial projects; more than 70 per cent of funds are earmarked for minority regions and poor areas of Central and West China. Subsidies to regional birth-planning budgets made up 24 per cent of the centre's expenditure in 1998. Money from the centre is also used to supply contraceptives free of charge (69 per cent of the centre's expenditures in 1998). Insistence on payment for contraceptives would further reduce their acceptance, but the sums from Beijing do not even suffice to include administrative costs and expenses for the distribution of contraceptives. These items have to be shouldered by the provinces.[72]

The regional differences in per capita appropriations for birth planning, the dramatic increase of financial resources since 1965 and the new push for raising the budget since 1990 are shown in Table 17. The fact that the majority of

Table 17 Birth-planning budget allocations per capita by provinces 1965–94 (yuan per total population, 1989–90 only regional budget without central allocations)

	1965	1972	1978	1989	1990	1992	1994
Beijing	0.10	0.37	0.24	1.06	2.50		2.78
Tianjin	0.08	0.20	0.52	1.25	1.78	1.97	
Hebei	0.06	0.54	0.66	1.01	1.07	1.29	1.96
Shanxi	0.04	0.37	0.57	0.95			2.17
Inner Mongolia	0.05	0.35	0.52	1.24	1.28	1.73	
Liaoning	0.05	0.36	0.62	0.99	0.98	1.50	1.85
Jilin	0.06	0.34	0.62	1.07		1.57	2.20
Heilongjiang	0.08	0.31	0.58	1.04	1.15		2.00
Shanghai	0.12	0.22	0.25	0.72	0.99	1.59	1.97
Jiangsu	0.05	0.29	0.48	0.55	0.64	1.05	
Zhejiang	0.04	0.34	0.55	1.40	1.67	2.01	2.89
Anhui	0.02	0.21	0.51	0.60		1.11	1.38
Fujian	0.05	0.28	0.72	1.07	1.62		3.48
Jiangxi	0.01	0.13	0.67	0.69	1.19		
Shandong	0.06	0.34	0.71	0.74			
Henan	0.02	0.25	0.63	0.67			
Hubei	0.03	0.33	0.53	0.82	0.70	1.01	
Hunan	0.02	0.28	0.57	0.84	1.00		
Guangdong	0.04	0.28	0.57	1.46			
Guangxi	0.02	0.16	0.33	0.76		1.85	3.60
Hainan				1.12	1.42		3.95
Sichuan	0.02	0.22	0.64	0.76	0.93	1.33	1.80
Guizhou	0.01	0.11	0.57	1.33	1.43		1.50
Yunnan	0.02	0.11	0.44	1.17			
Tibet				0.25			0.13
Shaanxi	0.05	0.28	0.67	1.13	1.58		2.56
Gansu	0.02	0.33	0.75	0.92			2.05
Qinghai	0.02	0.22	0.40	1.08			
Ningxia	0.02	0.38	0.33	1.19		2.41	2.79
Xinjiang	0.01	0.05	0.21	0.83		1.82	
China	0.04	0.28	0.58	0.99	1.22	1.65	1.87

Sources: For 1965–78: Peng Xizhe 1991, 32–33, 39; 1989–94 according to provincial reports in ZJSN 1987–; ZJSQ 1997, passim. Own calculation for Tibet 1994 based on population total in ZRTN 1995 and budget figure in RY, No.1/1996, 42.

resource allocations are decided at the province and county level clearly contributes to the different degree of birth-planning implementation at local level. The figures for 1965 document a clear gradation from highly urbanized provinces in the East to the large agrarian hinterland and the minority regions in the West. This mirrors the persisting urban bias of the second birth-planning campaign and the exemption of minorities from fertility control. Interpretation of the figures for the later period has to take note of the fact that above-average expenses are recorded for affluent regions such as Tianjin as well as for backward areas with high fertility levels such as Guizhou province. However, there is no longer a coherent pattern, since the wealthy Shanghai municipality paid below-average sums, while the poor Ningxia region exceeded them. Figures for Tibet are puzzling. For 1994, they placed the region in the customary lowest position of the ranking list. The difference in the 1989 figure remains unexplained. Reflecting these anomalies, regressions of provincial budget figures on a number of socio-economic variables thus do not yield significant results. Neither funding in proportion to social product, nor differential allocation according to perceived need can be detected. This latter principle is applied only in the distribution of central subsidies. Moreover, without analysing demand, cost structures and usage of funds, the data do not seem to be sufficiently valid. They simply document once again the wide range of birth-control implementation at regional level.

The item of birth-planning expenditure does not include expenses for national research projects and large-scale state investments related to birth control. These are budgeted as two separate items, and in 1996 amounted to 14 million and 380 million yuan, respectively. In the 1980s, investments for buildings and technical appliances usually involved a cost-share between the provinces and central government on an approximate 80:20 basis. Only key projects such as the establishment of county birth-planning stations have drawn larger investments from central government. Until 1989, it contributed under 7 per cent of the construction costs for new buildings of birth-planning institutions throughout the country. This share was substantially raised for the eighth five-year plan for the period 1991 to 1995, when the State Planning Commission set apart some 72 million yuan for the construction of new rural birth-planning stations. From these funds, each new station was to receive 0.1 million yuan. A further 0.1 million yuan of construction funds were to come from the provincial planning commissions, while a third amount of 0.1 million yuan for medical and technical appliances was assigned to various central and regional budgets. All other expenses for the newly built birth-planning stations had to be borne by the counties themselves. Conditions for stations at town and township level are even tighter. In the ninth five-year plan central government contributions to large-scale investments for birth planning seem to have declined again. In 1996 they amounted to 60 million yuan, under 16 per cent of the total. Again, the lion's share of 320 million yuan had to be shouldered by local governments.[73]

Funding contributions of provincial administrations, prefectures or municipal regions vary. Responsibility for various items is laid down in regulations from 1983 and in the resolutions of a conference on birth-planning finances in 1991. Generally, the counties have to shoulder the main liabilities of birth planning, since the majority of expenses are encountered here. This pertains to costs for sterilizations, IUD insertions, abortions and related medical treatment, expenses for transportation, food, and subsidies paid for leave of work due to contraceptive surgery, as well as to bonuses for part-time personnel, wages and training costs for grass-roots cadres. Urban birth-planning commissions have to bear the burden of paying for contraceptive operations and one-child bonuses for non-employed or self-employed persons. In the case of urban workers and staff in state, collective or private work units, such items have to be shouldered either by public health schemes or private employers. In rural areas, however, contraceptive surgery is paid out of the birth-planning budget. In principle, one-child bonuses or insurance fees should be settled out of the remaining collective income of rural communities. This creates problems if annual per capita figures remain below the level of bonus or insurance payments.[74]

Table 18 summarizes the few available figures on the structure of state expenditure.[75] The free supply of contraceptives listed in the table is mainly borne by central government allocations. Its percentage of total expenditure has shrunk considerably due to the massive investment in birth-planning stations, the shift to selling more sophisticated contraceptive devices, and the growing stress on long-term contraception by way of IUD insertions and sterilizations. Contraceptive operations and abortions, wages for grass-roots cadres and running costs are paid locally; they make up the lion's share of expenditure. Another main item are the newly established birth-planning stations at county, town and township level, which are largely financed by the lower levels, too. The one-child bonus is not listed in the table of state budget expenditure as it is largely paid out of the welfare funds of enterprises or communities. Subsidies for those practising birth control only enter the budget in cases where they are paid by the birth-planning commissions. Similarly, wage costs for cadres at county level and above are kept artificially low, because they are partly paid out of the general administrative budget.

For many years, remuneration for grass-roots personnel stayed outside of budget allocations. Before some limited state support was introduced in the early 1990s, it had to be entirely settled through the resources of people's communes, towns, townships, urban street committees and enterprises. As long as the funds of state enterprises and large collectives in the cities can be tapped, this may be a working proposition, but, as always, the real problems arise in the countryside, where, even today, the vow of the state to contribute at least half of the expenses for medical personnel is often not realized. A 1997 survey of birth-planning stations in townships and towns of seven provinces highlighted the fact that 80 per cent of the units concerned had not received the promised state subsidy.[76]

Table 18 Birth-planning budget allocations by expenditure items 1980–96 (% of central and regional budget allocations)

	All China				Jiangsu
	1980	*1981*	*1994*	*1996*	*1992*
Free contraceptives and devices	16	14	8	2	9
Free contraceptive operations and abortions	45	34		8	23
Wages for grassroots cadres	14	18		16	11
Insurance payments for single children				4	7
Expenditures for birth-planning stations				22	17
Cadre training				8	2
Research	1	2			
Subsidies for persons practicing birth control				6	
Other running expenses	23	32		34	30

Sources: Sun Muhan 1987, 273; ZJSN 1993, 1995, 1997; ZJSQ 1997, 1024

For administrative personnel at grass-roots level the situation is worse. Combined with the constant calls to improve enforcement and raise the number of grass-roots cadres, this creates a vicious circle. Typically, townships with the lowest level of birth-control compliance face the most stringent demands for expanding organization. Yet high birth numbers there are often connected with economic poverty and geographic isolation, cultural tradition-alism and weak government. Requiring such areas to foot the bill for steep rises in birth-planning expenses creates heavy burdens. Ultimately, it boils down to raising fees and contributions from peasants, who are asked to pay people who threaten them with unpopular policies and severe punishments. Severe strains in the relationship between cadres and populace result from such circum-stances.[77]

In view of such problems, a conference on birth-planning finances convened in November 1991 voted against increasing local contributions to the township or collective. In order to meet the widespread criticism of fleecing peasants with ever-increasing fees, it resolved to limit such charges to a maximum of 5 per cent of household income. However, the conference decided to allow townships to spend existing fees for birth-planning purposes.[78] In Tibet, where finances are particularly tight, even urban state enterprises, institutions and departments charged with birth planning have to rely on funding sources such as student enrolment fees, budgets for reading materials or running expenses. But the difficulties are widespread in other parts of the country, too. As of 1994, only half of all Chinese townships and towns were capable of settling their birth-planning expenses within the normal budget.[79]

The situation can be alleviated by recourse to birth-control fines, which constitute extra-budgetary income and are to be spent exclusively for birth planning. A rough calculation on the basis of the few figures available results in an annual total of 2.3 to 2.5 billion yuan of penalty payments. This surpasses budgetary appropriations for most years, but in 1996 extra income from birth-control fines declined steeply, worsening the problems of financing contra-ceptive surgery.[80]

Shock campaigns with ensuing sterilizations on a mass scale or other disproportionally high expenses can further aggravate the financial situation and run the birth-planning commissions into debt. Greenhalgh documented a number of pertinent cases in her investigations of Shaanxi villages. During 1983 to 1986 the number of sterilizations there massively increased, so that the birth-planning commissions owed a large debt to the health departments managing the local hospitals.[81] As testified by an accumulated debt nationwide of more than 2 billion yuan for contraceptive surgery during 1991 to 1995, this has continued to be a major problem. Under such conditions, it is possible that more persons are mobilized for surgery than can be borne by the funds available. Consequently, peasants either have to pay for such operations themselves, or the number of operations is markedly decreased. This seems to be one reason for the drop in contraceptive surgery and the cancellation of about a quarter of planned operations in recent years.[82] Moreover, rising outlays and wage claims have led to constant haggling about the charges for contraceptive operations.

The central authorities have found it necessary to issue repeated reminders of the instruction that such operations should be performed at standard cost prices.

The permanent lack of funds has also led to a general preference of IUDs and abortions over the more expensive female sterilizations. While standard costs in 1981 amounted to 1 yuan for IUD insertion and 6.50 yuan for abortion, they rose to 20 yuan for tubal ligation. Even a late abortion rated at only 13 yuan. Similar cost structures were reported for county hospitals in 1984, and from a 1987 list of Hubei tariffs that was circulated as a model to other provinces. Low figures for condom usage are likewise related to high costs. Official estimates for 1985 budgeted an annual 6 yuan for users of condoms, compared with 3 yuan for users of suppositories and oral contraceptives. In the 1990s, calculation of costs has become more refined by including wages, building expenditures and other overheads, as well as spending for pre- and post-operative check-ups or treatment of side-effects, in the bill. This factor, plus the general increase of prices, raised the 1993 calculations to an average 328 yuan for tubal ligations (plus about 7 yuan for annual check-ups), 230 yuan for implants (plus about 11 yuan for annual check-ups), 219 yuan for vasectomies (plus about 4 yuan for annual check-ups), 190 yuan for IUD insertions (plus about 10 yuan for annual check-ups); expenses for oral contraceptives and condoms amounted to approximately 18 and 55 yuan per year, respectively. Average expenses for a couple practising contraception were reckoned as 58 yuan.[83]

Seeking additional financial resources, economizing on expenditures and devising incentive structures for better cost-effectiveness have therefore been the main subjects for leadership deliberation. It is against the background of such problems of public funding that private financing for higher-quality contraceptives and various forms of responsibility systems with contracting for predefined items have been introduced since the mid-1980s. In the early 1990s, payment of expenses or deductions from budgetary items became linked to plan fulfilment. Financial mechanisms were introduced that favour long-term contraceptive surgery over abortions. In addition, lower-level birth-planning stations have been given the right to earn additional income by providing other medical services and selling higher-quality contraceptives.

The fiscal reforms of 1994 do not seem to have changed the basic dilemma of a mandated programme without sufficient funding. Although by 1998 central government had succeeded in pressuring nearly 75 per cent of all townships and towns to establish guaranteed items for birth-planning expenditure through their own fund-raising, and legal obligations for funding have been written into many newly revised birth-planning regulations, public deficits at county level and below remain large. Muddling through and makeshift solutions, unpaid services for 'voluntary' mass organizations and constant searching for income-generating schemes therefore continue at the grass-roots level. Although the latest birth-planning regulations explicitly require all governments from province to township level to establish a birth-planning item in the regular budget, a possible future transition from state-financed to privately paid contraception is appearing on the horizon.[84]

8 Planning and evaluation

8.1 The planning process

Since 1971, population targets have been incorporated into the five-year plan and the annual plans. In the following years the practice was widened to include population plans for all lower-levels units from the provinces to the counties. This ushered in a veritable mass movement for drawing up local population plans in 1972 and 1973. However, as no reliable population data were available at the time, the plans were strong on ideological propaganda and political mobilization but largely devoid of precise targets and concrete projections. At most, they could employ approximate figures for births and natural increase and some numbers for contraceptive supplies.[1] The increasing complexities of the one-child policy, the census of 1982 and the renewed emphasis on scientific planning quickly made the earlier procedures obsolete. They were replaced by a new concept of state-controlled fertility decline that all too clearly betrayed its design by engineers working within a framework of a command economy.

When the inventors of the one-child policy laid down the goals for Chinese birth planning in 1983, they also furnished a blueprint for plan formulation and the political prerequisites connected with it. Song Jian and his co-authors expressed the opinion that China was the only country in the world that had succeeded in establishing a model of organized demographic transition resting on two main pillars: a universal social consensus on the necessity of fertility reduction, and the government's power to enforce decisions for the well-being of the nation. The authors therefore concluded that population growth could be checked in the same way as mortality and migration during the past decades. It was to rely on a number of plan indicators, prescribing a fixed limit of children for each Chinese family. Furthermore, the propagators of the one-child policy outlined the following mechanism for population control:

> A large-system model can also be established to register, project, control, and administer China's population. This large system may be broken into vertical and horizontal structures. ... The central control layer directly administers, co-ordinates, and controls the provincial centers. Population statistics are collected from all the provinces. The data are analyzed, projections are made, programs are designed, and population policies are

formulated. In the meantime the center co-ordinates activities among the provincial centers. Information may be interchanged between provinces. Similar relations exist between provincial and county centers. Technically, this large system can be operated by means of computer and communication network, so that data can be collected, exchanged, stored, and treated.[2]

This concept of a large-scale model controlled from above has also guided the design of the planning process, which has undergone numerous changes over the years. Since the early 1990s it has become linked with schemes for regular cadre evaluations, incentives for plan adherence and sanctions for failure to do so. The following procedures evolved in the 1980s, with modifications laid down in Provisional Rules for the Formulation of Population Plans dating from 1992 and 1993.[3]

At the highest level, the State Planning Commission has been responsible for integrating demographic and economic planning. On the basis of guidelines from the Politburo, it has fixed the overall population target for the year 2000, which in recent years has been augmented by target figures for 2010 and projections for the period up to 2050. In its calculations, the Planning Commission emphasizes the balancing of labour force developments and fixed-asset growth. This is designed to secure full employment and to prevent the creation of a large-scale excess of labour. In addition, the Planning Commission also tries to harmonize population development and the production of consumer goods, in order to balance supply and demand and to secure a continuous raising of living standards. The third macro-relationship stressed is the proportion of urban and rural population. Here, the supreme goal is to facilitate a sufficient supply of labour for urban industries, while checks on migration are to promote a rise in labour productivity. Finally, the Planning Commission also strives for a balanced age and sex structure, with a minimum dependency ratio and maximum savings and investment potentials.[4]

Problems already arise in this early phase of population planning, for while it is relatively easy to use present age structures for calculating future labour supply, it is much more complicated to project future labour demand. Such projections have to involve assumptions about future economic development, taking domestic and international constraints, technological advances, wage standards and competitive advantages into account. Since there are many unknown factors in this picture, harmonizing population and labour force development has continued to be superficial. The situation with regard to planning for health, education and social services is similar.[5]

In practice, plan targets for the five-year plans have been calculated by the Birth-Planning Commission, which forwarded them to the Planning Commission for final control and promulgation. Since 1991, formulation of the national population plan has been completely vested in the Birth-Planning Commission, with promulgation made contingent on a final check by the State Council and a vote by the People's Congress. At provincial level, though, the planning commissions keep their prerogative of plan balancing.[6] As calculation requires projection of both likely and desirable population developments, and figures have to be harmonized with supplementary plans for birth-control implementation, this process starts well in advance of the new plan period and usually takes one year to complete. The time required is longer if new census or survey results necessitate adjustments of the original numbers. Annual plans are derived from the five-year plan on the basis of mid-term targets and a continuous assessment of marriage figures, policy changes, social and economic transformations. While they are very precise for the present and coming year, margins grow successively wider for the following period. This leads to a system of consistently shifting plan formulation.[7]

Absolute target numbers for the population at the end of the plan period used to be set only at national and provincial level. On the assumption of stable mortality levels, they served as the basis for deriving rates for natural increase and births. In recent years, these have been specified in absolute numbers too. Furthermore, per capita grain production has been added as another planning target for all administrative units from the counties up to national level. Augmenting these crude figures, total fertility rates are used for projections at the national, provincial and prefectural level. By estimating the hypothetical number of children born in the reproductive age of women, this indicator may be split into component age groups and treated as a variable for calculating birth numbers. Because total fertility is a standardized value, it is suitable for interregional comparisons and linkages between and macro- and micro-analyses. At the same time, however, it is hard to calculate, since, as a synthetic construct, it requires sufficiently large populations, plus rather detailed census and survey data. Alternatively, Chinese projections have employed parity progression ratios, which indicate the probability that women with a given number of children give birth to yet another child. Such indicators require even more refined data. Different scenarios are employed to estimate the consequences of a varying number of children per woman. The projections are used to derive a number of second children within given quotas. Finally, a margin for births out of plan is added.

A similar relationship is expressed by the birth-planning rate, which indicates the percentage of authorized births within the total number of live births during the current year. Because birth-planning regulations vary in different parts of the country, and conditional permits for second and higher-order births are granted, the rate does not indicate the degree to which the one-child ideal is realized. In small administrative units it also tends to be biased by changes in population structure. While the upper-level organs prefer larger margins to obtain sufficiently reliable plans, lower authorities often insist on birth-planning rates of 98 or 99 per cent. These are utterly unrealistic assumptions that lead to many false data and effect the reliability of the birth-planning rate.

Below the national level, provinces, prefectures (or municipal regions), cities and counties constitute the second to fourth planning levels. Differences in population structure here are much larger than on the higher planes of aggregation. In particular, this applies to percentages of women of reproductive age, the shares of minority nationals, as well as the averages for marriage age and fertility. The political, organizational and financial capacity for birth planning is different, too. Many cities and counties therefore use percentages for first, second, and higher-order births to complement the indicators mentioned above. They are also requested to take their economic circumstances, especially labour market conditions, into consideration. This applies also to the in-migration of young peasants with high fertility levels, which presents knotty problems. City plans are often confused when it comes to distinguishing birth-planning indicators for *de facto* and *de jure* population. Because of the widely differing local conditions, target rates for natural increase at this level are no longer uniform.

At the grass-roots level of townships, towns or urban street committees, only target figures for the number of births and absolute population totals at the year end are set. These are augmented by birth-planning rates and percentages of deliveries by birth order. Target numbers for births are calculated in the following way. The grass-roots organizations collect figures for the number of marriages between April the previous year and March the current year, which are then used for deriving a potential number of first births during the review period. The number of married women without a child may be checked by recourse to registration data from the local police districts. Furthermore, the grass-roots organizations keep track of married women who hold a second-child permit. These data are calculated for reports to the upper level on the potential number of births and the quota required. The county birth-planning bureau then uses these figures to calculate projected birth and birth-planning rates. After squaring them with the planned target numbers, a total number of authorized births is transmitted to the townships. In the final phase, the townships draw up name lists of women with authorized births, which are finally handed out and publicized in the villages.

The time required for these steps varies locally, but the following rhythm seems to be prevalent. Townships start to tabulate new marriages and the number of women eligible for second-child permits in January. The numbers reach the county bureaux one month later, after which they are balanced and revised by the provincial birth-planning commissions in March and April. The State Birth-Planning Commission in Beijing then collects the provincial reports, which serve as the basis for further revisions and the drafting of the next birth plan. This is followed by a phase in which the provinces are given the opportunity to plead special reasons for yet another round of revisions. The final birth plans for provinces, prefectures, cities and counties are transmitted between January and March of the following year. After counties and townships have matched their numbers once again, the birth plans are publicized by the rural townships and urban street committees in March or April. It is on the basis of these plans that pregnancies with dates of delivery in the following year are authorized.[8] Target numbers are not always restrictive. Although the authorities urge planning on the basis of local investigations on the spot, in many cases the targets seem to be based only on extrapolation of present birth rates. Because this can result in higher birth quotas than are commensurate with the regulations, such procedures may even stimulate fertility.[9]

Over the years, the influence and control exercised by the centre seems to have varied. Since the population data available in the late 1970s were very patchy, the first population plans from Beijing employed only approximate standard values for natural increase and birth rate. Until the late 1980s, the centre limited itself to stipulating five-year plans and a long-range plan for 2000, leaving the drafting of annual plans and the handling of second-child permissions to the provinces.[10] On the controversial question whether planned population targets should be treated as fixed limits or flexible guidelines, their interpretation of figures as a relaxed form of indicative planning prevailed. Since the early 1990s elements of centralism have become stronger. This is indicated by the demand that lower levels should report projections on expected birth numbers to their superiors by the middle of the year. It also appears that the centre has become involved in deriving annual targets from the five-year plan. Plan adjustments are allowed only after obtaining proper authorization, and units that do not respect their population plans are asked to submit a report on the reasons, together with a proposal for remedial measures.[11]

During the 1980s, there have also been a number of procedural changes at the lower levels with rather different effects on the distribution of planning rights. In the early period from 1979 to 1982, for instance, counties received the annual birth quota in absolute numbers. This rigid form of planning was discarded after 1982 but revived with the Provisional Regulations on Population Planning in February 1991. In the intervening period, birth planning at county level worked by calculating birth-planning rates and birth-order percentages. Districts within the county have always received different birth quotas. Practices for the townships and villages have vacillated between uniform and diversified planning.[12]

Moreover, the widely differing conditions within China and the varying organizational capacities have produced divergent practices as far as the density of planning indicators is concerned. The average figure for 1992 amounted to eight or nine indicators employed at provincial level. The highest number was in Fujian, which used twenty-four different indicators. At the opposite end of the spectrum, Hainan and Guangxi used only three. The most widely employed measure was the birth-planning rate. Nearly as popular were the birth rate and the percentage of third- and higher-order births among all current deliveries. Only a quarter to one-third of the provinces used absolute numbers for births, for natural increase or for the population total. In the early 1990s such absolute numbers have been made compulsory at all planning levels, thereby curtailing their margins of action.[13]

In addition to demographic indicators, a number of provinces also set planning targets for the number of sterilizations after the second child. While this practice has not yet extended to all regions, supplementary plans for cadre recruitment and training, medical operations, production, distribution and use of contraceptives, propaganda work, fine collection and budgetary development are universal.[14] Target rates for late marriages and late births are also employed. Conversely, the rate of one-child certificates, which was popular in the early 1980s, has decreased in importance. This has been caused by its changing definition, its sensitivity to age structure, and by the fact that one-child certificates can be handed back after obtaining a second-child permit.[15] Under such conditions, the usefulness of this indicator for assessing programme performance and projecting future population trends is limited.

8.2 Statistical controls

Birth-planning statistics function as the counterpart of planning. It is their objective to produce a realistic picture of demographic developments in the various regions of the country and to provide the leadership with the necessary information for decisions on population policy. At the same time, however, the statistical figures are used to evaluate the performance of the very same bureaucracy that collects them. This has produced foreseeable conflicts and impaired data quality. The leadership has reacted by controlling controllers but has registered only limited success.

At the basis of most statistical data are report forms regularly transmitted to upper levels. In the 1950s such special forms for birth-control figures were non-existent. Regular information was restricted to the birth numbers hailing from the household registration system that had been established between 1951 and 1958. Built on the model of antecedents from the republican era and centuries of coercive household registration during the imperial period, it meshed police and census work and curtailed the freedom of movement. In its practical application, it also reintroduced collective liabilities for the reporting of vital events. When more determined efforts for birth planning started in the 1960s, additional information was passed upwards only erratically. Intermittent reports from the grass-roots level were limited to exemplary cases, birth numbers, plus a few figures on contraceptive use; only Shanghai supplied better data. In the 1970s this situation did not change much. The only exceptions were production figures for birth-control devices and numbers provided by the health system, which since 1971 also files annual reports on contraceptive operations and abortions in its subordinate clinics and health stations. To these are added birth and vaccination records.[16] No reliable information was available from the census or from sample surveys, since the political class indulged in savouring political models and fabricated figures from largely pre-selected 'typical examples'. The patchy data therefore did not permit any coherent evaluation relying on time series and structured reference data.

Regularized report forms for birth planning were first introduced in 1981, when the newly established Birth-Planning Commission began to set up its own statistical apparatus. At that time, these forms comprised two sheets with eleven indicators on fertility and contraception, respectively.[17] After revisions in 1984 and 1987 the report forms contained columns for the following indicators: (1) absolute numbers for present population, births and deaths, as well as birth rates, death rates, and natural increase derived from them; (2) target numbers for the annual plan and the five-year plan; (3) fertility indicators such as the total number of married women of reproductive age, the number of births within and outside plan, the birth-planning rate in percentage form, and deliveries by birth orders; (4) data on new marriages, the total number of married women, the number of first marriages and late marriages, as well as rates derived from them; (5) figures on contraceptive measures, specifying planned measures, actual performance and different methods; (6) the number of one-child certificates in absolute terms and as a rate. The provinces acquired the right to collect additional data, which they, for instance, employ for breakdowns of births by nationality status.[18] The most recent ordinances on birth-planning statistics hail from 1989 and specify four report sheets: (1) providing information on births and deaths with altogether fifteen indicators; (2) providing five indicators on one-child certificates and the first marriages of women; (3) providing fourteen indicators on contraceptive use; (4) providing four items on age-specific fertility.[19]

Since the 1980s all grass-roots organizations such as villages, neighbourhood committees and industrial enterprises file cards of women of reproductive age. These cards list the name, birthday, work unit, occupation and educational level of the women, the contraceptive measures taken by them, the number and dates of pregnancies, abortions, live and stillbirths, information on the issuing of one-child certificates, as well as marriage dates, the name of the spouse and his work unit. The data are aggregated by townships, towns or urban street committees and then condensed into statistical reports of the counties or city districts. Counties or city districts transmit their numbers to the birth-planning commissions of cities, prefectures or municipal regions on a monthly basis. These administrative units then aggregate the numbers for monthly reports to the provincial birth-planning commission, which in turn files half-yearly reports to the State Birth-Planning Commission in Beijing. Altogether, there are six successive steps in aggregating numbers to higher-level figures.[20]

This procedure has its inherent difficulties. Although counties can easily compare the planned and actual numbers of births, which are transmitted by the reports in absolute terms, higher-level units have often faced rates permitting no direct comparison of plan targets and programme performance. Random checks are made twice a year to verify the number of birth permits, pregnant women and women taking contraceptive measures. They are also used to investigate unreported births from past years if there is suspicion of large-scale data falsification. In recent years, unannounced controls by provincial investigation teams have increased. Anonymous informants are a further instrument used to combat manipulation at the grass-roots level. But it is not only intentional falsification that is affecting data quality. The under-reporting of births is also often connected with the disorganization of statistical offices, high migrant numbers, or a lack of birth registration in collective households. Other recurrent flaws are wrong dates due to use of the lunar calendar or infant deaths registered as stillbirths.

Since double-checking within the same bureaucracy proved unsatisfactory, the Statistical Bureau was charged with an annual sample survey on population dynamics starting in 1982. This stratified sample survey covers 1.3 million cases or 0.1 per cent of the population. It is organized at provincial level, where it serves as an instrument for checking the numbers hailing from the household registers or the statistical system of the birth-planning commissions. In 1991, a systematic comparison of numbers highlighted the fact that the birth-planning statistics under-reported the number of births by a margin of 18 per cent. The discrepancies in Hebei, Hunan, Guangxi, Guizhou and Yunnan, Qinghai, Ningxia and Xinjiang were disproportionally high. Guangxi must have been a particularly striking case, since this region was the only one whose leadership was forced to deliver a written self-criticism in 1991. The situation in other years was worse. In 1992, China's leading statistician, who was transferred from the university campus to become Vice-Chairman of the Birth-Planning Commission, still reckoned with an average under-reporting of 30 per cent, rising locally to 50 per cent. A year later, this continued to be the margin in unannounced investigations of Hebei and Hubei villages. Check-ups conducted in the rural areas of Gansu and Hainan provinces during 1995 resulted in the startling figures of 30 per cent and 75 per cent under-reported or unauthorized births, respectively. And on the eve of the fifth census of November 2000, a county in the Sichuan basin with a 1990 population of nearly 1.4 million discovered that more than 0.4 million unreported births between 1991 and 1998 had to be added to this figure.[21]

Even greater deviations were discovered in the course of the 1988 national fertility survey. This large-scale investigation discovered a nationwide under-registration of births by more than 30 per cent if results were compared with the regular birth-planning reports. In two provinces, the number surpassed 40 per cent. A comparison of the 1997 national birth total, when obtained from the birth-planning reports and from the annual sample survey, documents that the discrepancy between both systems has grown to more than 45 per cent.[22] The national fertility surveys of 1982, 1988 and 1992 have worked with a sample of 1 per thousand to 2 per thousand of the population. Together with the census and micro-census, they serve as the main instrument for data validation. Although they gained recognition for their high standards of internal consistency in the 1980s, data quality seems to have fallen in recent years. The reliability of the last national fertility survey in 1992 is sharply contested since, data from that survey resulted in a total fertility rate for 1991 which may be 30 per cent too low.[23] This occurred despite repeated prior admonitions that 'no unit or individual is permitted to change survey numbers at will, to strike at staff for truthful reporting to upper levels, or to settle accounts with truthful respondents after the survey has passed'.[24]

Not surprisingly, the frequent differences between numbers reported by the birth-planning commissions and figures from the Statistical Bureau have created friction between the two bureaucracies. In 1987, the Birth-Planning Commission set up a second information system in order to augment the regular report numbers and to deflect criticism of its defective data. The second information system consisted of a permanently rotating sample survey in sixty prefectures or municipal regions of the country, a number equal to 20 per cent of the administrative units at this level. Because of a lack of funds, this system could not be extended further. In the late 1990s it seems to have been replaced by the practice of conducting two provincial check-ups with unannounced visits to rural households each year. The political consequences of such systems started to show up in 1990, when Shandong province rewarded seventeen local committees for respecting the birth plans, while publicly criticizing eleven and degrading four of them. Under-reporting of births had again reached up to 30 per cent. Eight years later, random checks in rural areas of Shanxi produced even more startling results. The discovery that nearly 20 per cent of all marriages were entered by young women under the legal marriage age and that almost 60 per cent of all births were unauthorized prompted sanctions with personal approval by Premier Zhu Rongji.[25]

Such consequences of truthful reporting turn obstruction and manipulation into the crux of all surveys. The centre thus faces a permanent conflict of goals. If it desires honest reports, the direct comparison of planned and actual numbers and the accountability of cadres have to be ruled out. Conversely, if it emphasizes strict adherence to birth plans, data must be suitable for direct comparisons, and cadres must accept responsibility. However, experience shows that data quality slips in such cases. Because these mechanisms are well known, the last two fertility surveys of the Birth-Planning Commission purposefully adopted a standard time not suitable for direct comparisons with reported birth numbers.[26]

Slightly better than the defective data from the birth-planning commissions are the birth numbers as reported by the household registration system. The registers are kept by the police stations existing at the street committee, town or township level and operating under the Ministry of Public Security. Figures are aggregated and transmitted to the Ministry in four steps via urban district or rural county, city and provincial departments. Before the onset of annual sample surveys in 1982, this was the only regular and nationwide source for birth numbers. However, it has always suffered from the problem of incompleteness. For the years between the first census in 1953 and the second in 1964, the undercount has been calculated as 38 per cent of all deaths and 16 per cent of all births. For the years between 1964 and the third census in 1982 these figures shrank to 16 per cent and 9 per cent, respectively,[27] but once again the one-child policy reversed the trend. Between 1987 and 1988 under-reporting of births in the registers amounted to a national average of nearly 17 per cent. A comparison of the 1989 household data with birth numbers adjusted by use of census results produces an undercount of 25 per cent for the whole of China. After the last census such a comparison was also undertaken in Ji'nan city, the provincial capital of Shandong. This resulted in 25 per cent of all births being under-reported by the birth-planning reports and 13 per cent under-reported by the household registers. In some rural counties subordinate to the city these figures rose to 52 per cent and 44 per cent, respectively.[28] In the following decade, the quality of registration data has remained problematic. The 1996 Chinese population total as shown by the household registers is 25 million (= 2 per cent) less than the total reached by the annual sample survey of the population.[29] The main reasons for this deviation are under-registration of births and deaths and incomplete records due to migration.

Birth numbers hailing from the annual sample surveys of the Statistical Bureau equally are not immune from undercounts. In line with its duties, the

Statistical Bureau emphasizes objectivity, the gathering of data in anonymous form, and the renunciation of penalties for births that show up in the survey but were not reported before. Nevertheless, all parties realize that spectacularly high numbers of above-quota births cause a tightening of birth planning later on. Broken promises of confidentiality, such as occurred in Anhui after the last census, have also hindered honest reporting. This creates a permanent incentive to manipulate the selection of survey points and to include more positive than negative cases. A rare documentation of this bias is available from the materials of the 1992 fertility survey, which clearly show an over-representation of sample units with above-average standards of birth-planning performance. This survey has also been blamed for under-reporting due to the off-putting wording of the questionnaire and reliance on local grass-roots cadres.[30] The annual sample survey of the Statistical Bureau has under-reported births by approximately 11 per cent during the last intercensal period between 1982 and 1990. Recent surveys necessitate a further upward revision of past figures. A closer look at critical age groups and provincial results reveals many inconsistencies. Discrepancies between survey figures and other demographic evidence have been such that a major check-up in 1989 also involved the Central Disciplinary Commission and the Ministry of Supervision. Since then, the Bureau has been reprimanding lower units for concealment of data in an unending number of instances. In 1995, one of its cadres publicly uttered this sentiment:

> Some people say: 'Birth planning is the Hardship Number One Under Heaven.' But after their experience with population surveys in recent years, population statisticians have acquired a still newer common understanding: 'The hardship of hardships are population surveys.'[31]

The best data should be contained in the national population counts which are staged every ten years, and the 1 per cent micro-census of the population which is held at mid-point of the intercensal period. Both serve as regular checks on the annual sample and report figures. Comparing the population counts with micro-censuses permits internal data verification by the calculation of survival rates for cohorts enumerated previously. As mortality takes it toll, such computations would ordinarily result in survival rates of less than 100 per cent. In fact, however, since the 1980s there have always been more than 100 per cent survivors for persons aged 0–2 at the time of the preceding count. Excess amounts to about 5 per cent in the 1987 micro-census, as compared with the 1982 census, and 7 per cent in the 1990 census, as compared with the 1987 micro-census. In the micro-census of 1995, it increases to approximately 13 per cent for persons born between 1988 and 1990. Even more irritating, present cohorts of persons born in the period 1979 to 1987 are also in excess of the respective age groups enumerated in the 1990 census.

The biased infant mortality rates, the ever more distorted sex ratios of births and discrepancies with the annual population surveys from later years similarly point to the need for an upward adjustment of the 1990 birth rate. This must be interpreted as births eluding even the large-scale population counts with their meticulous planning and preparation. Once again, it demonstrates the continuous downsliding of data quality in reaction to the tightening of policy.[32] The same conclusion may be reached for the fertility rates resulting from the last micro-census in 1995. Despite constant appeals for truthful reporting, it resulted in an extremely low current fertility rate, which the State Statistical Bureau finds necessary to adjust upwards by nearly 30 per cent. In a reversal of the customary division of roles, the Birth-Planning Commission has opted for an even larger adjustment by nearly 40 per cent.[33]

Summing up these glimpses of schemes for obtaining regular demographic information in China, an extremely complicated system of birth statistics emerges that is characterized by overlapping jurisdictions, double work and data confusion. There are five different administrations collecting fertility numbers by seven different methods. The Ministry of Public Security with its subordinate police districts continues to run the household registers which contain numbers for births and deaths. These numbers suffer not only from the problems discussed above. Because mobility has been rising incessantly over the past decade, registers have consequently become riddled with faults. Nevertheless, during an intercensal period, these and the birth-planning figures are usually the only population data available for territorial units below the province level.

Even more defective are the numbers hailing from the Birth-Planning Commission. For all purposes, the Commission has had to admit defeat of its regular statistical reporting system. However, the system continues to be maintained, because discarding it would impair accountability and evaluation of birth-control performance even more. The glaring flaws of the report system are the reason why the Birth-Planning Commission set up its systems for unannounced check-ups and the harsh controls referred to above.

The assessment of fertility levels also requires numbers on marriage patterns. Here, data from the Birth-Planning Commission compete with data from the Ministry of Civil Administration, which is responsible for marriage registration and keeps its own records. Data for infant mortality are collected by the Ministry of Health, which also tabulates the number of births, vaccinations, contraceptive operations and abortions. These data again do not conform to similar data from the other bureaucracies.[34]

The Statistical Bureau with its annual sample survey of population dynamics has become the main source of current figures on demographic trends at the provincial and national level. Yet even these data have been shown to suffer from under-reporting of births and have been repeatedly adjusted. Finally, there are the attempts at a complete population count, which serve as benchmarks for evaluating annual registration and sample figures yet are defective in themselves. While becoming ever more refined, fertility data from China have also become ever more muddled.

8.3 Other information systems

The administration has to make decisions on population policy on the basis of unreliable and contradictory information from statistical reports. This is why a number of other internal controls have been introduced. The regular cadre evaluations with their standardized sheets for checking performance are among them and have already been discussed above.[35] Another instrument is an internal communication network, which is designed to furnish the leadership with implementation reports, accounts of popular attitudes and information on political incidents, as well as analyses of current trends and new problems in birth control.

In 1987, all lower echelons from the provinces to the villages were asked to appoint correspondents responsible for regularly sending special accounts in addition to the routine statistics and work reports. Two years earlier, a vice-minister of the Birth-Planning Commission had already recommended some topics of interest to the centre: information on problems and complaints concerning contraceptive surgery; family size preferences of new social groups such as migrants, rich peasants, rural workers in village and township enterprises; and popular reaction to birth-control policies. Further topics of interest are recommended by the State Birth-Planning Commission in regular 'Outlines for Current Information Requirements'. Reports received are then edited by its General Office and transmitted to leadership organs in a system of finely graded information privileges. While some classified reports are restricted to the Central Committee, the State Council and the Standing Committee of the People's Congress, another class of documents also circulates to the National Committee of the Political Consultative Conference (the highest organ of the united front), to ministries and central departments, provincial Party committees, the birth-planning groups of the Army and of the armed police forces. Directives issued in 1990 and 1993 prescribed a monthly minimum of two reports from the provinces and one from the sub-provincial units, with copies of lower-level reports being directly forwarded to Beijing. Information on political incidents is to be passed on immediately.[36]

The effectiveness of this system depends on the truthful and regular reporting of lower units – a delicate matter, since honesty can entail reprimands and punishment. Under such circumstances, reports are always in danger of internalizing a professional optimism, rehashing political slogans and becoming self-congratulatory. The accounts of provincial birth-planning efforts submitted for official compendiums such as the yearbooks of the Birth-Planning Commission or the *Encyclopaedia of Chinese Birth Planning* convey a taste of such formalized reporting with little critical content. It is indicative of the situation that lower levels have been constantly reminded to fulfil the minimum requirement of one or two reports per month, that an excess of non-specific, generalized reports and the evasion of sensitive topics is bemoaned, and that bonuses are used for encouraging reluctant correspondents.

Such incentives do not have to be applied to complaints and petitions from the population, which constitute yet another means of retrieving information from the grass-roots level. They are collected, archived and processed by a special section of the Birth-Planning Commission's General Office, which then edits and issues regular excerpts for the benefit of the leadership. As with the petition sections in other bureaucracies, the General Office also keeps a monthly statistical report on the number of complaints received. This helps to gauge popular acceptance or refusal of present measures and may instigate policy changes. An example is the extremely high number of complaints in 1983, which seems to have contributed to the relaxation of birth control a year later.[37] The petition sections of the birth-planning commissions can thus provide an input for policy formulation. However, as in the case of statistical information, work reports and communication from correspondents, it is an input vulnerable to distortion, as representativeness, trustworthiness, selection and editing of complaints are hard to judge. Moreover, use of information is largely left to the discretion of cadres, and popular demands not in line with policy can be easily stifled. Procedures are particularly vulnerable to power relations within the bureaucracy, and the willingness of subordinate cadres in the complaints sections to become embroiled in cases against leadership personnel.[38]

Planning and evaluation are therefore far removed from the idealized visions held by the propagators of birth planning. In contrast to their assumptions on the internal integrity of the system, there neither exists the supposed consensus on policy, nor a sufficient governmental capacity, nor a smooth flow of information. While the political leadership is flooded with a host of contradictory statistics, as many as four public periodicals and six internal tabloids from the Birth-Planning Commission, plus innumerable materials from other specialized government institutions and academic institutes, ensure that reliability and validity of information is always in doubt.

This is why many compromises and inconsistencies characterize the birth-planning procedures, which cannot be adequately subsumed under the great rubrics 'centralized' or 'decentralized'. Elements of centralism may be detected in the population limits for the country as a whole and for the provinces, which are set by the State Planning Commission and the State Birth-Planning Commission. Centralism is also implied by the periodical rulings of the Central Committee Secretariat on the global percentage of second-child permits and by the calculations of the average number of children per woman. If upper levels decree target numbers in absolute terms, or if they employ a battery of more than twenty birth-planning indicators, the leeway for lower units is severely limited.

But these strong interventions from above are countered by other factors. For once, the practice of upper organs to reckon with low birth-planning rates results in more flexibility for the subordinate bureaucracy. Although upper limits for population numbers are fixed, it is largely left to the discretion of the lower levels how these targets are met. In practice, second-child permits are decided by the provinces with a great diversity of procedures. The system of transmitting different target rates to the cities and counties also takes account of the existing differences within China. Population plans are even more relaxed if they operate with only a few target numbers, which are interpreted as guidelines only. All these different aspects have been coexisting for some years. They have had to struggle with the problem of defective statistics and distorted reports and been subject to a permanent process of procedural change. Generalizing on the process of birth planning is therefore perfunctory. Like many other features of China, it has to be understood as a 'system' *sui generis*.

Part IV
Popular response

9 Gender roles, family size and sex preferences

The discussion so far has analysed policy goals and implementation problems, focusing on the perspective from above. It has touched more than once on difficulties of enforcement. The picture, however, would be biased and highly incomplete if the perspective from below were not be taken into consideration. In the final analysis, only this view from below can explain why birth planning has not been a complete success.

There is no better starting point for discussing the discrepancies of both perspectives than an investigation of family size preferences. Unfortunately, many studies from China on family size preferences are rather limited; they either contain overt generalizations or unsatisfactory survey results. In most cases sample sizes are small, and case distribution uneven; randomization of interviewees has often not entered the survey design, and questionnaires are sometimes full of questions inviting conformity to prescribed norms. Because of different survey designs and varying territorial coverage, numbers are therefore not strictly comparable. Only the 1997 survey on population and reproductive health and the two rounds of the in-depth fertility survey in 1985 and 1987, whose results from nine provinces are presented in the upper part of Table 19, managed to interview larger and more representative samples of women. Most other survey results introduced in Table 19, though, are from small, localized studies and have to be treated with some degree of caution. An obvious case are the Beijing soldiers interviewed in 1980. The fact that 90 per cent of them opted for only one child, probably reflects more military drill than personal opinion. The 1983–85 results from Jiangsu, which show 45 per cent of the interviewed peasants indicating a preference for one-child families, similarly strain credulity. They most likely mirror the strong normative pressures emanating from the propagation of one-child families in that province with its strict fertility policies, its heavy concentration of collectively owned rural enterprises, and the ensuing clout in blocking promotion for violators of birth control.

The province-level figures for both rural and urban regions show that, on the whole, childlessness has not developed into a viable alternative lifestyle as yet. Only in highly urbanized areas does this group of the population slowly gather strength. Over the last years, China's cities have seen the appearance of childless woman teachers, academics and secretaries as the harbingers of new gender roles and a Western way of life. Recent surveys indicate a marked rise in the number of well-to-do urbanites preferring to remain single. If the results of a 1995 Beijing survey of women born after 1960 prove trustworthy, the adherents of such a lifestyle will have significantly expanded in the 1990s. A Harbin survey staged a year later showed that they made up 17 per cent among the age group 20–29, dropping to 10 per cent and under for older respondents. In the same vein, percentages for a one-child preference in the cities and highly urbanized regions such as Beijing, Shanghai and Liaoning are invariably higher than in the countryside, but rural women, too, display higher one-child preferences in the younger age groups with a linear decrease for older cohorts. Panel studies are needed to determine whether this indicates a lasting change of attitudes among the younger generation or gives way to the more traditional preferences on reaching later stages of life.

More interesting than preferences for single households or one-child families are the percentages of families with two, three or more children. Whoever indicated such a preference documented his open disagreement with the Party line. Generally, Table 19 documents the expected fact that urbanites prefer smaller family sizes than do peasants. In particular, the percentages of three-child families or even larger family sizes are very low. The dependency of urban employees on the state in matters of work, housing and social security, the political pressures resulting from such circumstances, as well as rising demands for consumer goods, higher educational levels, new patterns of living and the prevalence of women in work all favour small urban family sizes.[1]

Nevertheless, observing such developments may lead to a disregard of proportions. In the mid-1980s most urban surveys recorded more than two-thirds of respondents with a preference for two children. Outside the big cities, an absolute majority of one-child women between the ages of 30 to 39 continued to hold on to the idea of bearing a second child. Even for women aged 40 to 49 such percentages ranged up to 40 per cent. This documents the low degree to which the one-child norm is internalized. If surveys investigated women's lifestyle ideals more fully, they would most probably still result in a majority predilection for traditional family arrangements, with a husband in work and a wife staying at home to care for the children. Survey results differ depending on the formulation of questions. Generally they document a high verbal consent to the Party's one-child policy, an already lower degree of satisfaction with the present one-child family status, a prevailing will to have another child, if policy permits, and nearly 70 per cent of respondents viewing the two-child family as the ideal. It remains to be seen if the drop in such figures shown in some recent surveys proves to be representative. Although the 1997 survey for the whole of China seems to indicate a move towards smaller family sizes, it may also be read as a continuing majority vote for a two-child policy.[2]

The rejection of one-child norms in rural areas is even clearer. The variations in average numbers reflect an urban–rural gap that, instead of

Table 19 Surveys on family-size preferences 1980–97

Year	Region	Number of children wanted (% checked)					Average	Sample size
		0	1	2	3	4+		
Rural and urban areas								
1985	Hebei	0	4	53	25	18	2.6	5080
1985	Shanghai	0	25	69	5	1	1.8	4143
1985	Shaanxi	0	3	51	27	19	2.7	4084
1987	Beijing	1	41	52	4	2	1.7	5157
1987	Liaoning	0	31	57	7	4	1.9	4477
1987	Shandong	0	15	65	14	6	2.1	3900
1987	Guangdong	0	3	36	31	25	2.9	4293
1987	Guizhou	0	4	32	27	37	3.1	2958
1987	Gansu	0	6	41	29	25	2.8	2562
1997	China		29	59			1.8	12305
Rural or suburban areas								
1980	Beijing	2	24	73	2		1.8	206
1983			9	77	9	5	2.1	480
1985	Tianjin		5	80	15		2.1	549
1990		0	3	49	14	34	2.5	
1992	Liaoning	1	34	63	2	2	1.6	
1985	Jilin		16	78	4	2	1.9	5405
1990	Heilongjiang		11	65	5			
1981	Shanghai		20	56	20	4	2.1	1509
1984			5	50	36	9	2.5	648
1983–85	Jiangsu		45	55			1.6	2693
1991							1.8-2.3	1100
1991							1.8	
1983	Zhejiang		5	51	17	27	2.7	460
1983	Anhui		3	81	14	3	2.1	490
1992			4	56	28	9	2.4	420
1983	Shandong		28	72			1.7	141
1989			15	79	2	4	2.0	100
1989			5	65	25	5	2.3	100
1991	Henan						2.0	
1981	Hubei		5	51	28	15		
1984	Hunan		2	78	17	3	2.2	2576
1991							2.3	
1982	Guangdong		7	90	3		2.0	148
1980	Sichuan	1	23	73	3			135
1984			16	81	3		1.9	839
1991–92		1	30	69	3			3825
1985	Shaanxi		22	74	4		1.8	
1997	China		25	62				9610
Urban areas								
1980	Beijing	6	58	36	1		1.3	1071
1983		3	25	70	2		1.7	370
1992			21	55				457
1995		28	43	25				2162

Year	Region	Number of children wanted (% checked)					Average	Sample size
		0	1	2	3	4+		
1994	Tianjin	7	66	27				100
1992	Shenyang		38	49				400
1996	Harbin	12	63	25	.		1.3	2785
1985	Shanghai	1	30	60	8	2	1.8	861
1990			44	64	.			
1983	Jiangsu	2	47	52			1.5	240
1984	Zhejiang	12	62	27			1.2	1079
1986	Hefei		65	20	1			
1984	Wuhan		33	67			1.7	510
1988	Hubei		20	77	4			1293
1984	Sichuan		25	70	5		1.8	822
1997	China		42	52				2695
Special groups								
1980	Beijing soldiers		90	10			1.1	12109
1992	Liaoning peasants		39	57	1	3		
	Liaoning peasant-workers		32	68				
	Liaoning peasant-retailers		40	54	2	2		
	Liaoning urban peasants		56	22				
1982	Fujian fishermen		1	12	47	41	3.2	282
1991–92	Sichuan peasants		25	65	3			
	Sichuan peasant-workers		35	51	1			
1984	Guizhou minorities			7	19	74	3.9	850
1990	Dalian migrants			52	33	15		231
1993–94	Peasant migrants, 6 provinces	2	34	58	6	1	1.7	1125

Sources: Zhang Ziyi *et al.* 1982; Li Xian 1985; Guo Shenyang 1985; Zhong Sheng 1986; State Statistical Bureau 1986, Vol. 1, 93; Whyte and Gu 1987; State Statistical Bureau 1989, Vol. 1, 160–161; Lu Li 1990; Feng Xiaotian 1991; Kua shiji de zhongguo renkou: Tianjin juan, 122; Kua shiji de zhongguo renkou: Heilongjiang juan, 172; Huang Runlong 1994; *Xinhua*, 23 January 1995; *Zhongguo funü bao*, 3 March 1995; Wei Jinsheng and Wang Shengling 1996, 297–346; Peng Xizhe and Dai Xingyi 1996; Wang Jianmin and Hu Qi 1996; Milwertz 1997, 69; ZRN 1997, 257; Zhongguo weilai renkou fazhan yu shengyu zhengce ketizu 2000; www.cpirc.org.cn/e-view1.htm

narrowing, may have actually widened over the years. With the exception of areas within the reach of major cities, and a few provinces with particularly strict policies, under 25 per cent of peasant respondents desire a one-child family. Only provinces with very strict rural birth-control policies such as Liaoning, Jiangsu, Shandong or Sichuan show higher shares. Remarkably enough, the group of provinces with very low percentages of a one-child preference does not only include backward areas such as Hebei, Guizhou, Shaanxi or Gansu but also rich and modernized Guangdong province on the

South China coast. Whereas the two-child family draws most of the votes in the rural areas of the country, up to a quarter of rural respondents continue to opt for three children. Moreover, percentages of those wanting four children or more are anything but negligible; besides readily expected cases such as Anhui, Hubei and Hunan they even involve the rural hinterland of Tianjin and Shanghai. As the available data only reflect the situation after 1979, it may be speculated that preferences for a larger number of children were higher during earlier decades.

Not all surveys offer a breakdown of the desired children by gender, but if such a breakdown is provided, it immediately produces the expected son preference. Controlling figures for place of residence brings out another urban–rural gap: in some regions a majority of urban respondents indicate no sex preference for the first child. In Shanghai and Beijing this is particularly marked. Sex preferences in the countryside are unequivocal, though. About two-thirds of the respondents there would prefer a son if they are forced to respect the one-child norm. Together with the fact of rural residence, the sex of the first child is thus the most important predictor for assessing the likelihood of having another child. Educational level does not lead to significant differences in this regard. If the first child is a girl, nearly 90 per cent of the peasants wanting another child aspire to a boy. After two girls this share climbs to almost 100 per cent. This strong preference for sons can lead to many children, even among couples declaring agreement with the one-child norm. For if a son is not born in the first instance, he must be produced at the second, third or more attempt. Women who give birth to one or two girls have a particularly difficult time sticking to the official norms, since they suffer from considerable social discrimination.[3]

Despite the unsatisfactory data, all surveys indicate that the preference for two children in most cases implies the wish to have one son and one daughter. The percentage of respondents preferring such a constellation always amounts to a very large majority. The same tendency shows up in adoption practices and in retrospective data on the likelihood of women having yet another birth. It is higher for women with a number of sons but no daughter than for mothers who have both sons and daughters. This can be taken as the expression of traditional gender role expectations, which require energetic efforts from sons in raising family fortunes, while they expect daughters to be obedient, sympathetic and helpful at home. If people are asked for the preferred gender distribution in three-child families or even larger households, the well-known bias for sons emerges again.[4] The national fertility survey of 1982 also related the strong sex preference to contraceptive prevalence and the holding of one-child certificates. The children of couples holding such a certificate were predominantly male; contraceptive rates among families with a son were markedly higher than for the parents of one daughter, while in abortion rates the opposite situation prevailed. The sex ratio of new-born children, which mirrors the number of new-born boys in proportion to new-born girls, diminished with the number of children.[5]

More differentiated data specified by various social groups are hard to obtain, but the few available figures included in Table 19 point to the fact that the birth-planning norms have good reasons to make concessions to national minorities[6] or groups with raised manpower needs such as fishermen, miners and peasants in mountainous areas. The record for preferences of peasants in non-agricultural pursuits seems to be mixed. Survey figures from Liaoning show the surprising result that the percentage of rural peasant workers embracing the one-child ideal was even lower than among peasants working the fields only. Peasant peddlers working mainly in trade and service jobs showed less inclination to have a second child than villagers in small-scale industries. Very high percentages of peasant migrant workers working in the Northeastern port city of Dalian inclined towards the ideal of having two, three or more children. Liaoning peasants living in suburban areas with urban household registration, however, showed the least preference for two children – an expected result, since they are subject to much stricter fertility restrictions than villagers elsewhere.

But the Liaoning figures do not need to be representative. The 1993/94 survey on peasant migrants produced clearly lower shares for respondents desiring more than one child. By including villages and urban areas in six provinces, this survey aimed at greater representativeness. Nevertheless, it still remained small and did not rely on random design. The results must therefore be treated as extended local case studies. The same applies to a Sichuan survey staged two years earlier, where peasant workers in village and township enterprises clearly showed smaller family-size preferences than peasants mainly working in agriculture. This is also the conclusion of most general discussions and descriptive studies, which add that most peasants who are engaged in commercial activities opt for more children. The picture of a rural society in transition without sufficiently clear changes in family-size preferences is further complicated by the question of whether employment opportunities outside agriculture are controlled privately or collectively. For while state or collective enterprises can exclude violators of policy from hiring, private companies often demonstrate a bias in favour of employing relatives. This would tend to serve as an incentive for bearing children. The markedly higher consumer and income orientation of private entrepreneurs, plus the technical and legal difficulties for migrant workers wanting to raise more children, are standard assertions for opposing this line of reasoning. Few materials are to hand for checking the validity of either argument.

Information on the motivational structure at large varies too, but its general thrust is less ambiguous than the surveys on preferred family sizes. A more extensive 1992 survey on family economics and fertility in the rural and urban areas of ten provinces, which asked for the main motive for childbearing and did not permit multiple checking, resulted in an average 22 per cent of all respondents answering with the perpetuation of family line; 21 per cent chose the desire for old-age support, 18 per cent wanted primarily to increase labour power, 17 per cent checked risk minimization and handing down heirloom, 12 per cent regarded protection against disorder as their main reason, and only 9 per cent considered this to be the spiritual enjoyment of having a child. The rural–urban divide showed up in similar tendencies as in the figures discussed below.[7]

Table 20 summarizes the results of a survey of 1100 men and women living in an urbanized rural county in a remote corner of Hubei which boasts a huge hydropower-station. These people were asked to associate children with specific advantages and disadvantages. Again, this is a limited sample in a distinct regional environment; moreover, its method of allowing multiple checking makes the results incompatible with more recent studies. Nevertheless, it has the benefit of listing both advantages and disadvantages and offers quite a large choice of items. Its tendencies fit well with other investigations on the motives for family-size preferences in China.[8]

Some of the items listed in the survey may differ considerably in other regions. The desire for more labour power, for instance, varies with the economic situation and the man-land-ratio of villages. As demonstrated in Table 20, old-age security often takes pride of place among peasant motives for preferring sons or a larger number of children. Given the fact that in the mid-1980s less than 5 per cent of peasants above age 60 relied mainly on some form of pension, while more than 50 per cent received most of their income from continued work, and 38 per cent were mainly dependent on support from children, this is perfectly understandable. Even greater is the number of old peasants still actively working. In the census of 1990 this amounted to 89 per cent of the agricultural population above age 65. In this respect, peasants differ markedly from urban citizens, the majority of whom retire and are entitled to

Table 20 Advantages and disadvantages of more children: survey from Danjiang County, Hubei, 1986 (% checked, multiple checking permitted)

	Rural	Urban
Advantages		
Economic support in old age	82	43
Continuity of family line	58	33
To increase labor force	48	21
To add power to kin group	22	11
To add to spouse bond	28	54
For enjoyment of parents	28	89
Disadvantages		
Financial cost	78	64
Fatigue	56	69
Less time for spouse	8	9
Health hazards	30	42
Problems in neighborhood	8	17
Concern for children's future	70	9
Concern for overpopulation	24	52

Source: Whyte and Gu 1987, 484

old-age pensions. In the mid-1980s this was the main income source for more than 70 per cent of city dwellers above age 60; conversely, income from continuing work and support from children rated at only 11 per cent and 15 per cent, respectively.[9]

Many urban families in China have already reached a moderate standard of living with a consecutive rise of expenses for educational and recreational activities. Although city children continue to contribute to the living expenses of their retired parents, the principle of separate book-keeping becomes more and more dominant. Conditions in the countryside are different, though, where average household expenses are still overwhelmingly dominated by basic needs such as food, clothing and housing, with only limited structural changes in favour of other interests. Rural households mostly operate on a common budget, and children, in particular sons in work, directly contribute to family income. After decollectivization and the decline of collective revenue, this trend has increased still further. When children raise the allotment of land, they contribute to household income once more. Again, this strengthens gender-specific discrimination as out-marrying girls may reduce family landholdings. Even young women who stay in their native village and enter one of the highly propagated uxorilocal marriages do not usually receive land allotments and income shares from village enterprises.[10] Finally, the help of children is indispensable when elderly peasants fall ill and cannot afford medical treatment because there is no health insurance. These factors are either non-existent or of secondary importance in urban settings, where private and emotional motivations for having a child play a much larger role.

It is also not surprising that the wish to continue the family line or to add power to the kin group is much more potent in rural than in urban settings. Cultural traditionalism here correlates closely with the economic and social motives for having children. One of the best Chinese studies on peasant fertility culture, which is based on a recent comparative survey of villages in three widely differing regions, tried in vain to establish a clear pattern of correlations between the desired number of children and a long list of individual socio-economic attributes. Most statistics produced only hazy results, and local differences were far more important than individual choice. The sole constant factor was preference for sons and the urge to continue the family line. In high-fertility areas more than 70 per cent of all female respondents perceived this as their main responsibility in life; families without sons were considered to be 'finished', 'ruined', or 'unfit for human life'. The motive of family line continuation was reinforced in those rural areas where the erecting of clan temples and the compilation of pedigrees has been revived over the past decade. Some case studies have also shown that the desire to add power to the kin group is dependent on the clan composition of villages, the degree of clan feuding and local insecurity. Closed rural communities with clannish structures, a large pool of excess labour, few employment alternatives outside agriculture and a consequent problem of juvenile hooliganism seem to be particularly affected by feelings of insecurity.[11]

The fact that peasants rate child-raising costs higher than urban households seems rather to reflect their hard-nosed attitude towards having offspring than the actual expense. In addition, because village children are far less pampered than in urban areas, fatigue does not play the same important role as it does in the cities. The very few checks in Table 20 for children having the disadvantage of leaving spouses with less time for each other once again demonstrate how far Chinese ideas of marriage life are removed from the ideals and patterns of behaviour in Western marriages. Finally, the table also demonstrates the rural–urban gap in regard to concern for the children's future. This has to do with the economic hardships of many peasant families. Whyte and Gu also explained it with high expectations of the children's future. According to their data, the majority of peasants aspired to a university education for their offspring with subsequent employment in industry – in most cases a rather unrealistic assumption.[12]

All investigations into family size preferences have tried to establish a link to income and educational levels. They have highlighted the expected fact that women with more years of schooling tend to prefer a smaller number of children than those with less education. However, although the importance of the educational factor for gender roles and family size preferences clearly emerges, the connection to population economics remains problematic. It has been demonstrated that child-raising costs in urban areas surpass those in the villages by a margin of 4:1. Comparing rural towns with villages, this margin shrinks to 3:1 or 2:1.[13] It is also shown that the general excess of labour on the urban job market implies a decisive role of quality over quantity in job searching. This raises childrearing costs in the cities, where old-age pensions paid by the work units further lower the utility of offspring. The same rules apply in the villages, where higher developed counties or non-agricultural enterprises feature higher demands for educational levels with consequently higher costs of childrearing. With regard to the labour participation of children and youth, interesting comparative figures are available from both a wealthy and a poor county in Shandong province. While in the wealthy county only 3 per cent of all youth in the age groups 13 to 17 regularly joined in the main earning activities of the family, in the poor area this share rose to 5 per cent of 13-year olds, 22 per cent of 14-year olds, 25 per cent of 15-year olds, 40 per cent of 16-year olds and 50 per cent of 17 year-olds.[14]

Such figures suggest that rising costs and lowered utility of children also diminish the desired family size. But the surveys available from China so far confirm this basic assumption of Western theories of population economics only to a limited degree. Confirming a general increase of costs over the years, they result in a clearly negative balance of childrearing expenses and revenues for the cities. Urban families aspiring to a higher education for their offspring have come to face prohibitively high costs. In the rural regions, however, the balance is blurred. In some regions it has also turned negative with costs incurred by children exceeding their utility, while in others it stays positive. The 1992 nationwide survey on family economics and fertility resulted in a slightly negative balance for the rural areas if direct childrearing expenses, opportunity costs and income contributions from children were taken into account. The balance turned positive once the utility of children for old-age support and other ends factored in the calculations. Under these circumstances, clear preferences for a small number of children are indicated only by families living above a certain income level.[15]

Most surveys thus result in only weak negative correlations between family-size preferences and income levels. A situation is sometimes met where both the poor and rich prefer higher numbers of children and only the middle group indicates a preference for reduced family size.[16] The Party has reacted to this state of affairs with a correction of its own propaganda line. After long internal controversies it revoked the advertising of rich peasants with hard-working sons. Veteran cadres and conservative politicians such as Chen Yun and Bo Yibo had already protested against this promotion campaign in 1982.[17]

Circumstantial evidence points to the rule that fertility levels are declining beyond a critical margin of income only. An investigation conducted in rural areas of Liaoning province in 1989 to define this critical threshold showed that only rich peasant families with an annual per-capita income of more than 1000 yuan voluntarily renounced a second-child permit. These were rural households which predominantly believed in their ability to manage old-age support themselves. Half of them owned a washing machine or radio, and one-third possessed a colour television and refrigerator, respectively. More than half of these rich peasant households shared the opinion that children would lower standards of living. Did this indicate propitious developments for the policies of the Party? Probably not, for the few rich peasants who voluntarily renounced a second child comprised only 0.8 per cent of rural one-child families in that area.[18]

Five years earlier, a survey conducted in the rich Shanghai region did not produce even this ray of hope. It recorded a slightly negative correlation of incomes and family size preferences only in the urban districts of Shanghai. In the rural areas, however, the correlation was strongly positive: the higher the income, the larger the number of desired children. The correlation between family-size preferences and educational attainment was equally weak. Only academics displayed a clearly reduced desire for children.[19]

Studying the evidence leads to the following conclusion. Family-size preferences have clearly dropped, if they are compared to fertility decisions prior to the 1970s. In this sense, the propagation of birth control has been a success. Reducing the number of children further beyond the already low level of the 1970s remains a major problem, however. The Party has good reasons to doubt the spontaneous decline of birth numbers in the wake of economic growth. Investigations dating from 1992 confirm that family-size preferences of most parents continue to remain at an average level of two children.[20] The strong bias in favour of sons can easily turn this into a real average of more than two births. Once again these are strong indications that until now rural birth planning in China predominantly relies on administrative control rather than on spontaneous changes due to socioeconomic developments. Only in the cities does the balance seem to be different.

As far as gender roles are concerned, the situation is highly ambivalent, too. For while the arrival and continuing increase of young women with different family values and lifestyle preferences can be clearly documented, the one-child policy has made the burden of traditional sex preferences for the majority of women even more onerous. Although this is predominantly a rural phenomenon, further analysis of sex-specific birth figures shows that even in the cities the evidence for fundamental changes is not as clear-cut as it may look at first sight.[21]

10 Strategies and evidences of non-compliance

Propaganda in favour of one-child families has not succeeded in changing the basic contradiction between numbers and sex of children desired in private life and in state policies. At least in the rural areas of China, with the vast majority of the population, a massive conflict between state and family interest persists. Whereas in most parts of the world this antagonism would erupt in violent clashes, in China it mostly leads to passive resistance and cunning strategies of non-compliance. Many birth-planning norms and a host of circulars from the Birth-Planning Commission, various ministries and the Supreme Court contain a list of contextual acts punishable under criminal or administrative law. It may be surmised that they are sufficiently widespread to justify their specific inclusion in the regulations. Indicating that opposition against the one-child policy remains a major problem, recent regulations show a tendency to enlarge this list.[1] In this sense, Chinese administrative documents also hint at the kind of non-conformist behaviour met in social life. Further information is provided by case reports in the Chinese press that illustrate the conduct penalized in the regulations.[2] Finally, statistical data on births outside plan provide a chance to gauge the overall extent of non-compliance.

Bracketing the various acts of non-compliance under broad categories results in the following picture. There seems to exist widespread sabotage of contraceptive measures by spouses or third parties, the latter most likely being the parents of a couple. Guangdong, Shanxi and Anhui make such sabotage liable to prosecution. Other provinces include the mistreatment of or discrimination towards women who bear daughters in the list of offences. Husbands who sue for divorce after the birth of a daughter may also be liable. Patchy accounts from the early 1990s suggest that even in suburban areas of big cities such as Tianjin such cases comprise more than 50 per cent of all divorce suits. Husbands, mothers-in-law and other relatives have been reported to beat, scold and maltreat infant girls and their mothers, chasing them away from home to live in chicken coops. Already in the early 1980s violence must have been sufficiently widespread to cause CC Secretary Hu Qiaomu to urge firm action in a letter to the Minister of the Birth-Planning Commission dated November 1982.[3]

Non-compliance with marriage regulations is another sensitive area. Between 1982 and 1992, the number of marriages below the legal age is supposed to have risen from 4.5 to more than 9 million. As traditional Chinese society did not practise any official marriage registration by the state and most women married in their late teens, the idea that one is committing an offence in concluding an early marriage is rather tenuous. But there are also other reasons. The large number of adoptions indicates that in the 1980s early marriages were also entered with the intention to escape birth planning by means of an unregistered union. Early marriages in the villages have also been ascribed to a revival of traditional marriage forms such as non-registered customary unions, child brides or arranged weddings; the decrease of household sizes with an ensuing lack of manpower plays a role, too. Furthermore, the small cohorts of marriageable women from the Great Leap (1959–61) may have forced bachelors to turn to younger brides. Other reasons advanced are rising peasant incomes, making weddings affordable, the weakening of rural grass-roots organization after the introduction of household farming, earlier puberty and the increase of premarital sex in the course of social changes during the reform period. Since most unmarried women are refused access to contraceptives, and childbearing outside wedlock is considered illegal, they have to undergo an abortion if they become pregnant. This is the situation in China's cities, but in the countryside, many youngsters have to marry immediately under such circumstances.[4]

Against this background, most provincial birth-planning regulations and a number of pertinent circulars threaten sanctions for unregistered marriages with resulting early pregnancies. Implementation of this ban in the villages, however, meets problems of jurisdiction. Frequently, the local branch of the Women's Federation limits itself to propaganda work, while offices of the civil administration, the judicial organs or the birth-planning commissions take responsibility only for marriage registration, divorce cases and pregnancies. Many early marriages have therefore been silently condoned due to lack of suers seeking redress. It is only in recent years that regulations have become stricter. The State Council guidelines of September 1992 and the new implementation rules for the marriage law of February 1994 abolished the subsequent recognition of non-registered marriages. Some counties nowadays threaten fines of 500 to 1000 yuan for early marriages even without evidence of a birth.[5]

Nearly all regulations mention resistance to activities of the birth-planning bureaux, rumour-mongering, disturbance of public order, incitement of unrest or physical assaults on cadres. Destroying the personal property of birth-planning personnel and molesting their families are also listed under the acts liable to prosecution. Such passages, and the increasing reports of violence against birth-planning cadres, explain why a special insurance covering accidents and damage to their household effects has been implemented. In the late 1980s, instances of harassment, wounding or even murdering birth-planning personnel spread through many provinces, prompting the Birth-Planning Commission to issue a special report form for fatal incidents. An internal circular issued in June 1987 acknowledged that assaults were frequently provoked by cadre misconduct such as corruption, arbitrariness and coercion in regard to abortions, sterilizations and the administering of penalties. Similar reports have continued throughout the 1990s.[6]

Although incidents of violence and protest are not reported in the official press, there are rare instances when a glimpse of the situation becomes possible. One example is the account of rioting in the Guangdong city of Gaozhou in September 1997, when a rally of about a thousand protesters opposed the arrest of three informants, who had leaked news about the imminent arrival of an inspection team to check contraceptive measures. In addition, the protesters deplored high birth-control fines and the death of a young woman caused by an IUD insertion. The demonstrations led to a clash with police and paramilitary forces, and the protesters were quelled only by a promise of leniency for 'trouble-makers'.[7]

Quieter forms of resistance are evident from application forms. The increasingly complicated conditions for second-child permits require a lot of paperwork to prove eligibility to such special favours. Falsification of documents that have to be presented with applications has increased accordingly. Forgery of medical certificates testifying to chronic ailments of the first child and misreporting of nationality status are particularly popular. Many minority nationals enjoy childbearing preferences, even if they are highly assimilated or hail from mixed marriages with Han-Chinese, which is why declarations of ethnic status invite manipulation. In the past, such ruses were difficult to prove, since arguments relying on family history were hard to check. The new rules for declaration of nationality status promulgated in 1990 have therefore erected high barriers against random changes. Nowadays, it must be clearly shown that one parent holds minority status.

The spread of modern ultrasound B machines for gynaecological check-ups introduced a new era of modern technology. These machines have been manufactured in China since 1979, and a large number were also imported between 1985 and 1989. Today, ultrasound B machines are available in all counties, and they have also been increasingly introduced at township level.[8] The machines were originally intended for monitoring pregnancies and checking IUD insertions, but they are frequently misused for prenatal sex identification with consequent abortion of a female foetus. Since there is no reliable method of sex determination before the fifth month of pregnancy, such abortions are induced rather late. In view of the strong preference for sons, medical personnel are strictly warned to refrain from sex identification.

Since 1986 the Ministry of Health and the Birth-Planning Commission have repeatedly banned the misuse of ultrasound machines. Many birth-planning regulations contain relevant passages that in recent years have increasingly specified penalties. Supplementary regulations to combat corruption and bribery have also been drawn up and are liable to prosecution. Fujian, Shandong and Henan provinces have even passed special laws against sex screening, threatening the revocation of licences for the doctors concerned. For women who illegally abort after sex determination, the laws stipulate delayed birth permits for the first child and none for a second child. A number of other provinces have integrated similar provisions into their birth-planning regulations. The new Law on Population and Birth Planning of December 2001 explicitly prohibits sex screening and threatens hefty penalty sums, too.[9]

Such rules are well intentioned but difficult to enforce. Personal relations, corruption and the manifold ways of non-verbal communication via secret signs make it easy to circumvent the ban. Financial burdens on Chinese hospitals due to massive cut-backs in public funding create further incentives for generating additional income. In addition, the pressures of responsibility schemes have led some grass-roots cadres to conclude that open promotion of sex-specific abortion is the best way to reconcile the demands of the government and the anxieties of the peasantry.[10] An estimate for 1990 put the number of sex-specific abortions at approximately one-third of the abortion total. This share is likely to have risen since.

The birth-planning documents also contain references to illegal midwifery and assistance to pregnant women hiding for childbirth in secret places. This indicates other widespread methods of evasion. If relevant passages in the regulations are accepted as circumstantial evidence, this practice seems to be particularly prevalent in Shanxi, Zhejiang, Anhui, Guangdong and Gansu. Other problems faced by the authorities are changes of residence with no records of out-migration at the place of origin and no registration at the place of destination. In these cases there is a vacuum in jurisdiction which migrants exploit for having unauthorized births. The number of unauthorized births seems to be particularly large in remote areas, in regions straddling the borderline of administrative units with different birth-planning norms, in urban squatter settlements and among boat people. All these areas at the margins of Chinese society afford freedom of movement to the 'birth guerrilla'.[11]

Making unauthorized children available for adoption is another practice that has caught the attention of the authorities. In most cases these are non-registered infant girls born illegitimately. Giving them away for adoption offers the parents a chance to try again for a son after marriage. As childless couples view children, especially sons, as valuable, a black market for illegal trading in children has emerged. This concerns largely backward areas with lax birth control, which have become notorious as 'producers' of adopted children. Some peasants in 'specialized households' have thus developed a new appreciation of their wives who are cherished as a 'little bank', providing high sideline incomes from children sold shortly after delivery. In 1989, prices were said to range from 500 to 3000 yuan, depending on local conditions and the sex of the child. Ten years later these figures had more than doubled.[12] The national fertility survey of 1988 brought out the fact that the number of adoptions rose from 0.159 million in 1980 to 0.562 million in 1987, 75 per cent of whom were infant girls.[13] Cross-checking with figures supplied by the notaries reveals that in 1987 more than 95 per cent of the adoptions were not certified[14] and probably relied only on customary conventions – thus allowing for easy circumvention of birth-planning guidelines.

Against this background, a large number of later birth-planning regulations explicitly prohibited the unauthorized fostering of infants and young children. A new national adoption law of December 1991 with additional implementation rules of April 1994 requires written adoption contracts with additional registration for orphans from welfare institutions or abandoned foundlings. It permits such steps only for childless couples above age 35. Moreover, adopted children have to be either foundlings, orphans, or offspring from parents who can prove particular hardship. In emulation of the one-child policy, only one child may be adopted according to the original regulations. The restrictions may be relaxed for the last two categories; but for abandoned children they had to be strictly applied. This law has turned adoption from a social convention into a legal step and has kept the number of notarized legal adoptions within a range of 20,000 to 30,000 cases per year. Adoptions in disregard of the law's stipulations have been promptly added to the list of penalized acts contained in many birth-planning regulations. Fines have increased to the equivalent of one year's earnings or more. While enforcement of the minimum age for foster-parents seems to have been handled leniently and was lowered to age 30 in 1999, adopted children were treated as unauthorized births if the adoptive parents already had another child. In view of the rising numbers of orphans, this latter rule became highly controversial. It is a positive sign that it was revoked in 1999.[15]

The re-increase of traditional practices of abandonment and infanticide by neglecting, drowning or suffocating new-born children was noted by the Politburo in 1982. They were first listed as a crime in the birth-planning norms of Shanxi, Anhui, Zhejiang, Guangdong and Gansu; indictment has since spread to all other provincial regulations. Conspicuous accumulations of such cases have been reported in 1983 by Chinese newspapers from Liaoning, Anhui and Guangdong. These reports have given rise to widespread accounts on infanticide, which in former times was common in some rural areas of Europe, too. In particular, speculation was fuelled by the abnormal sex ratios of new-born children. As of today, the situation does not seem to be quite as dramatic. The high number of infant girls who are not registered or who are given away for adoption, and the many cases of sex-specific abortions after prenatal ultrasound examinations, seem to explain much of this bias.[16]

However, this does not signify that archaic forms of birth control have vanished. Although survey figures on this subject remain a well-guarded secret and are almost certainly inaccurate, a careful examination of the 1990 census results shows 140,000 or so infant girls born in 1989 who may have died during that year in excess of the normal infant mortality rate. This would have been equal to approximately sixty-five cases per county, or 1.2 per cent of all infant girls born in 1989. The estimate depends on a number of assumptions, and may not be correct; but it gives an idea of the dimensions involved.[17]

Instances of abandoning new-born children have been rising in direct proportion to the intensity of birth-planning campaigns. Generally, abandoned children are left at roadsides, at entrances of public buildings or on the doorsteps of possible foster-parents in the certain knowledge that they will be found. Most cases do not involve first-born daughters, but are girls from families who have already two other daughters and who fear losing the chance of producing a son. It is therefore not surprising that, according to the State Birth-Planning Commission, approximately 98 per cent of abandoned infants in the early 1990s were girls. Abandonment has become sufficiently widespread for Chinese studies to speak of a 'rampant' practice with 'an unbearable burden for orphanages everywhere', and disturbing reports about rising instances of fatal neglect in Chinese welfare institutions have leaked out. Chinese sources for the total number of orphans, including foundlings, range from 140,000 for 1990 to 100,000 in 1995. According to Chinese dimensions, these figures are low. While in 1994 approximately 17,000 of all orphans and abandoned children were taken in by urban orphanages and welfare institutes, the majority continue to be accommodated through private arrangement.[18]

Since all parties involved have vested interests in obscuring the real situation, it is wellnigh impossible to disentangle the jumble of legal and illegal adoption, abandonment, infanticide, sale of children and unregistered births in constant fear of discovery that exists on the dark side of the one-child policy. The continued and probably growing presence of these problems may be gleaned from a document issued by Fujian province in July 1992 and circulated around the country ten months later by order of the central authorities. The circular reiterated that infanticide and abandonment will be prosecuted under criminal law. It threatened conniving midwives with punishment, urged an immediate registration of births, and warned all parents unable to prove the whereabouts of their child that no new birth permits would be granted for at least seven years. If the case in question had been a second birth, a further birth permit would be completely withheld. In a similar way, recent birth-planning regulations from Liaoning and a number of other provinces expressly deny second-child permits to persons who cannot prove the cause of death of their first child.[19] An additional rule introduced by Shaanxi province in 1998 has a similar thrust: it requires immediate reports of infant deaths, and medical certification as to the cause of death.

Private interests coincide with cadre concern if one-child families do not report a second or higher-order birth, and birth-planning cadres refuse such registration for fear of punishment or wage deductions. In the judgement of Chinese experts, this is the most prevalent and hard to tackle act of non-compliance. The extent of undercounts caused by such overlapping interests may be gathered from the fact that unreported births made up one-third of all deliveries on the eve of the last population count in 1990.[20] Records are further falsified when above-quota births are registered as in-migrations, or deaths are not reported, in order to keep up large household sizes and to conceal unauthorized births. In recent years, unreported deaths in rural areas have amounted to up to 12 per cent of all deaths.[21]

With regard to the duties of birth-planning personnel, the administrative documents frequently raise the charge of 'lax work'. The misuse of authority and corruption are also mentioned. Examples include the following: selling or handing out second-child permits in unjustified cases, preferring penalty sums over abortions, and misusing and embezzling funds. Such practices can entail a creeping mutation of birth-control fines, which may become transformed into non-budgetary income from extra-birth fees, stimulating rather than limiting fertility. If local authorities with few regular revenues come to depend on this extra income, contradictions are particularly acute. All birth-planning norms prescribe a proper use of penalty sums, which should be used only for birth-planning purposes. It is a well-known fact, however, that many bureaux use such sums for the construction of housing or office space, for banquets, presents, recreational activities, and other types of consumption. But even regular birth-planning expenses often rely on substantial contributions of fines. Recent birth-planning regulations expressly confirm this. In such instances, rich peasants who are able to afford high fines can effectively finance birth prevention for the less well-to-do.[22]

The regulations deplore abortions, IUD insertions and sterilizations that are reported but have not been performed. Such cases involve both the motives of unauthorized pregnancies as well as the embezzlement of funds. In June 1988, a circular of the Birth-Planning Commission criticized the following practices within the bureaucracy: issuing second-child permits for friends and relations, registering second children as twins, or falsifying statistical reports and medical certificates, among them the documents required for proving disabledness of the first child.[23] Ten years later, the report of a birth-planning cadre from one of the densely settled rural areas of the Sichuan basin contained the following graphic list of twelve prevalent implementation problems and evasion techniques at the end of the 1990s:

1. Young girls move out for work and business elsewhere. They cohabit illegally and give birth to a child that is not recorded in the households books. After returning home, they officially register a marriage, ask for a first-birth permit and give birth to a second child. ... 2. A couple or a whole household moves out for many years without leaving any information. They hide outside and do not return home for a long time, in order to prevent their births from getting registered. ... 3. Place of living and place of household registration are different, so that marriage and birth records are in disorder. ... 4. A birth is neither entered in the household register, nor is it reported in the birth files. ... 5. Laid-off workers and staff have different places of household registration and work, so that it becomes hard to follow up changes in their marriage and birth affairs. ... 6. Annual wages or incomes of laid-off workers are hard to determine, so that fixing penalties for childbearing outside plan becomes difficult. ... 7. Abandoning infants. ... 8. Divorces with earlier birth permits being kept. ... 9. Divorces without actual separation in living and housing. ... 10. Factual unions of women from outside with local men. ... 11. Letting other women step in for gynecological examinations, in order to avoid contraceptive measures and detection. ... 12. Paying some other woman for having an abortion on behalf of oneself, obtaining her abortion certificate and passing the test.[24]

Some of these ploys are pursued against the opposition of cadres, others are practised with their silent consent, but, no matter how grass-roots cadres ultimately feel, they always fear the penalties of the responsibility systems. Check-ups and controls by the upper levels therefore often turn into games of hide-and-seek. A popular ruse are 'explanatory letters' from a middle-level to a lower-level authority, in which the latter is asked for cooperation with an inspection group arriving from the capital. The middle-level organs use these letters to transmit in a perfectly neutral tone the number of births for verification – thus causing the lower levels to produce exactly the same follow-up figures. This method has become modernized in the advanced coastal regions. It then ends up in a race of time between inspection teams arriving without notice and warnings of their approach via portable phones. Generally, there is a tendency of falsification and fraud to grow in proportion to the increasing strictness of birth-planning rules. An example is the case of a township committee accused of printing a booklet with twenty stratagems for handling unwelcome investigations and evaluations.

A final group of cases mentioned in the birth-planning regulations points to criminal acts and other offences in medical treatment. Above all, this involves fake contraceptive operations, abortions and unauthorized IUD removals. Other items in the list are malpractices in contraceptive surgery, already mentioned in a circular of the early 1980s and which, because of the unsatisfactory equipment of township clinics, do not seem to be rare.[25] While all other cases singled out for punishment reflect state interest in birth control exclusively, redress for medical malpractices is the only instance in which individual rights are protected.

Although in most cases no information on the pervasiveness of these various acts against the birth-planning policy has been publicized, Chinese birth-planning materials permit an estimate of the overall extent of the problem. Chart 1 outlines the extent of non-compliance with regulations by comparing birth-planning rates, indicators used for expressing the percentage of planned, authorized births among all childbirths of the running period. The rates take into account changes in plan formulation and locally varying regulations. They are presented in their inverse form as percentages of births outside plan. While these include some first births not authorized within the current year, they exclude second- or higher-order births with an appropriate permit. Most cases of unauthorized births seem to involve couples with only one daughter. According to some Chinese specialists, these make up more than 90 per cent of all births outside plan.[26]

While the report numbers in the chart hail from the regular report forms of the birth-planning commissions, the alternative figures were collected by the national fertility surveys of 1988 and 1992. As the survey for 1992 displayed serious defects in the enumeration of recent births, results for 1991 and 1992 may be too favourable. The chart discloses the dilemma of Chinese population policy in the 1980s. The official reporting system of the birth-planning apparatus recorded a continuously falling degree of non-compliance with birth

Chart 1 Percentage of births outside plan by birth order 1979–99

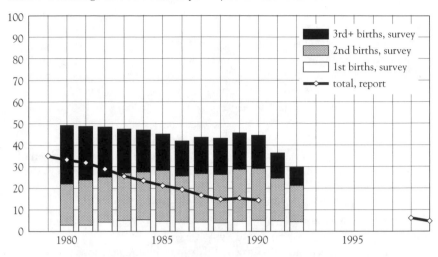

	% all births outside plan, BPC report	% all births outside plan, survey		% 1st births outside plan, survey	% 2nd births outside plan, survey	% 3rd + births outside plan, survey
	34.9					
1980	(33.4)	48.9		2.3	20.1	26.4
	31.9	48.5		3.0	21.0	24.5
	(28.9)	48.2		4.2	21.5	22.5
	25.8	47.3		5.0	22.3	19.9
	(23.7)	46.8		5.3	22.4	19.1
1985	(21.6)	45.0		5.0	23.8	16.2
	(19.5)	42.2		4.2	21.8	16.2
	17.3	43.9		4.6	23.2	16.1
	15.3	43.4		4.2	22.7	16.5
	15.8	46.2		5.3	24.5	16.4
1990	14.9	45.1		5.6	24.0	15.5
		36.9		5.5	19.8	11.6
		30.5		5.1	17.0	8.4
1995						
	6.9					
	5.9					

Note: Figures in parenthesis by linear interpolation

Sources: Report figures from the Birth-Planning Commission (BPC), 1988 and 1992 fertility survey data in: ZJSN 1986–91; Liang Jimin and Chen Shengli 1993, Vol. 3; Jiang Zhenghua 1995; Cai Fang 2000, 4

planning down to a margin of less than 15 per cent in 1990. The national fertility survey of 1988 shattered this belief in the success of the programme, while the 1990 census and the 1992 survey dealt it a final blow. The difference between reported and actual figures for non-authorized births has steadily grown since 1981 and amounted to more than 30 percentage points in 1990. During the period from 1981 to 1990, the percentage of above-quota births has always hovered between 42 and 49 per cent. The extent of the drop thereafter is questionable.

Table 21 with provincial rates for births outside plan pinpoints the regions with the greatest problems of non-compliance. It also helps to assess the extent of data falsification and to reveal the glaring contradictions between population policy and people's aspirations in the 1980s. The gap in the enforcement of regulations is extremely wide. Although the data are defective, they clearly point to those provinces with the greatest enforcement problems. In 1979, these have been Inner Mongolia in the North, Zhejiang, Fujian and Jiangxi in the East, as well as large parts of the hinterland in Central, Southwest and Northwest China. The common denominators of these areas are always a high percentage of rural population, a predominantly low development level and cultural traditionalism. The report numbers from the lagging provinces convey the message that they began to step up enforcement in later years, but the fertility survey squarely contradicts this claim. Even worse, provinces with seemingly stable birth-planning efforts such as Jilin, Shandong and Guangdong are revealed as serious violators of policy as well as falsifiers of reports. In 1988, the greatest margins of under-reporting show up in all these regions. Although the differences between report and survey numbers diminished in 1992, and reported rates for 1997 reached spectacular lows, past experiences and the incongruities of present birth statistics counsel for scepticism. Upward revisions of the 1995 micro-census results averaged more than 20 per cent for the country as a whole; provincial units with adjustments of more than 30 per cent included not only familiar problem areas but also new cases such as Beijing and Hebei, Hainan and Xinjiang.[27]

In 1992, nobody less than the Minister of Birth Planning herself has spoken of the growing 'sophistication' in data concealment and furnished a concise description of cadre psychology:

> The grassroots cadres have a difficult mentality. First of all, they are afraid that nonfulfillment of the birth plan will spoil everything, that they will get punished, demoted, or even dismissed. But then they also fear that honesty does not pay and that realistic figures meet censure. Some of them just take chances. They bet on luck for not getting caught in such a big country with so many townships and villages. And then there is still another type of behavior: if plan targets or demands are transmitted by the upper levels, these are in no way trespassed. These people feel that they make the leadership happy and earn fame by reporting exactly the numbers required.

Table 21 Percentage of births outside plan by provinces 1979–97 (%)

	1979	1981	1988		1992		1997
	Report	Report	Report	Survey	Report	Survey	Report
Beijing	16.0	10.7	4.7	24.5	1.0	11.3	2.2
Tianjin	28.9	16.7	3.2	24.5	2.7	11.3	1.7
Hebei	22.2	28.2	20.9	48.7		19.3	3.3
Shanxi	34.4	36.4	18.2	43.6	13.4	47.3	11.0
Inner Mongolia	48.6	35.1	8.9	39.1	16.7	19.4	1.8
Liaoning	25.6	19.5	1.3	6.6	1.1	2.4	0.3
Jilin	33.0	20.5	5.1	52.4	7.6	29.2	5.9
Heilongjiang	26.5	27.9	10.7	28.6	9.7	8.2	3.0
Shanghai	12.4	6.6	0.6	24.5	0.2	11.3	4.8
Jiangsu	26.6	25.4	13.0	33.0	5.9	16.0	4.9
Zhejiang	40.3	29.1	6.2	33.1		7.4	2.2
Anhui	38.0	30.9	23.9	39.4	29.7	34.4	4.0
Fujian	53.5	41.2	32.3	71.8		52.0	6.9
Jiangxi	46.7	29.1	23.6	55.9		49.1	6.8
Shandong	19.7	23.5	6.5	48.1	18.6	20.1	1.0
Henan	37.4	37.9	16.1	51.0	30.0	35.2	2.1
Hubei	18.0	25.7	15.8	46.3	27.1	40.2	5.6
Hunan	36.8	32.9	26.0	43.8	30.3	22.6	2.9
Guangdong	37.3	34.6	14.8	51.2		36.9	22.1
Guangxi	47.7	42.4	18.1	39.4	43.0	42.7	10.0
Hainan				47.1		47.3	30.7
Sichuan	24.9	30.1	8.7	34.2		20.8	6.2
Guizhou	51.1	47.6	23.7	54.6		48.5	14.4
Yunnan	44.7	47.3	22.6	33.1		27.1	9.0
Tibet				47.1		47.3	1.3
Shaanxi	38.2	34.8	17.0	43.4	12.2	37.2	5.7
Gansu	38.0	39.6	13.8	59.1	25.0	52.5	15.0
Qinghai	72.8	56.5	23.0	47.1	29.7	47.3	13.8
Ningxia	60.3	36.8	15.0	47.1	12.2	47.3	18.8
Xinjiang	29.7	23.6	21.7		13.9		1.9
China	34.9	31.9	15.3	43.4		30.5	

Note: 1988 and 1992 survey figures for Beijing, Tianjin and Shanghai as one average for these three municipal regions; for Hainan, Tibet, Ningxia and Qinghai as one average for these four regions; all data as inverses from birth-planning rates

Sources: report figures for 1979 in Peng Xizhe 1991, 43; for later years in ZJSN 1986–; 1992 fertility survey data for 1988 and 1992 in Jiang Zhenghua 1995

... We have discovered that in some provinces all levels raise plan targets in order to be on the safe side, until at the end a high number results in the villages. If this target number is not fulfilled, only two ways out remain: you either start commandeering, use simple and crude measures, and do not hesitate to employ all means available, or you just falsify the figures. If we pass on a target number to such a person, he just reports it as fulfilled or nearly fulfilled. In this way we have a hard time getting down to reality.[28]

This is the perspective from above, where the state authorities do their best to keep track of the shrewd evaders of birth control. But there is also the perspective from below. In 1988, an internal survey among birth-planning cadres in six provinces produced depressing results: 92 per cent of respondents felt that birth planning was incompatible with the cultural tradition of their area, 63 per cent found the situation of birth planning prevailing at that time unsatisfactory, and 45 per cent deplored the lack of a sufficient birth-planning budget.[29] While some of these figures may have since improved, it is unlikely that the basic contradictions mirrored by them have vanished.

Part V
Demographic results

11 Female marriage trends

11.1 Marriage rates and marital status

Analysis of the demographic results of birth-control policies starts with a discussion of female marriage patterns. To an even greater degree than in other cultures, Chinese traditions of universal marriage and premarital chastity make wedlock a prerequisite for childbirth. Fertility levels are therefore closely tied to the annual number of marriages, which again depend on legal and customary rules for marriage age, as well as on the age structure of the population. Large cohorts of women entering marriageable age, as they arrived on the Chinese scene during the 1980s, are obviously increasing marriage numbers and subsequent births. This is why rates relating absolute numbers to the size of different age groups are clearly the preferable indicator for measuring marriage intensity. Furthermore, political interventions and economic developments can also bring about a general delay in weddings during certain periods or a compensatory glut later on. In China's case, this occurred during the Great Leap Forward and the Cultural Revolution. Subsequently, the late-marriage rules of the 1970s, the sudden lowering of the permissable marriage age in 1980, and the re-emphasis on late marriage in the 1990s also led to abrupt changes.[1]

Table 22 First-marriage rates of women of reproductive age by generations 1930–73 (women marrying at specified age as % of all women born in the reference period)

Period of Birth	10–14	15–19	20–24	25–29	30–34	35–39	40–44	45–49	Sum
1930–35	4.9	64.5	26.1	3.7	0.6	0.1	0.1	0.1	99.9
1935–40	3.4	59.6	31.3	4.9	0.5	0.1	0.1	0.1	99.8
1940–45	1.4	56.1	35.7	6.0	0.6	0.2	0.1		99.9
1945–50	1.3	45.4	43.8	8.4	0.9	0.2	0.0		99.8
1950–55	0.6	30.5	49.7	17.9	0.9	0.1			99.6
1955–60	0.4	15.4	68.3	14.7	0.3				99.0
1960–65	0.2	19.8	65.2	2.7					87.7
1965–70	0.2	16.1	14.7						30.9
1970–73	0.1	0.9							1.0

Note: Rates are cumulated for five-year cohorts from average figures. Periods of birth refer to midyear dates. Missing values signify non-completed life periods in 1988.

Sources: 1988 fertility survey results in: Liang Jimin and Chen Shengli 1993, Vol. 2

Long-term marriage trends may be gleaned from Table 22 with generation-specific marriage rates for women aged 10 to 49 who married between the founding of the People's Republic in 1949 and the survey date in 1988. The survey also supplied figures for older women born between 1895 and 1930. Although these figures may be biased by faulty memory and selective mortality, the pattern does not greatly differ from the 1930 to 1935 cohorts. Summing up these longitudinal data results in the percentage of women ever married. Since this reaches nearly 100 per cent for those beyond reproductive age, it once again demonstrates the universality of female marriage in China. The table also shows the secular trend away from wedlock in young age and the widening spread of the peak period of marriage. Nevertheless, the number of women who marry between 15 and 19 years of age continues to be anything but negligible.

The clearly discernible social changes taking place under the influence of modernization forces such as rising female education, employment and self-determination are reinforced by strong governmental intervention. While there has been a regular increase in marriages at age 20 to 24, those born in the 1950s who reached marriageable age during the late-marriage campaign of the 1970s evince a further shift towards marriage at age 25 to 29. This is paralleled by an equally conspicuous drop of early marriage figures in these generations, with a slight rebounding for their successors. Cross-sectional period data show that this was primarily caused by the rising incidence of marriage among those aged 17 to 19 during 1962 to 1963 and those aged 18 to 19 after 1980. Both setbacks were attributed to prior upheavals and the release of pressure at the end of political campaigns.

Table 23 Marital status of women of reproductive age 1982, 1990, 1995 (%)

Status	15–19	20–24	25–29	30–34	35–39	40–44	45–49
Single							
1982	95.62	46.45	5.27	0.69	0.28	0.20	0.18
1990	95.32	41.35	4.20	0.64	0.30	0.24	0.18
1995	97.94	47.44	5.53	0.82	0.34	0.22	0.18
Married							
1982	4.33	53.33	94.32	98.56	98.21	96.66	93.36
1990	4.63	58.35	95.05	98.44	98.41	97.20	94.73
1995	2.01	52.24	93.75	98.03	98.08	97.38	95.48
Widowed							
1982	0.00	0.00	0.18	0.47	1.21	2.84	6.12
1990	0.00	0.00	0.19	0.39	0.84	2.13	4.71
1995	0.00	0.08	0.23	0.46	0.85	1.78	3.81
Divorced							
1982	0.02	0.17	0.24	0.28	0.29	0.30	0.33
1990	0.05	0.23	0.47	0.53	0.45	0.43	0.39
1995	0.04	0.25	0.48	0.69	0.73	0.62	0.52

Sources: 1982 and 1990 census, 1995 microcensus results in: Zhongguo 1982 nian renkou pucha ziliao; Zhongguo 1990 nian renkou pucha ziliao, Vol. 3; 1995 nian quanguo 1% chouyang diaocha ziliao

The more recent census figures on marital status in Table 23 show the cumulated effect of age-specific marriage patterns and furnish further detail in considering the influence of widowhood, divorce and remarriage. The figures demonstrate an increasing concentration of married women in the age group 20 to 24 during the 1980s with renewed decrease in the 1990s. In addition, the doubling or even tripling of divorce rates caused by individual emancipation and social strains in the reform period emerges. These changes do not affect the main message, however. The overwhelming majority of women marry in their mid-twenties; at 30 years of age married status continues to be almost universal; the overall effects of mortality or divorce on the fertility potential of women of reproductive age remain minuscule; and staying single has yet to develop into an alternative lifestyle and mass phenomenon. These factors show that despite a reduction of marriage among the very young and first signs of changes to come in the future, basic elements of traditional marriage patterns persist and continue to constrain birth control.

11.2 Average age at marriage

As an easily comprehensible measure of central tendency and a shorthand for the more refined age-specific marriage rates, the average marriage age of women deserves particular attention. It correlates closely with fertility rates. The few retrospective calculations from scattered genealogical materials for the sixteenth to eighteenth centuries have resulted in values between 17 and 20 years of age. First, more reliable, statistics from the republican period give it as slightly above 17 years around 1930, increasing to more than 18 years up until 1940. Longitudinal analysis documents a slight backsliding for the generations born between 1930 and 1934, before a sustained rise sets in for those who married after 1955. Cross-sectional data pre-date the beginning of the ascent to 1949. They show the average marriage age rising slowly by less than 0.1 annually until it reached more than 20 years in 1970. The late-marriage policies of the following decade then rapidly push it upwards to more than 23 years by 1979.[2] In the cities, a steep ascent already takes place during 1964 to 1966.

Data in Chart 2 confirm the reversal due to the slackening of policy in the 1980s; national figures for 1985 are back to the level of 1975. Despite a renewed emphasis on late marriage ever since, it seems that until 1995 such unions had not yet regained the frequency of 1979 before the lowering of the permissable marriage age. In contrast to these figures, recent reports from China claim that by 1997 the average marriage age had risen to between 23 and 24 years. The annual sample survey on population dynamics gives it as 23.6 years for 1998.[3] Like many other data for the 1990s, this awaits confirmation from a new census.

Chart 2 also documents the distance of approximately 1.5 to 2.5 years between rural and urban areas – down from nearly three years in the 1970s. The drop in the average marriage age for the urban areas was longer and steeper than for the villages. This seems to have been caused by the abolition of special urban rules demanding even later marriage than in the countryside. Urban averages also oscillated more in the 1960s and early 90s. Besides the urban–rural

Chart 2 Average age of women at first marriage 1949–98

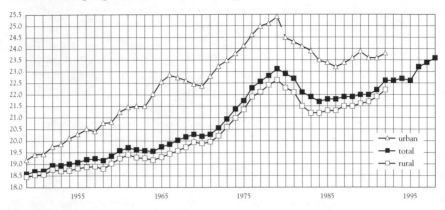

	Total	Urban	Rural
1949	18.6	19.2	18.4
1955	19.1	20.3	18.8
1961	19.7	21.5	19.4
1963	19.6	21.5	19.3
1965	19.7	22.6	19.3
1970	20.2	22.4	19.9
1975	21.7	24.1	21.4
1978	22.8	25.1	22.4
	23.1	25.4	22.6
1980	22.9	24.5	22.3
	22.7	24.3	22.1
	22.1	24.1	21.5
	21.9	23.9	21.2
	21.7	23.5	21.2
1985	21.8	23.4	21.3
	21.8	23.2	21.3
	21.9	23.4	21.5
	21.9	23.6	21.5
	22.0	23.9	21.6
1990	22.0	23.6	21.7
	22.2	23.6	21.9
	22.6	23.8	22.2
	22.6		
	22.7		
1995	22.6		
	23.2		
	23.4		
	23.6		

Note: Average age at first marriage here signifies the mean age from a cross-section of women marrying during the same year. Data for the 1949–79 period are for all women at and above age 15, by urban and rural areas; later data are for women in age groups 15–44, by agricultural and non-agricultural status

Sources: 1982, 1988 and 1992 fertility survey data in: Quanguo qian fen zhi yi renkou shengyulü chouyang diaocha fenxi 1983; Liang Jimin and Chen Shengli 1993, Vol. 2; Jiang Zhenghua 1995; ZRTN 1995; 1995 microcensus data from Zhang Weimin, Yu Hongwen and Cui Hongyan 1997, 58; 1996–98 birth-planning report data from: Cai Fang 2000, 10–11

Table 24 Average first-marriage age of women by provinces and place of residence 1978–92

	1978	City	Village	1987	City	Village	1992	Urban	Rural
Beijing	25.3	25.8	24.4	24.0	24.6	22.5	24.8		
Tianjin	25.2	25.9	24.4	23.6	24.3	22.5	24.0		
Hebei	23.3	24.7	23.0	21.9	22.6	21.7	22.8	23.5	22.1
Shanxi	21.5	22.6	21.3	21.4	22.7	21.0	22.2	23.9	21.4
Inner Mongolia	22.0	23.3	21.6	21.8	22.8	21.5	22.6	23.6	21.9
Liaoning	23.6	24.4	22.8	22.8	23.5	22.0	22.8	23.5	22.3
Jilin	22.6	24.1	22.0	22.2	23.2	21.7	22.9	22.5	21.4
Heilongjiang	22.2	23.7	21.6	22.0	23.0	21.5	22.9	23.9	21.0
Shanghai	25.0	26.1	23.9	25.0	26.3	22.8	24.5		
Jiangsu	23.1	24.3	22.9	22.2	23.7	21.8	23.1	23.7	22.9
Zhejiang	22.3	23.2	22.0	22.4	23.2	22.2	23.3	23.6	23.1
Anhui	23.0	24.3	22.7	21.6	22.1	21.5	22.8	23.8	22.7
Fujian	21.2	23.2	20.9	21.0	22.8	20.8	22.4	22.3	21.4
Jiangxi	20.9	21.8	20.7	21.1	21.9	21.0	22.0	24.1	21.3
Shandong	23.6	24.5	23.4	22.3	23.1	22.2	24.2	23.3	23.1
Henan	23.3	24.5	23.2	22.0	22.9	21.9	22.8	24.4	22.7
Hubei	23.0	24.4	22.6	21.8	23.0	21.4	22.6	23.6	21.7
Hunan	22.4	23.4	22.3	21.4	22.6	21.2	22.5	24.0	21.7
Guangdong	23.0	24.7	22.8	22.9	24.8	22.6	23.6	24.4	24.1
Guangxi	23.0	23.8	22.8	22.1	23.5	21.9	23.2	23.0	22.0
Hainan	22.7	24.8	22.5	22.2	24.0	21.9	22.4		
Sichuan	23.2	23.7	23.1	21.4	22.2	21.2	21.8	22.7	21.3
Guizhou	22.2	22.9	22.1	21.5	22.4	21.3	22.1	24.4	21.3
Yunnan	21.3	23.3	20.9	21.2	22.4	21.0	21.5	23.0	21.7
Tibet	21.7	21.6	21.6	21.6	22.0	21.7	23.5		
Shaanxi	22.2	24.1	21.9	21.6	22.9	21.3	22.1	24.1	22.0
Gansu	21.3	23.0	20.5	20.5	22.0	20.0	21.8	24.0	20.7
Qinghai	19.8	22.5	18.9	20.7	23.0	20.1	21.8		
Ningxia	20.9	22.1	20.7	21.0	22.3	20.3	22.0		
Xinjiang	19.6	22.8	19.0	21.0	22.9	20.4	22.1	23.2	21.4
China	22.8	24.0	22.5	21.9	23.1	21.6	22.7	23.7	22.1

Note: 1992 data for urban and rural areas signify non-agricultural and agricultural population.

Sources: 1988 fertility survey data in: Liang Jimin and Chen Shengli 1993, Vol. 2; 1992 fertility survey data in: ZJSN 1994

differential, educational standards influence the marriage age independently. Both within the urban and the rural population, marriage age rises almost invariably according to the number of years in school.

As shown in Table 24, regional differences in the average marriage age have decreased since 1978. For the total population of the various provinces, the range between maximum and minimum figures diminished from 5.7 years in 1978 to 3.3 years in 1992. Between 1978 and 1987 this was due mainly to a levelling out of the averages for rural areas; in the period 1987 to 1992 it was rather the variation of urban averages that diminished. The lowering of the average marriage age was most pronounced in some areas of North and Central China. These were regions with forceful marriage policies in the 1970s that were relaxed in the 1980s. In contrast, most backward western provinces with particularly low marriage ages saw either only minor changes or continued their incremental move to higher levels for marriage age. Policy changes played a less important role there.

11.3　Early- and late-marriage rates

For administrative purposes, early- and late-marriage rates are the clearly preferred indicators for measuring compliance with marriage rules. The former are defined by reference to the legal marriage age of 20 years for women. In principle, the cut-off point should be changed to 18 years for earlier periods in which the rules of the old marriage law of 1950 applied, but in order to facilitate comparison, the present definition has often been extended backwards. Because marriage of extremely

Table 25 Early-marriage rate and age-specific marriage rate 1978–97 (early-marriage rate as women marrying at ages 15–19 in % of all current first marriages, age-specific marriage rate as women marrying at ages 15–19 in % of respective age group)

| | Early-marriage rate | | | | Report China | Age-specific marriage rate at 15–19 years |
| | 1988 survey | | 1992 survey | | | |
	China	rural areas	China	rural areas		
1978	13.1	17.1				
	12.5	16.9				
1980	15.5	21.0	18.0	22.0		2.6
	19.3	27.4	22.1	27.4		4.4
	28.0	36.1	30.8	37.7		4.5
	25.6	33.4	28.3	34.6		3.9
	23.7	31.4	27.1	31.8		3.0
1985	21.4	27.9	25.1	30.1		3.1
	21.2	27.1	24.5	29.5		3.5
	20.0	25.9	23.6	28.0		4.2
	18.8	24.2	23.4	27.8		4.7
			22.2	26.6	2.9	4.8
1990			20.5	23.8		4.8
			16.8	20.2		
			12.9	16.1		
					2.3	
					1.2	
1995					0.9	2.0
					0.8	1.6
					0.7	1.7
					0.7	1.1

Sources: ZJSN 1988–93; ZRTN 1995–; Jiang Zhenghua 1995; Yu Xuejun, *et al.* 1994, 27

young girls under age 15 has dwindled to negligible proportions, it is largely ignored. Also neglected are the lower age limits for minorities in some regions of the country. This is how data are presented in Table 25.

Early-marriage rates should be easily computable by making use of marriage registration and birth-control files. Retrospective data for the 1940s document figures of more than 70 per cent, decreasing to an average of 58 per cent in the 1960s. It was only after 1973/74 that there was a sharp drop to under 20 per cent. When state control eased during the first half of the 1980s, the prevalence of early marriages rose significantly. Some 90 per cent of these were concluded in the countryside, where people's communes were dissolved.

However, Table 25 shows that such report data are seriously flawed by non- or misreporting. Control figures from life-table calculations and the 1988 and 1992 national fertility surveys establish that the real rates were up to ten times higher than the reported rates. Just as in other areas, the success stories proved to be grossly exaggerated but difficulties in pinning down the real extent of early marriage remain. It has also been demonstrated that the early-marriage rate is not immune from bias. Changes in the age structure of the total population with a concomitant variation in the number of first marriages affect the rates. This emerges in the comparison with marriage rates for women aged 15 to 19 during the period 1984 to 1989: whereas the early-marriage rate fell, the age-specific marriage rate of the relevant age group increased. It indicates that the drop of the former was primarily due to the rising number of first marriages and not to a diminishing incidence of early wedlock.[4] It is only for the 1990s that all indicators point to a decline in the prevalence of early marriage by more than half, documenting the vigour of the new drive for law enforcement. It remains to be seen whether this will be substantiated by a new census.

Table 26 gives an overview of the situation at provincial level. The resurgence of early-marriage figures in the 1980s was uneven. It largely affected populous Sichuan province and a number of other agrarian hinterland regions. But even in coastal Jiangsu of the wealthy Lower Yangzi region the increase was dramatic. For many years both provinces had been at the forefront of Chinese birth control. As in the case of the average marriage age, early-marriage levels in the backward western regions, that were high from the outset, did not change very much. This also pertained to Fujian and Jiangxi, also regions with extremely high early-marriage rates. The situation improved at the end of the 1980s, and a massive drop in the rates is being claimed for the 1990s. The glaring differences between report and survey data for 1989, however, counsel caution in regard to the extravagantly low report figures of recent years. Reported cases of early-marriage rates that remain markedly above average are primarily related to high minority shares of the population to which reduced age limits for marriage apply. One of the most prominent examples has been Xinjiang Autonomous Region, where Muslim customs have always favoured very early marriages that were tolerated only grudgingly. The sensational drop in the figures for this Chinese part of Central Asia implies either a repeal of former policies or large-scale fraud.

Finally, Table 27 sums up the available figures on the percentage of late marriages in China's provinces. Again, the unreliability of data from the highly defective report system of the birth-planning commissions emerges. Although they seemed to decrease over the years, the discrepancies between report and survey data still remained large in 1990, no matter if hinterland or coastal regions were involved.

Table 26 Early-marriage rate by provinces 1980–99 (women marrying at ages 15–19 in % of all current first marriages)

	1980 survey	1985 survey	1989 report	1989 survey	1992 survey	1993 report	1999 report
Beijing	1.3	5.5	0.0	8.8	6.9	0.0	0.0
Tianjin	1.3	1.3	0.1	8.8	6.9	0.1	0.1
Hebei	14.0	19.1	1.8	16.7	14.8	0.8	0.1
Shanxi	23.3	30.3	4.4	30.9	15.2	2.9	1.7
Inner Mongolia	18.2	19.5	1.5	24.1	11.6	0.6	0.2
Liaoning	8.5	12.4	0.1	8.5	7.6	0.0	0.1
Jilin	16.3	27.7	2.2	28.7	17.3	1.9	1.7
Heilongjiang	19.5	19.1	5.0	27.9	16.1	1.5	1.5
Shanghai	1.3	5.5	0.4	8.8	6.9	0.0	0.2
Jiangsu	5.9	18.4	0.8	17.8	6.2	0.2	0.2
Zhejiang	13.1	19.8	0.8	15.6	8.1	1.0	0.6
Anhui	29.7	22.9	4.3	16.1	9.9	0.2	0.2
Fujian	32.3	40.0	4.6	30.9	15.2	0.7	0.5
Jiangxi	39.8	43.0	3.4	35.9	21.4	10.7	0.5
Shandong	7.1	14.0	0.7	17.1	2.9	0.0	0.0
Henan	13.5	20.2	2.2	13.7	7.8	0.4	0.2
Hubei	10.6	20.8	4.0	24.5	14.4	1.4	0.3
Hunan	25.4	28.1	4.1	24.9	14.3	1.6	0.4
Guangdong	18.9	17.1	2.6	16.8	6.7	1.7	0.5
Guangxi	19.6	28.8	3.0	10.8	17.6	0.8	0.1
Hainan	42.9	44.4	7.8	30.1	30.3	4.5	1.2
Sichuan	19.6	36.0	1.0	29.3	17.0	0.5	0.4
Guizhou	41.1	41.6	12.4	28.3	22.1	3.9	0.5
Yunnan	32.7	33.1	9.9	27.4	13.8	5.9	4.6
Tibet	42.9	44.4		30.1	30.3		15.2
Shaanxi	16.8	27.9	4.3	29.6	12.5	1.4	0.1
Gansu	39.2	49.4	5.7	35.3	28.8	5.0	0.4
Qinghai	42.9	44.4	10.8	30.1	30.3	10.1	10.1
Ningxia	42.9	44.4	16.0	30.1	30.3	12.1	6.9
Xinjiang	47.6	47.1	1.9	47.4	18.2	3.0	0.2
China	18.0	25.1	2.9	22.2	12.9	2.6	0.7

Note: Survey figures for Beijing, Tianjin and Shanghai as one average for these three municipal regions; survey figures for Hainan, Tibet, Ningxia and Qinghai as one average for these four regions.

Sources: survey data from 1992 fertility survey in Jiang Zhenghua 1995; birth-planning report data in ZJSN 1990; ZJSN 1993; ZRTN 1995–

Table 27 Late-marriage rate by provinces 1980–99 (women marrying at ages 23 and over in % of all current first marriages)

	1980 report	1980 survey	1985 report	1985 survey	1990 report	1990 survey	1999 report
Beijing	92.4	79.5	71.9	57.5	74.5	54.5	86.5
Tianjin	96.5	79.5	63.3	57.5	58.0	54.5	61.7
Hebei	96.8	41.1	52.8	20.1	44.3	28.6	50.2
Shanxi	88.0	24.4	59.3	18.3	61.4	27.8	63.7
Inner Mongolia	74.7	40.3	64.1	32.5	71.7	37.3	72.2
Liaoning	95.3	57.7	48.4	27.7	49.4	33.6	61.3
Jilin	93.2	45.0	60.9	19.3	49.2	13.0	42.4
Heilongjiang	87.7	40.7	67.5	27.0	56.3	21.4	45.8
Shanghai	2.4	79.5	76.8	57.5	59.9	54.5	63.8
Jiangsu	94.4	59.3	67.9	27.6	65.4	29.2	57.6
Zhejiang	84.6	40.3	54.9	18.9	64.2	36.8	67.2
Anhui	90.9	41.5	66.9	16.5	67.5	29.5	52.6
Fujian	74.9	17.7	42.2	13.0	42.0	17.5	53.1
Jiangxi	76.7	23.7	37.8	12.1	35.9	23.0	41.8
Shandong	92.5	60.3	68.1	27.0	76.1	39.7	99.0
Henan	90.2	53.7	80.4	20.6	75.2	30.2	64.1
Hubei	88.2	55.9	59.7	24.5	49.8	37.8	46.9
Hunan	85.6	35.5	46.1	12.3	39.2	15.2	48.6
Guangdong	84.3	44.8	67.9	38.2	68.3	50.2	74.3
Guangxi	77.2	41.1	41.9	27.3	55.0	38.8	64.9
Hainan		26.5		9.7	67.4	10.3	44.7
Sichuan	95.0	45.5	29.4	8.8	30.1	15.5	45.5
Guizhou	77.4	26.0	48.7	13.6	53.5	25.8	54.5
Yunnan	65.5	34.6	33.4	19.4	38.8	27.3	43.2
Tibet		26.5		9.7		10.3	81.5
Shaanxi	89.1	39.7	56.5	16.4	53.3	21.1	62.2
Gansu	80.1	17.7	24.7	13.3	36.7	25.2	51.3
Qinghai	25.2	26.5	31.7	9.7	46.0	10.3	50.9
Ningxia		26.5	31.3	9.7	35.1	10.3	45.9
Xinjiang	85.8	33.3	42.5	11.8	58.5	29.7	82.6
China	87.5	45.6	55.2	21.9	54.2	29.0	60.1

Note: Survey figures for Beijing, Tianjin and Shanghai as one average for these three municipal regions; survey figures for Hainan, Tibet, Ningxia and Qinghai as one average for these four regions.

Sources: Birth-planning report data in ZJSN 1986; ZRTN 1995–; survey data from the 1992 fertility survey in Jiang Zhenghua 1995

In 1949, late marriages of women aged 23 and older did not exceed 7 per cent of all first marriages in that year. Up until 1970, this share gradually increased to 14 per cent, with a wide margin between urban places (40 per cent) and the countryside (10 per cent). Afterwards the rates sharply increased due to the efforts of the third birth-planning campaign. According to reports from the late 1970s, late marriages had become almost universal in some areas. This was not vindicated by the retrospective surveys, which resulted in a national average of only 45 to 50 per cent. The 1978 figures amounted to 84 per cent for urban areas and 41 per cent for the villages.

Annual survey data – not reproduced in Table 27 – highlight the expected fact that in 1982, one year after the new marriage law was enacted, late-marriage rates dropped dramatically by some 7 percentage points. They continued to decrease until 1985, when a plateau of 22 per cent was reached, after which time a slow ascent set in again. Judging by the figures from 1998, this increase accelerated considerably in the 1990s. The rates climbed particularly steeply during 1992 to 1994 when a new late-marriage campaign was initiated. In the process, the urban–rural gap has diminished. In 1992 the rate stood at 58 per cent for the non-agricultural population and 30 per cent for the agricultural one.[5] Today, provinces with percentages still markedly below the national average tend to be the same for which high early-marriage rates were recorded in the past. This shows that enforcement of the legal marriage age has become tighter than action on the late-marriage recommendation. Nevertheless, most current figures have surpassed the level of the survey data for 1980. If this is borne out by later census results, it would signify that in terms of late-marriage levels Chinese birth control is almost back to the state of affairs in the mid-1970s. If it is falsified, it would necessitate corresponding adjustments in the average age at first marriage.

12 Fertility levels

12.1 Absolute numbers, birth rates and proportions of birth orders

In spite of ever more statistical sophistication, absolute birth numbers continue to be an indispensable item in the demographic record. Having the advantage of concreteness, they constitute an immediate datum for all population-related policy arenas. Chart 3 summarizes official figures from China since 1978. Although hailing from a period of stringent birth control, their size rivals that from former peak periods of births (average annual birth numbers 1950 to 1958: 20.49 million; 1963 to 1971: 27.00 million). This, of course, is connected to the growth of the female population of reproductive age, which offsets the drop of individual fertility to a large degree.

Chart 3 documents how complicated the enumeration of births has become. Although the registration records of the public security offices have been discarded as unreliable since 1982, even the annual sample surveys of the State Statistical Bureau do not succeed in establishing a sufficient degree of certainty. The fourth population census of 1990 highlights the fact that approximately 10 per cent of all births between 1982 and 1989 were not covered by them. This figure rises to approximately 30 per cent if the adjusted birth numbers are compared to the original reports of the birth-planning or household registration systems. Under-reporting was continuously high during the 1980s, only to decrease on the eve of the 1990 census. Between 1985 and 1988, the number of new-born children escaping the net of birth-planning reports reached the staggering level of 33 to 37 per cent. A comparative study of population data from the 1990s hints at continuing under-registration of births on a grand scale of 25 to 33 per cent.

In order to convey a sense of proportion, absolute birth numbers have to be linked to population size. This is the purpose of crude birth rates, which relate the number of births during a given year to the total population at mid-year. Obviously, the calculations suffer if numerator or denominator in the equation is wrong. Under-registration has been a feature of Chinese birth statistics in the past. Calculations by Ansley Coale and Judith Banister put it at approximately 20 per cent in the 1950s and 10 per cent in the 1960s and 1970s. In the early years, it was primarily due to the defects of a household registration system under construction; additional distortions caused by political influences may also have played a role.

Chart 3 Absolute birth numbers and crude birth rates: original and revised figures 1978–99

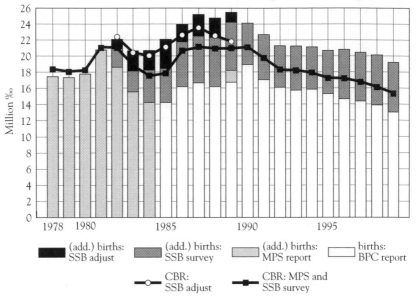

	Million births BPC report	Million births MPS report	Million births SSB survey	Million births SSB adjust	CBR: MPS report, SSB survey	CBR: SSB adjust
1978		17.45			18.34	
		17.27			17.90	
1980		17.79			18.21	
		20.69			20.91	
		18.68	21.26	22.38	21.09	22.28
		15.41	18.59	20.58	18.62	20.19
		14.26	18.02	20.55	17.50	19.90
1985	13.93	14.16	18.51	22.02	17.80	21.04
	15.98		21.83	23.84	20.77	22.43
	16.55		22.40	25.22	21.04	23.33
	16.15		22.47	24.57	20.78	22.37
	16.71	18.07	22.88	24.07	20.83	21.58
1990	18.95			23.91	21.06	
	16.97		22.58		19.68	
	15.96		21.19		18.24	
	15.70		21.26		18.09	
	15.75		21.04		17.70	
1995	15.21		20.63		17.12	
	14.55		20.67		16.98	
	13.88		20.38		16.57	
	13.83		19.91		16.03	
	12.77		19.09		15.23	

Note: Absolute birth numbers from 1985–99 reports of the Birth-Planning Commission (BPC), from 1978–81 and 1989 reports of the Ministry of Public Security (MPS), from 1982–99 SSB surveys and 1982–90 SSB adjustments are original figures; the same applies to 1978–81 crude birth rates (CBR) from the MPS reports, the 1982–97 birth rates from the annual sample surveys of the State Statistical Bureau (SSB) and the 1982–90 birth rates adjusted by the SSB on the basis of the 1990 census. All other figures are calculated from birth rates and the official population totals

Sources: Own calculations and basic data from ZJSN 1986–; ZRTN 1988–; ZTN 1992–; Nygren and Hoem 1993; Zeng Yi 1995; Cai Fang 2000, 12

Despite glaring discrepancies between registration data, survey and census results, vital rates for the period 1949 to 1977 have never been adjusted by the State Statistical Bureau. A corrected time series since the founding of the People's Republic points to high fertility in the 1950s, with an average birth rate of nearly 43 per thousand between 1949 and 1957. This equalled or even surpassed the upper margin of local surveys in the countryside from the late 1920s and early 1930s. A sharp decline in the crisis years of the Great Leap Forward between 1959 and 1961 (average birth rate for these three years fell to 26 per thousand) and another peak period of births (average for 1962 to 1970 rose to nearly 40 per thousand) followed. Leaving aside the anomaly of the Great Leap, these figures point to a high natural fertility that remained essentially unchecked. Introducing birth control in the urban areas barely affected the national averages. It was only after 1970 that birth numbers and birth rates diminished regularly due to the third birth-planning campaign: the average birth rate for 1971 to 1979 stood at 26 per thousand. On the eve of the one-child campaign in 1979 it fell to below 18 per thousand according to the official reports, and to more than 21 per thousand in an independent computer reconstruction.[1]

Instead of being lowered further, this level increased slightly in the following decade of tight one-child policies. Only in the 1990s did it decline again consistently – a trend awaiting confirmation from a new census. Since the new wave of births in the second half of the 1980s, debate has centred on the question to what degree this development was linked to the emergence of large cohorts of women of reproductive age from the peak period of births in the 1960s or due to a renewed increase in fertility levels. Although the figures in Chart 3 do not answer this question directly, they do show that despite intensified birth control and a very low birth rate in the 1990s, absolute birth numbers continue to be almost as high as in earlier high-fertility periods. This hints at the continuing influence of age structure. All projections point to the fact that the number of women in the high-fertility age group 20 to 34 continued to increase until 1997. However, as there were shifts in the internal composition of this group,[2] the sudden drop in birth numbers between 1991 and 1992 and the slight downward trend thereafter must be attributed either to misreporting or to birth-control measures lowering birth parities, delaying marriage and increasing intervals for childbearing. A combination of all these factors probably is involved.

Chart 4 takes up the story of the one-child campaign from another angle. It presents percentages for second and higher-order births among all births of the running year. By implication, the percentage needed to reach 100 per cent signifies the proportion of first births. Known as first-, second- and multiple-child rates in Chinese usage, these figures are an easy-to-grasp indicator of birth-control performance. Once again, the chart reveals wide statistical discrepancies, which increased by leaps and bounds after 1983. Between 1982 and 1990, first births only made up approximately 50 per cent of the current birth total – a far cry from the one-child ideal. While some of the second-order births were covered by the permits granted after 1983, their proportion far exceeded the

Chart 4 Proportions of second and higher-order births 1980–99 (% of current births)

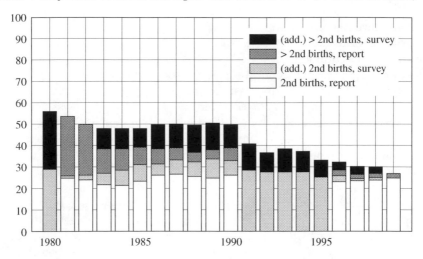

	% 2nd births BPC reports	% 2nd births surveys		% > 2nd births BPC reports	% > 2nd births surveys
1980		28.3			27.5
	25.4	26.2		28.1	25.4
	24.2	26.1		24.2	23.3
	22.4	27.2		11.7	20.7
	21.7	28.2		10.3	19.9
1985	23.9	31.0		8.5	17.0
	26.9	31.4		7.3	17.9
	26.6	32.9		6.2	17.3
	25.4	31.9		5.3	18.0
	25.2	33.3		5.0	17.7
1990	26.4	32.8		6.4	16.3
		28.4			12.4
		27.3			9.6
		27.5			11.2
		27.6			9.5
1995		25.6			7.4
	23.4	25.6		2.8	6.6
	23.6	24.0		2.1	5.1
	24.0	25.0		2.0	4.7
	24.9			1.6	

Note: report figures form the Birth-Planning Commission (BPC) for 1985–90 according to original, unrevised numbers

Sources: Own calculation from data in ZJSN 1986–; ZRTN 1996–; Liang Jimin and Chen Shengli 1993, Vol. 3; Jiang Zhenghua 1995; ZJSQ 1997, 26, 887; Zhang Weimin *et al.*, 1997, 47; Cai Fang 2000, 3

limits of 10 to 20 per cent indicated in contemporary Party guidelines. Only in the 1990s was the proportion of second births supposed to have been reduced to the desired levels – and rather suddenly. Even more disturbing is the high percentage of third- or higher-order births. Although it has continuously diminished, it has still been way above the margin permissible by special policies for the national minorities. Because penalties for non-authorized higher-order births are rising steeply, under-reporting has been even larger than in the case of second births. It may be assumed that this also holds true for the figures from the post-1990 period, which have not been validated by a new census.

The elevated proportions of second and higher-order births in the 1980s have sounded alarm bells. Nevertheless, the indicators are biased once more. High proportions of first births may signal compliance with the one-child policy, but they can also be caused by marriage policies or the age structure of the population, resulting in an increase of first marriages with attendant childbearing. This would drive down the share of second and higher-order births without a real drop in fertility levels. The large cohorts of newcomers to the Chinese marriage market between 1982 and 1995 exactly fit such a scenario. The already high proportion of second and higher-order births in Chart 4 therefore disguises still higher fertility levels. During the 1990s, a rise in the marriage age and extended birth spacing have slanted the figures once again.

12.2 Age-specific, duration-specific and total fertility rates

Although birth rates relating births to the total population are widely accepted in popular usage, they are biased by age and sex structure. Obviously, populations with a high share of women of reproductive age have higher birth rates than those with a preponderance of elderly or juvenile members. Defining a proper reference group is therefore a core problem of measurement, turning the construction of appropriate fertility indicators into a long-standing occupation of demographers.

At first sight, women in the reproductive age group 15 to 49 seem to be the immediate solution. However on closer scrutiny, this reference group is problematic, since it lumps both married and unmarried women together. In China, where illegitimate childbearing is virtually unknown and where frictions between social, political and legal conventions lead to sharp variations in marriage age, it again produces bias. The composition of birth orders and birth spacing complicate the picture further and furnish sufficient reasons for calculating still more refined statistics. To make matters worse, both longitudinal data for completed fertility of women from the same period of birth and cross-sectional period figures from various generations are collected, in order to distinguish long-range cohort patterns from more recent changes in external conditions. Of course, all these data are again marred by the manifold problems of defective registration. The resulting jumble of frequently contradictory figures is usually left to the demographic profession and other experts. However, under the stiff Chinese birth-control regime it has become a subject closely watched by politicians and the many citizens affected by birth control alike. Academic debates on fertility data hence immediately turn into controversies on programme performance. They also bring about a constant refinement of indicators in order to distinguish the effects of different policy elements. Refinement is also required to make up for the fact that the usual set of indicators seems to be inadequate for measuring oscillations on a low fertility level.

Age-specific fertility rates, which give the number of births by women in a certain age group as a standardized figure per 1000 women in that age group, convey a more precise picture. As they relate to women of reproductive age only, they are untainted by the age structure of the total population. For brevity's sake, the table beneath Chart 5 presents them as period averages for

Chart 5 Age-specific fertility rates 1957–99

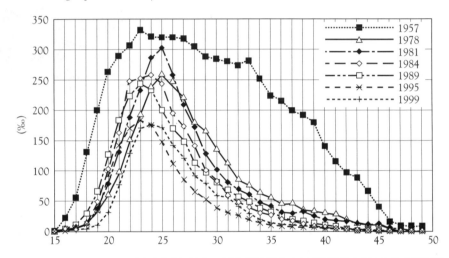

	1957	1978	1981	1984	1989	1995	1999
TFR	6261	2724	2647	2353	2250	1427	1452
15–19	83.60	12.78	15.10	17.00	21.99	10.89	2.6
20–24	302.80	151.42	183.58	187.00	198.81	154.07	122.0
25–29	308.80	216.24	214.08	166.00	155.55	91.84	118.8
30–34	273.60	96.22	70.82	53.00	55.74	26.50	40.0
35–39	201.40	44.18	30.82	17.00	19.56	5.71	9.8
40–44	100.40	20.66	12.76	7.00	5.67	1.58	1.3
45–49	14.40	4.38	2.20	1.00	1.63	0.63	0.4

Note: TFR = total age-specific fertility rates in ‰; age-specific rates in ‰ as means for five-year age groups

Sources: 1957: National fertility survey 1982 in Quanguo qian fen zhi yi renkou shengyulü chouyang diaocha fenxi 1983, 152
1978, 1981: National fertility survey 1982 in ZJSN 1986
1984: National fertility survey 1988 in Liang Jimin and Chen Shengli 1993, Vol. 3
1989: Census 1990 in ZRTN 1992
1995: Microcensus 1995 in: 1995 nian quanguo 1% renkou chouyang diaocha ziliao
1999: Annual sample survey 1999 in ZRTN 2000

five-year age groups. The graph, however, is based on the full record for one-year cohorts.

Chart 5 shows how after promulgation of the new marriage law in the early 1980s, the most active period of childbearing moved from the age group 25 to 29 to 20 to 24. The highest increases were recorded for ages 21 and 22, immediately after the attainment of the legal marriage age. The decade also saw an accompanying rise of fertility rates for the age group 15 to 19, mostly for women aged 18 to 19. This is also the group most affected by under-registration. In 1989, age-specific fertility rates for women aged 15 to 19 years, as recorded by the birth-planning system, missed nearly 90 per cent of the level reached by census results. Rates for women aged 35 to 49 also went underreported.[3]

Since the start of the one-child campaign, births have become ever more bunched within a small life-cycle period. Whereas in 1978 age-specific fertility rates above 100 per thousand extended to all cohorts between 21 and 31 years of age, such high levels had become confined to the age groups 20 to 28 by 1989. The micro-census of 1995 showed a further concentration in the age groups 21 to 26. These contribute 65 per cent of total fertility; for cohorts between 20 to 29 years of age the share rises to around 85 per cent.

The reduction in higher age groups has been much larger than that in the younger age brackets, but its recent extent in comparison to the 1990 census strains credulity. Rival data from the annual sample surveys in the period 1994 to 1999 suggest that, above all, births from women aged 25 to 29 were overlooked; these would tend to be mainly second births. If results from the annual surveys between 1994 and 1999 were verified, they would imply that very early childbearing had been successfully checked and that the peak period of childbearing had again shifted to the higher age group. A comparison of the curves with earlier data for 1930, 1957 and 1965 underlines the extent of long-term changes in childbearing patterns. Formerly, fertility rates above 300 per thousand peaked in the age groups 23 to 27. Rates above 200 per thousand extended over a prolonged life-cycle period in the age groups 19 to 37. They increased early at age 17 and decreased slowly after 37. Both skewness and peakedness in this 'natural' distribution of births were much less marked than today.[4]

Of course, the consistently high fertility plateau of former years was caused by the larger number of births per woman, which prolonged the period of childbearing. With the reduction of birth numbers the rates have had a natural tendency to cluster in the age groups below 30. This development started immediately after the beginning of the third birth-planning campaign in 1970. Moreover, age-specific fertility rates have become closely linked to the incidence of marriage. Correlation with age-specific marriage rates for the same and the preceding year has become extremely high (r = 0.7 and 0.9, respectively, for 1989). However, it is precisely this close connection to marriages that invalidates the age-specific fertility rates to a certain extent. For age groups with a low incidence of marriage they are necessarily low. Sudden changes in the average marriage age or in the timing of births thus increase or reduce the rates for some age groups in a given year without yet leading to compensatory changes in other age groups. This creates distortion and impairs comparability.

It is against this background that duration-specific fertility rates have been devised. They relate births to married women only and are structured by years after marriage. Under conditions of birth control, marital fertility decreases markedly once the desired or permitted number of children has been reached. As the age distribution of marriages and births in China virtually rules out fecundity problems in later stages of life and marriages of older women beyond reproductive age are virtually unknown, the duration-specific fertility rates are largely free from the influence of changes in marriage age. If the latter is rising, they are higher than age-specific rates and vice versa. Only changes in birth intervals remain as a factor of bias.

With the exception of a brief period after the founding of the People's Republic and the deep plunge of the Great Leap, average rates of more than 300 births per thousand women for zero to four years after marriage have remained stable over the years. Some peaks (1981–82, 1987–88) and troughs (1980, 1983–86) occurred. Average rates for five to nine years after marriage have generally been lower, an anomaly of the immediate postwar period 1945 to 1951 apart. Between 1952 and 1969, their behaviour more or less paralleled that of the earlier five-year interval, but, from 1970, they began to plummet, diminishing from their former level of more than 300 per thousand in most of the 1960s to a low of 100 per thousand in 1988. Births after ten years of marriage showed similar developments and were down to an average of 50 per thousand in 1988. Overall, the fertility decline as judged by duration-specific rates has been more pronounced than in other types of measurement.

The same conclusion emerges from the comparison of the crude birth rate (CBR) and various formulas for the total fertility rate in Chart 6. It demonstrates how, despite convergence in the long run, assessments for separate periods can differ. A case in point is the reform period of the 1980s, where the indicators convey rather conflicting trend signals. Although the CBR increases slightly, the total fertility rate does not communicate a clear message. This rate is a hypothetical construct indicating the average number of births per woman, provided all women follow the present fertility schedule in their future years of reproductive age. Easy conceptualization and use, integrative and prognostic properties turn the total fertility rate into a popular indicator. In reality, however, future birth histories never wholly follow present patterns, and actual numbers of children can only be calculated after present cohorts have completed their reproductive period. Generally, the rate is reached by calculating the total of age-specific fertility rates (TAFR). It then acquires all their problems of linkage to the ages of marriage and childbearing.

Other means of calculation are more robust, but they require more demographic data that are not always available. One is the total duration-specific fertility rate (TDFR), which is calculated analogously by summation, too. A further alternative is the total parity progression rate (TPPR).[5] In a simplified explanation, this latter indicator combines the proportion of women who marry with period probabilities for all women progressing to childbirth and thenceforth from one birth to another. Only those women who experience the prior event enter the calculations. Total fertility is then defined as the product of these factors, allowing a close scrutiny of the effects of birth number reductions.

The long view shows the familiar picture of high fertility in the 1950s. The total fertility rates from retrospective surveys move on to a level of approximately six children per woman between 1949 and 1958 (average TAFR 5.70 by the 1982 fertility survey, 6.07 by the 1988 fertility survey; TDFR 6.07). Instead of showing a beginning fertility decline, they indicate a trend of increasing birth levels during the first decade of the People's Republic. They fit birth averages in pre-communist China (1926–30 TAFR from the rural Haishan area of Taiwan 5.70, adjusted TAFR from the 1929–31 Buck survey in twenty-

Chart 6 Crude birth rate (%) and total fertility rates (children per woman) 1949–90

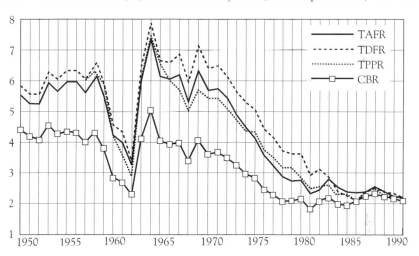

	CBR	TAFR	TDFR	TPPR
1949	4.40	5.54	5.90	
1957	4.33	6.21	6.66	6.37
1961	2.24	3.28	3.59	2.83
1963	4.98	7.41	8.02	7.16
1965	3.90	6.02	6.61	5.96
1967	3.39	5.25	5.89	4.98
1970	3.70	5.75	6.46	5.43
1975	2.48	3.58	4.48	3.73
1979	2.14	2.77	3.65	2.88
1985	2.10	2.39	2.10	2.13
1990	2.11	2.24	2.18	2.09

Note: CBR = (adjusted) crude birth rate; TAFR = total age-specific fertility rate; TDFR = total duration-specific fertility rate; TPPR = total parity progression rate

Sources: Banister 1987, 352; ZRTN 1988–; Feeeney and Yu Jingyuan 1987; Feeney *et al.* 1992; Chen Shengli and Coale 1993; Jiang Zhenghua 1995

two provinces 5.50–5.80, 1931–35 TAFR from Jiangyin County in Jiangsu 6.40). They also conform with cohort fertility rates around 5.6 for all women born between 1927 and 1932, who experienced their most active period of childbearing between 1947 and 1966 and completed their reproductive age in the 1980s. But these figures are up to 20 per cent higher than retrospective data for the civil war period before the founding of the People's Republic (1945–49 average TAFR 5.08 or 5.66).

The total fertility rates drop slightly at the height of land reform in 1953 and during collectivization in 1956. They nearly halve during the Great Leap (1959–61 TAFR average 3.83), only to show a spectacular compensatory increase in 1963 and a return to their former level until the mid-1960s (1962–66 TAFR average 6.35). In 1967 to 1969 the Cultural Revolution brought another, albeit smaller oscillation with it (TAFR average 5.76). Many traces of man-made disasters, but little evidence of birth control, may be found in the aggregated figures of the 1960s.

A final downward trend sets in after the beginning of the third birth-planning campaign in 1970, and it leads to an unprecedented rapid decline of total age-specific fertility. This was caused by both a reduction in the number of children per woman and by the quickly rising marriage age. TDFRs (1971–79 average 4.65), which surpass TAFRs (1971–79 average 3.80) by some 22 per cent throughout the period, furnish indirect proof of the important role played by this latter element. The TPPR (1971–79 average 3.90) in turn stays closer to the TAFR. However, since it starts from a lower plateau in 1970 and stands at a higher value in 1979, the fertility decline measured by it is not quite as dramatic as that evinced by the two other indicators. These differences may be important if they enter economic or demographic models. They do not change the overall picture, though. No matter how it was defined, China's fertility at the end of the 1970s was the lowest among all the developing countries of the world.[6]

Chart 7 views the developments since 1978 in minute detail. Besides survey and census numbers, it includes the original model calculations for lowering the TAFR that guided the one-child policy in its early phase before their revision in 1983. The graph shows that the attempt to push the total fertility rate further down to 1.5 started from wrong base numbers and was thwarted in the 1980s. As with the birth rates and absolute birth totals, the total fertility rates display a conspicuous peak in the period 1981 to 1982 after the lowering of the marriage age. This effect levels off in the three following years when fertility declines. All indicators document a resurge between 1986 and 1987, before another decline sets in. The sharpest oscillations are shown by the TAFR. Only at the end of the decade did it come down slowly, lowering the final average for 1980 to 1990 to around 2.45. Even then it was unclear whether this final downward trend was real or caused by the tendency of Chinese fertility behaviour and birth records to comply with regulations shortly before a new count.

The drop of the other two indicators was clearer and their oscillation less marked. Although they document greater effects of birth control than evinced by the TAFR, neither reach the envisaged target. Due to the combined effect of

Chart 7 Total fertility rates (children per woman) 1978–99: a comparison of survey and census figures

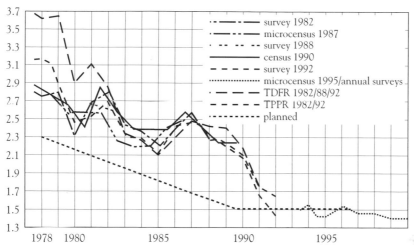

	TAFR Survey 1982	TAFR Microcensus 1987	TAFR Survey 1988	TAFR Census 1990	TAFR Survey 1992	TAFR Micro census 1995 + annual	TDFR 1982/88/92	TPPR 1988/92
1978	2.75			2.87			3.62	3.16
	2.80	2.77		2.77			3.65	2.88
1980	2.32	2.55	2.31	2.65			2.88	2.46
	2.71	2.58	2.61	2.42			3.15	2.54
	2.62	2.57	2.86	2.85			2.85	2.67
		2.25	2.42	2.57			2.33	2.30
		2.19	2.35	2.38			2.26	2.28
1985		2.20	2.20	2.39			2.10	2.13
		2.41	2.42	2.38	2.45		2.31	2.41
		2.49	2.59	2.57	2.55		2.48	2.48
				2.39	2.28		2.42	2.27
				2.24	2.24		2.40	2.24
1990				2.24	2.04		2.18	2.09
					1.65		1.70	1.75
					1.44			1.65
						1.55		
1995						1.43		
						1.55		
						1.46		
						1.45		
						1.45		

Note: Census and microcensus figures for mid-year, national fertility survey data for year-end; TAFR = total age-specific fertility rate; TDFR = total duration-specific fertility rate; TPPR = total parity progression rate

Sources (literature with alternate figures in parenthesis): Survey 1982: Coale and Chen Shengli 1987, 25. Microcensus 1987: ZRTN 1989; (Luther *et al.* 1990). Survey 1988: ZRTN 1989; (Feeney and Yuan Jianhua 1994; Chang Chongxuan 1991,78). Census 1990: Feeney *et al.* 1992; (ZRTN 1993; Zha Ruizhuan *et al.* 1996, 236). Survey 1992: Jiang Zhenghua 1995; Nygren and Hoem 1993; (State Family Planning Commission 1997). Microcensus 1995 and annual surveys: 1995 nian quanguo 1% renkou chouyang diaocha ziliao; ZRTN 1995–. TDFR 1982/88: Chen Shengli and Coale 1993, 120; (Jiang Zhenghua 1995). TPPR 1988/92: Jiang Zhenghua 1995; Feeney 1996. Planned: Liu Zheng *et al.* 1981, 31; Song Jian *et al.* 1982

the sharply decreasing marriage age and birth control, the TDFR declined rather sharply. It showed a much smaller peak in 1981, followed by another rapid decline until 1985. After the relaxation of second-child birth permits in the period 1984 to 1985 there was a new peak just as for the TAFR, but again it took a different form due to the influence of the marriage factor. The 1980 to 1990 average amounted to 2.49. The TPPR gives the same general trends. Its 1980 to 1990 average stands at 2.35, but the swings of the curve are less pronounced. This is the same effect as shown in the long-term trend chart for 1949 to 1990. It seems that this indicator is best suited to attenuate exaggeration due to factors outside fertility changes in the strict sense.

Besides showing discrepancies caused by different methods of calculation, Chart 7 also helps to gauge internal data consistency. The figures hail from the six nationwide counts between 1982 and 1995 that have been used to correct the defective birth figures from the bureaucratic report systems in Chart 3. The sources given for the six counts contain some variations due to methodological differences. Although the official time series are used in most cases, adjustments are preferred for the 1990 census. These rest on reconstructed birth histories and lower the figure for 1981 slightly by 6 per cent, while raising the figures for 1982 to 1985 by an average 11 per cent. Such corrections enter the figures based on parity progression ratios, too. Generally, the fertility survey data for the TAFR in the 1980s show a high degree of congruence. If half-year swings and the shift in the reference period are taken into account, survey figures also display a good consistency with census results. Most discrepancies stay within a margin of one to two decimal points of the rate, or approximately 1 to 2 million births per year. Only the 1987 micro-census results for the mid-1980s, which continue to be used in official publications, appear conspicuously low.

The figures after 1990 are a different matter. Their extremely low level is barely believable (1991–99 TAFR average 1.50). The figures are meanwhile challenged by specialist literature from China, too. While the TAFR for 1992 was first reported as reaching 2.1, it was later claimed to have dropped to 1.4.[7] Another striking element in the picture is the fact that all calculations of the 1990s end up with about the same depressed figures, and they more or less equal the target rate that would result once only authorized births are counted. Moreover, they are largely resistant to methods for the correction of defective population data. All attempts at substituting birth figures from the 1995 micro-census with a fertility estimate derived from the number of children ever born result in minor corrections only.[8] This points to internal consistency of cheating. An alternative explanation would stress the increase of the marriage age and of birth intervals over recent years. Correction of the total fertility rate for these factors would push it up sizeably in the 1990s, but again, this interpretation would rest on shaky ground, as reported marriage and parity data may also be falsified.

Since 1992, adjustments by the State Statistical Bureau have raised the TAFR to a stable level of about 1.8, but, although repeated checks of this figure have been undertaken, doubts as to its reliability remain. The fertility record of the one-child campaign therefore continues to be blurred to a certain extent.

Disaggregation of national-level figures is necessary to bring it into focus and to separate the factors involved.

12.3 Fertility by parity progression and sex of previous children

Disaggregation of total rates by birth orders is a first step in checking the various factors involved in the general fertility changes. This procedure may be performed for all three indicators introduced above. It then amplifies the effects associated with each of them. TAFRs by birth orders are particularly vulnerable. Those for first births suffer from postponements of childbearing, which can be made up later on by heaping, if delayed and ordinary births combine. This may create the statistical artefact of TAFRs for first birth-order amounting to more than value one, namely the paradox of women having more than one first child. This is exactly the situation for China in the 1980s. TAFRs for second birth-order are similarly distorted. For many years they suggest little variation or increases of second births – but as these trends do not account for changes in marital status they are to a certain extent spurious. TDFRs by birth-orders perform better but show a tendency to produce the opposite kind of exaggeration. Again, for many years all data have suffered from under-reporting. Comparing the census results for 1989 with contemporary figures from the report system of the Birth-Planning Commission shows that some 30 per cent of second births and up to 80 per cent of third and higher-order births were not recorded.[9]

Because they control for birth orders and relate them only to women of the appropriate parity (namely the correct number of previous births), parity progression ratios are a superior device for measuring the extent to which calls for limiting birth numbers have been heeded. Chart 8 presents such ratios with abbreviated information for earlier decades. Column 1 gives the proportion of women who proceeded to a first marriage and to bearing at least one child. With the exception of the Great Leap crisis years, this ratio of 96 to 99 per cent has been relatively stable over the years. It once again underlines the universality of female marriage and childbearing in China, even if its extremely high level is probably reached by the inclusion of adopted children. The percentage of women who progressed from first to second birth is similar. It went down from 96 per cent in 1978 to a low of 65 per cent in 1985, rose again to 84 per cent in 1987, and finally fell to circa 58 per cent in 1991. The share of women with a second child who progressed to a third child started to slowly decrease after 1969, but, even so, it was higher than 90 per cent until 1973. It fell by three to four percentage points annually for the rest of the decade and by almost fourteen percentage points in 1980. Uneven development between 1981 and 1988 was followed by a final decline. Nevertheless, in 1991 it still stood at 28 per cent. The ratio for higher-order births showed similar tendencies. In 1995 all ratios are supposed to have stayed at more or less the same level as in 1991.[10] Their sharp drop in 1992 may be spurious.

There are several conclusions to be drawn from these figures. They tell us that apart from the rising marriage age, the dramatic fertility decline in the 1970s was also caused by the reduction of higher-order births. This trend

Chart 8 Period parity progression ratios 1955–95

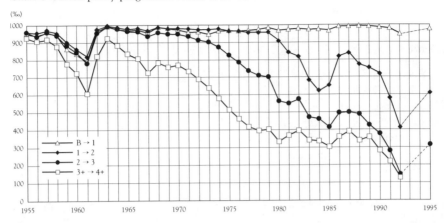

	B → 1	1 → 2	2 → 3	3+ → 4+
1955	956	962	960	925
1961	797	818	781	606
1963	994	996	992	924
1965	972	979	964	833
1967	960	966	935	726
1970	975	981	947	770
1975	969	964	825	515
	966	965	784	463
	970	957	736	417
	975	957	710	396
	985	959	700	403
1980	969	908	562	340
	974	841	558	388
	980	817	571	404
	974	681	465	339
	975	623	465	338
1985	967	653	423	312
	990	817	494	333
	992	837	499	390
	993	773	488	338
	990	752	425	358
1990	987	718	375	280
	980	579	278	219
	949	411	147	127
1995	977	609	315	

Note: B → 1 denotes progression from birth of woman to woman's first child, 1 → 2 progression from first to second birth, etc.

Sources: Calculations for 1955–92 on the basis of data from the 1982, 1988 and 1992 fertility surveys in: Feeney and Yuan Jianhua 1994, 387; Feeney and Wang Feng 1993; State Family Planning Commission 1997; figures for 1995 microcensus data from Zhang Weimin, Yu Hongwen and Cui Hongyan 1997, 49

accelerated at the start of the one-child campaign. Moreover, the figures confirm that the irritating rise of the TAFR in the period 1981 to 1982 was primarily due to earlier marriages, and to a small increase in third and higher-order births. Second births did not play a role: they just stagnated. Fertility plummeted in the mid-1980s, before socioeconomic developments and policy changes after 1984 drove it up again. As the smaller fertility peak of 1986 to 1988 was not accompanied by a further decline of the marriage age, it seems to have been caused mainly by an upsurge of second births, and to a lesser extent of third births. Overall, the parity progression ratios bear witness to a fall in fertility levels during the 1980s. However, this fall has been neither linear, nor did it reach the spectacularly low levels of the birth plans.

Retrospective studies on Chinese fertility before 1970 have also investigated the link between parity progression and the sex of preceding children. They come to the conclusion that the likelihood of women progressing to a further birth was highest if no son had yet been born. Interestingly enough, the second highest ratios occurred if there were sons but no daughter. The lowest were recorded for women with many sons and a few daughters, in which case women had their children stopped earlier. These results substantiate the prevalent son preference of Chinese culture, though not in an unmitigated form.[11]

Whenever recent fertility surveys have been analysed for the influence of the sex of a previous child on childbearing, they have confirmed the importance of the son preference. Between 1970 and 1990, the proportion of the TFR caused by sex preference increased from just 2 to 8 per cent. Parity progression differentials between families with and without sons have widened considerably, and the dislike of those who have exclusively sons has vanished – at least in the evidence to hand at national level. Invariably, parity progression is highest for families with only daughters. In this respect, there is no difference between urban and rural areas. Among the factors influencing the likelihood of having another child, son preference usually ranks third or fourth place, immediately after variables distinguishing urban–rural residence, different localities and policy phase. Depending on time, place and the overall fertility level, the likelihood of a second birth for women with one daughter can exceed that for women with one son by up to 160 per cent. The alarming rise of the sex ratio at birth during recent years points in the same direction. The overall effect of son preference in the 1980s has been calculated as raising the TFR by 0.2 points.[12]

12.4 Birth spacing

In terms of birth spacing, the record prior to 1970 again shows conspicuous regularities. Birth intervals are shortest for women who have had only daughters before and longer if only sons have been born before; they are longest where both sons and daughters are among the preceding births. This points to exactly the same kinds of preferences as discussed above, and corroborates the thesis of traditional forms of fertility control in China. It has been speculated that these have been connected to the near non-existence of premarital intercourse, low coital frequency afterwards, delayed co-residence of young couples and long periods of breast-feeding with differences for girls and boys. Such practices may also explain the rather low conception rates and long intervals between marriage and births that have been calculated for the period 1944 to 1972. They incidentally call into question the often advanced argument that cultural factors of long standing enforce swift childbearing after marriage. Before the advent of birth planning, the time between marriage and birth of a first child in China was prolonged. Although this declined from the lengths observed during the civil war in the late 1940s, it still amounted to almost three years in the mid-1950s. About the same time span passed between the birth of a first and second child; for the following birth interval it was slightly longer. During the Great Leap all intervals rose significantly; afterwards they fell again.[13]

The longer birth intervals propagated by the 'Later, Fewer, Longer' policy of the 1970s did not produce the desired results. Instead of being prolonged, the interval between marriage and first birth shortened; the following interbirth intervals changed only slightly. These developments were helped by the fact that there was no explicit requirement for the interval between marriage and first birth. Strict rules demanding adherence to a late-birth age of 24 were introduced only during the 1990s. One can only speculate on the reasons for these developments. They have been explained as the desire to counter official birth planning and to make up for late marriage, as low continuation of contraceptive measures, or rising marital intimacy due to more self-determination of partners. It seems that in the 1970s a currently valid norm to produce the first child shortly after marriage developed. A careful examination of the 1988 fertility survey also reaches the conclusion that premarital conceptions with consequent marriages noticeably increased in the 1970s and 1980s. Whereas they remained at a low level of less than 2 per cent throughout the period 1950 to 1975, they climbed to more than 5 per cent by 1987. The percentages for better educated urban strata were more than twice as large as among peasants.[14]

While the general trend of developments is uncontested, precise information on birth intervals, in particular on developments since the beginning of the one-child campaign, is contradictory, indicating greater problems of calculation. Table 28 assembles data from the last two national fertility surveys of 1988 and 1992. These show wide discrepancies for the years 1986 and 1987. In a comparison with the retrospective results of the 1982 survey, the 1988 survey arrives at the same time curve, albeit at a markedly higher level for the interval between marriage and first birth. Rival calculations for the 1980s largely parallel the 1988 results for the interval between marriage and first birth but show no downward trend for the first and second interbirth periods.[15] Reaching a definite conclusion on the basis of these unreliable data does not seem possible. In combination with information on the average marriage age and age-specific fertility however, they reconfirm that during the mid-1980s the late-birth recommendation of 24 years was not enforced and came to be widely disregarded. Spacing rules between first and second births were observed even less. Tighter enforcement of spacing requirements in the 1990s makes it likely that intervals increased over the past decade. The data from the 1992 fertility

Table 28 Average birth intervals 1950–92 (years)

	M → 1	1 → 2	2 → 3
1950	3.57	2.93	2.52
1955	2.92	3.09	3.17
1960	3.24	3.03	3.15
1965	2.58	2.74	2.92
1970	2.38	2.68	2.99
1975	2.05	2.87	3.14
1979	1.87	2.98	3.02
1980	1.88	2.91	2.78
1981	1.75	2.93	2.67
1982	1.79	2.85	2.65
1983	1.78	2.54	2.43
1984	1.72	2.23	2.28
1985	1.64	1.95	2.01
1986	1.50 (2.02)	1.55 (3.79)	1.57 (3.44)
1987	1.16 (2.01)	1.21 (3.81)	1.19 (3.51)
1988	1.99	3.83	3.64
1989	1.97	3.69	3.62
1990	1.90	3.75	3.45
1991	1.92	3.75	3.56
1992	2.07	4.14	3.50

Note: M → 1 denotes interval between first marriage of woman and woman's first child, 1 → 2 between first and second birth, etc. 1950–87 figures hail from the 1988 fertility survey, those for 1986–92 from the 1992 survey. Overlapping data for 1986 and 1987 come from both surveys with the latter one in parenthesis.

Sources: Liang Jimin and Chen Shengli 1993, Vol. 3; Jiang Zhenghua 1995

survey indicate an abrupt increase in 1986 or 1988. Rising intervals are also claimed by more recent surveys from the late 1990s. According to the Birth-Planning Commission, the percentage of women whose first birth was an infant girl and who gave birth to another child within four years fell from 61 per cent in 1990 to 17 per cent in 1997.[16] But the glaring inconsistencies of the data for 1986 to 1988 and the discrepancies in other retrospective calculations continue to constitute an element of uncertainty in the assessment of fertility levels.

12.5 Provincial differentials

Regional data document that birth control and socioeconomic developments have brought about an increasing variation of fertility levels in China. Until 1963, the total fertility rates[17] of the provinces generally moved within a well-defined band of an average four to eight children per woman. The Manchurian provinces, the Southwest and parts of the Northwest were at the high end of this range, and Qinghai and Xinjiang ranked lowest. In all regions fertility dropped sharply during the crisis years of the Great Leap Forward, before it recovered in 1962. The extent of the drop differed however, and regional variation in fertility levels increased. Shanghai was the only province-level area where a sustained decline of fertility commenced already in the 1950s. After 1957 the total fertility rates in this metropolitan region never regained their former level of approximately five to six children per woman.

When the second birth-planning campaign started to show effects in 1964 to 1965, Beijing and Tianjin joined Shanghai to become the lowest-ranking fertility areas in the country – a place which they have been occupying ever since. Other regions followed after some delay and noticeable variation. In 1968 to 1969 fertility increased everywhere. These were years immediately following the most violent phase of the Cultural Revolution, but administrative functions had not yet been fully restored. Again, Shanghai was the first place where the total fertility rate resumed its downward course in 1969. With the third birth-planning campaign after 1970, regional variation dramatically increased. Whereas modernized coastal regions registered a fast decline of fertility, the majority of the hinterland provinces moved at a much slower pace.

As demonstrated by Table 29, a great diversity of circumstances prevailed in the first half of the 1980s, too. Some provinces stabilized at low fertility levels, others recorded wild fluctuations, while yet others continued their slow descent from a high fertility plateau. It is only since 1986 that dispersion has again diminished, but it continues to remain distinctly higher than in the first two decades of the People's Republic. Its precise extent is hard to pin down, since provincial fertility indicators have been revised even more than the national figures, where regional adjustments can offset each other. Revisions of 1978 to 1981 data for Hebei, Jilin, Jiangxi, Guangdong, Gansu and Qinghai provinces have been particularly striking. Heilongjiang, Anhui and Fujian, Guangxi, Henan, Hubei, and all Southwestern and Northwestern provinces have also suffered from large-scale misreporting. In the 1990s, data problems spread to all the other provinces. The Birth-Planning Commission found it prudent to revise total fertility rates resulting from the 1995 micro-census upward by an average of 22 per cent. Such revisions even ranged between 30 and 40 per cent in eight provinces.[18]

This is why figures from the last 1990 census serve as the main point of reference for the following analysis. The overview is based on earlier studies of regional population dynamics in China; it takes contemporary pronouncements of Chinese politicians on birth-control implementation in the provinces as a starting point.[19] Grouping the provinces by both present and past birth rates, four different fertility areas may be discerned.

The first group of low-fertility provinces comprises the three municipal regions of Beijing, Tianjin and Shanghai, the three Manchurian provinces of Liaoning, Jilin and Heilongjiang in the Northeast, and the two provinces of Jiangsu and Zhejiang in the Lower Yangzi region adjacent to Shanghai. Altogether, 21 per cent of the Chinese population live in this area. More than 40 per cent live in cities and towns, and fewer than 5 per cent belong to minority nationalities.[20] The area as a whole boasts per capita figures for gross domestic product that are more than twice as high than the average for China. Other indicators of income and welfare also rank top among all Chinese

Table 29 Total fertility rate by provinces 1957–95 (children per woman)

	1957	1965	1973	1979	1981	1984	1987	1989	1992	1995
China	6.21	6.02	4.51	2.80	2.58	2.19	2.49	2.25	1.54	1.78
Beijing	6.07	3.50	2.55	1.41	1.55	1.39	1.64	1.42	1.54	1.11
Tianjin	7.17	4.39	2.30	1.51	1.41	1.45	1.69	1.73	1.54	1.41
Hebei	5.69	5.92	3.82	2.33	3.09	2.35	2.81	2.47	1.41	1.78
Shanxi	5.84	5.91	4.69	2.24	2.16	2.55	2.45	2.49	1.83	2.02
Inner Mongolia	6.70	6.38	4.20	2.49	2.56	2.28	2.23	2.13	1.63	1.94
Liaoning	7.29	5.54	3.35	2.15	1.94	1.11	1.89	1.55	1.30	1.49
Jilin	6.98	6.58	4.17	2.72	2.05	1.46	1.83	1.84	1.39	1.46
Heilongjiang	7.13	6.10	4.97	2.85	2.27	1.64	1.92	1.81	1.35	1.46
Shanghai	6.32	2.55	1.56	1.23	1.20	1.11	1.51	1.37	1.54	1.05
Jiangsu	6.09	5.39	2.67	1.93	1.97	1.51	2.04	2.05	1.05	1.49
Zhejiang	6.99	6.23	3.24	2.32	2.23	1.51	1.70	1.61	0.98	1.50
Anhui	5.40	5.47	4.87	3.52	2.98	2.35	2.73	2.63	1.51	1.71
Fujian	6.73	6.46	5.30	2.84	2.79	2.76	2.33	2.63	1.88	1.75
Jiangxi	6.08	6.54	6.76	4.01	3.34	3.07	2.88	2.68	1.32	2.11
Shandong	6.40	5.61	3.66	2.48	2.12	1.95	2.70	2.22	0.93	1.14
Henan	5.67	6.13	4.93	3.19	2.81	2.13	3.06	2.98	1.70	1.66
Hubei	7.22	6.18	3.98	2.95	2.50	2.51	2.98	2.59	2.01	1.91
Hunan	6.30	6.76	4.55	2.58	3.00	2.43	2.71	2.49	1.11	1.47
Guangdong	5.73	5.61	4.81	3.74	3.83	2.82	2.76	2.60	2.14	2.21
Guangxi	6.15	6.55	5.60	3.98	3.81	3.95	3.57	2.99	1.95	2.24
Hainan		4.64	5.06	4.35	4.43	3.59	3.08	3.10	2.40	2.64
Sichuan	6.12	6.29	5.43	2.03	2.61	1.66	2.24	1.92	1.17	1.74
Guizhou	6.25	7.04	6.72	4.18	4.46	3.68	3.65	3.24	2.44	2.62
Yunnan	6.17	6.71	5.54	3.99	3.73	3.27	3.19	2.78	1.91	2.39
Tibet		4.33	5.09	4.81	5.16	4.75	4.21	4.35	2.40	3.43
Shaanxi	6.74	5.33	4.43	2.93	2.42	2.55	2.98	2.74	2.10	1.92
Gansu	5.75	6.68	5.82	3.51	2.86	2.65	2.60	2.37	1.51	2.16
Qinghai	3.97	5.57	5.97	4.17	3.94	2.74	2.71	2.62	2.40	2.41
Ningxia	6.71	5.66	5.75	4.76	4.00	3.25	3.12	2.67	2.40	2.08
Xinjiang	5.12	6.66	5.43	3.70	3.58	4.15	3.71	3.37	1.77	2.35
Coeff. of Variation	12.0	17.4	27.2	33.1	33.0	37.0	25.3	26.2	26.6	28.5

Note: total fertility rate by summation of age-specific rates; 1992 figures for Beijing, Tianjin and Shanghai as one average for these three municipal regions; 1992 figures for Hainan, Tibet, Ningxia and Qinghai as one average for these four regions. Data for 1995 are adjusted figures differing from the microcensus results.

Source: Census, microcensus and national fertility survey data from Chen Shengli and Coale 1993; Jiang Zhenghua 1995; ZJSN 1997, 97–98

regions. Life-expectancy is up to more than 71 years. Educational levels are similarly two or three times above the national average, while illiteracy is at only 16 per cent. Most of this area is densely settled with an extremely high man–land ratio in the Lower Yangzi region. At the same time it also contains the wide, empty spaces of China's Northeastern frontier, the major destination of domestic migration streams in the twentieth century. A high degree of urbanization and industrialization is the common denominator between the Northeast and the Lower Yangzi region.

Birth control began early in most of these provinces and municipal regions: in Shanghai and other cities in the late 1950s, and in the Northeast and surrounding areas of Beijing and Shanghai in the first half of the 1960s. Other parts of Jiangsu and Zhejiang followed later; in these two provinces a regular decline of fertility rates commenced after 1969. Today, birth-planning regulations in this area tend to be rather strict, enforcement is tight and IUD use widespread. The fertility level of the whole area averaged 3.2 between 1970 and 1977. Since 1978 it has been constantly below the replacement level, leading to an ageing process far ahead of other regions. In 1989, the total fertility rate amounted to a weighted average of 1.8; it was lowest in Beijing and Shanghai, and highest in Heilongjiang and Jiangsu. Forty per cent of mothers with one child had progressed to a second, only 25 per cent of those with a second child to a third. The marriage age was nearly one year higher than the national average. Since 1992 the national surveys give an extremely low total fertility rate of supposedly 1.2 children per woman for this area.

The fertility indicators for the second group of provinces that includes Inner Mongolia, Shandong and Sichuan, with 19 per cent of China's total population, are slightly higher. Here, the total fertility rate for the whole area averaged 4.4 between 1970 and 1977; it was down to 2.1 in 1978, where it also remained in 1989. The latest results from the period 1992 to 1995 amount to an average of 1.3. In contrast to the first group of provinces, these three regions saw larger oscillations of birth rates in the 1980s. In addition, their marriage age is clearly lower and approximates the national average. According to the last census, nearly 60 per cent of mothers with one child had given birth to a second, 33 per cent of those with a second child to a third. Although indicators for plan compliance show less efficient enforcement, birth control is still judged to be relatively stable. To a greater degree than in the first group it relies on sterilizations. In Shandong and Sichuan, which have long histories of rural birth control reaching back to 1970, partially even to 1956, this also includes a larger share of vasectomies.

In itself, the area is rather disparate, ranging from populous and peasant-dominated Sichuan – with a poplulation of 115 million people the giant among China's provinces – to sparsely inhabited Inner Mongolia with a much higher urban element. Shandong is densely settled, too. In terms of urbanization it occupies the middle ground. Minority shares also vary widely between nearly 20 per cent in Inner Mongolia to under 1 per cent in Shandong. Per capita figures for gross domestic product are just half the size of the first group and somewhat below the national average, as are other indicators for economic performance, educational attainment and standards of living. Life expectancy is below 69 years.

With eleven provinces (Hebei, Shanxi, Anhui, Fujian, Jiangxi, Henan, Hubei, Hunan, Guangdong, Shaanxi, Gansu) and altogether 47 per cent of

China's population, the third group is the largest of the four fertility areas. It consists mainly of the agrarian hinterland of North and Central China, plus a few provinces of the South and the Northwest. All these provinces belong to the traditional core region of the country, and national minorities number under 3 per cent. Urbanization rates amount to an average 22 per cent – half the size of the first group and also less than the second. Population density in the agrarian areas can be very high. Other socioeconomic indicators are about the same as in the second group. The biggest deviant case is coastal Guangdong, one of the wealthiest and most modernized provinces of the country. Contrary to widely held assumptions on the link between economic and demographic development, it also features a rather elevated fertility level. Stubbornly, it has long held fast to the envied privilege of granting a universal second-child permit to its peasantry. High fertility also characterizes Fujian, another coastal boom region since the initial economic reforms.

With a few local exceptions in Hubei and Hunan, the eleven provinces started to implement rural birth control only in the 1970s. In a number of cases, percentages for second or third births started to fall only as late as 1978 to 1980. Even in 1989 some 80 per cent of women with one child gave birth to a second, 50 per cent of those with a second child followed up with a third. Against this background, it is not surprising that the decline of the total fertility rate for the area as a whole was slower than in the first two regional groups. It came down from an average 4.6 between 1970 and 1977 to 3.1 in 1978, wavered in the 1980s and stood at 2.6 in 1989. Dubious figures from the period 1992 to 1995 put it at approximately 1.5. It is in these still largely traditional provinces that the fate of Chinese birth planning is ultimately decided. Here the silent war between the state and peasant China is also waged in the toughest terms. Non-compliance with regulations and misreporting of data are highest in the country, as is the percentage of enforced sterilizations.

Eight provinces and autonomous regions on the Western and Southern periphery of China constitute the final distinct fertility area: Guangxi, Hainan, Guizhou, Yunnan, Tibet, Qinghai, Ningxia and Xinjiang. They make up only 13 per cent of the Chinese population total but occupy nearly half of the national territory. Within this area, national minorities figure prominently in birth-planning matters as they make up an average of 40 per cent of the population. The share is lowest in Hainan (17 per cent) and highest in Tibet (96 per cent). In many respects, the area is backward in development. Indicators for gross domestic product per capita, educational attainment or life-expectancy (66 years) trail noticeably behind the national average. Only illiteracy surpasses it. Urbanization levels are uneven, and industrialization is lagging behind.

Balanced by high infant mortality, fertility has always been high in this part of China. The total fertility rate for the period 1970 to 1977 averaged 5.5, in 1978 it had fallen to 4.0. Its 1989 level of 3.0 was based on largely the same parity progression ratios as in the third fertility area. Only progression to fourth birth was higher; it involved more than 55 per cent of all women with a third child. In relative terms, these are already depressed levels. Until the introduction of birth control for the national minorities in the mid-1980s the percentages were still higher. Equally conspicuous have been the low marriage ages in this area. Early-marriage rates of 30 to 50 per cent have been particularly prevalent in the Muslim regions of the Northwest. Since 1992 a total fertility rate of 2.0 for the whole area has been claimed. It is hard to determine to what extent this is caused by the concealment of births or by stiffer birth control for the minorities that is gradually replacing the more liberal policies of the past. Nevertheless, nearly all provinces in this group continue to uphold a general second-child permit policy for the rural population. Exceptions are Guangxi and Guizhou, which have tied this privilege to other conditions, or Hainan, where it is linked to a vague exhortation to demonstrate 'special circumstances'.

12.6 Urban and rural fertility levels

Disaggregation of national fertility data along the urban–rural divide provides further clues to China's population development. Although the precise share of the rural element in the total population varies according to different and rather complicated definitions, an approximation has it coming down from about 90 per cent in 1949 to an average 83 per cent between 1962 and 1978 and thenceforth to 70 per cent in 1998. Peasants thus continue to exert the dominant influence at the overall birth level. Urban fertility changes are not unimportant, though. In many respects they act as the harbinger of future developments in the rest of the country.

Moreover, different urbanization levels are one of the most important factors underlying regional fertility differentials. They can range from around 70 per cent in the case of the three centrally administered metropolitan regions Beijing, Tianjin and Shanghai to low levels of 15 to 18 per cent in some agrarian hinterland provinces. Multivariate analysis establishes the urban–rural divide as one of the most important variables influencing the likelihood of having another child. Measuring the distance between urban and rural fertility is therefore an essential step in understanding both trends in time and variation in space.[21]

There are no good disaggregated benchmark figures for urban and rural fertility from the pre-revolutionary period, but the data presented for the People's Republic in Chart 9 indicate that until the end of the 1950s an urban–rural fertility gap had not yet developed. In some years the urban figures equalled those from the villages, in other years they trailed only slightly behind. As far as the aggregated urban population of China was concerned, no impact of the first birth-planning campaign may be detected. In contrast to the fertility rates, urban birth rates of the 1950s may even have surpassed their rural equivalents.[22] This was probably caused by strong rural–urban migration, which helped to slant the urban age structure in favour of younger age groups and thereby raised the number of births.

In terms of fertility rates, the Great Leap Forward affected the urban areas just as much as the countryside – only the scope of compensatory childbearing in 1963 was smaller. Urban fertility began to fall in 1964 and, with a small deviation in 1968, it continued on a sustained downward course until 1980. The influence of the second birth-planning campaign starting in 1962 can be clearly

Chart 9 Urban and rural total fertility rates (children per woman) 1949–99

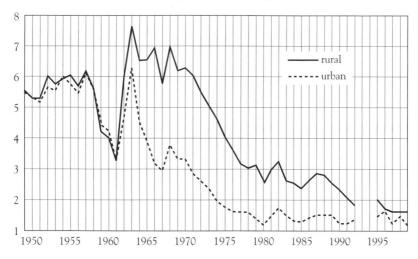

	Urban	Rural
1949	5.51	5.54
1957	6.17	6.21
1961	3.13	3.31
1963	6.34	7.65
1965	3.78	6.53
1967	2.90	5.78
1970	3.22	6.31
1975	1.76	3.97
1979	1.40	3.10
1985	1.27	2.36
1990	1.21	2.32
1995	1.48	2.00

Note: total fertility rate by summation of age-specific rates; 1990–92 as adjusted rates for agricultural and non-agricultural population; 1995 microcensus figures as adjusted by the State Statistical Bureau, the unadjusted results for urban and rural areas amount to 1.16 and 1.58, respectively; 1995–99 figures for urban areas as weighted averages for cities and towns

Sources: national fertility survey results from Chen Shengli and Coale 1993; Jiang Zhenghua 1995; 1995 microcensus and 1996–99 annual survey results from ZRTN 1997–; Zhang Weimin *et al.* 1997, 47

felt; after 1970 it merged with the third one. When urban birth-control activities were largely discontinued during the Cultural Revolution, a small resurge of urban fertility took place, but the limited extent of this resurge indicates that other developments in urban society also played a role.

Urban fertility rates of the 1980s show the familiar picture of oscillation with the two peaks of 1981/82 and 1986/87. The former is more pronounced than in the national-level figures. It is clearly associated with the abolition of particularly tight rules for late marriage in urban areas and with the consequent sharp fall in the average marriage age. As a result, the resurge of urban fertility during 1981/82 was mainly concentrated in the age groups 20 to 23.[23] In contrast, the second fertility peak of 1986/87 reached the urban areas in attenuated form only. This indicates that the resurgence of second births at the end of the decade was mainly a rural affair. Urban fertility data from the 1990s point to a further decline of birth numbers in the cities, even if some of the figures look spurious. For major cities of the country, natural population growth close to zero is claimed. Since 1994, Shanghai municipal region reports negative growth of its resident population.

Over the years, there have been some marked changes in the correlation of urban and rural figures. While urban fertility fell sharply after 1962, rural fertility remained high. Its overall level surpassed that of the 1950s, even if the ups and downs of the Cultural Revolution are considered. In this way, the 1960s witnessed the emergence of a large urban–rural gap in childbearing behaviour. It was only after 1970 that rural fertility levels started to fall dramatically. A further plunge is indicated for the period after 1990. Its precise extent is hard to measure; both adjusted and unadjusted figures vary spectacularly and await confirmation from a new census. The general trend, however, seems to be clear: despite some fluctuation in the 1980s, the urban–rural difference in fertility levels is shrinking. At the end of the 1990s it was reduced to little more than one child per woman. In some unconfirmed figures of the 1990s it almost vanished.

Chart 10 takes a closer look at the urban–rural fertility gap as far as component age groups are concerned. It demonstrates that at the turn of the 1970s to the 1980s urban fertility was largely concentrated in the age group 25 to 29. In the mid-1980s it shifted back to earlier childbearing at 20 to 24 years of age. Even in 1995 this trend was not fully reversed. There has been a constant drop of fertility rates among urban women aged 30 to 34; figures for the age group 35 to 39 have seen some slight upward movement, and those for women in their forties continue to be negligible. To a small extent, early childbearing in the age group 15 to 19 has reappeared even in the cities.

In the countryside the clustering of fertility rates in the age group 25 to 29 has never been as marked as in the cities. Childbearing at 20 to 24 years of age was still quite frequent in 1978; after 1981 it again increased, contributing more than half the total fertility in 1995. In a similar vein, until 1989 the comeback of early childbearing at ages 15 to 19 continued to be more pronounced in the countryside than in the cities. The contribution of older age groups to total fertility has continued to be greater than in the cities, too. Only the 1995 micro-census shows a sharp decrease, probably due to under-reporting of second and higher-order children. This pushes up the percentage of children born to women under age 30.

Chart 11 finally looks at the composition of the total fertility rate by birth order. It again points to the fact that urban fertility was already low at the outset of the one-child campaign. From its level in 1978 it vacillated only slightly downward or upward. The chart further demonstrates that second and higher-order births diminished sizeably in the early 1980s, increased in the second half of the decade, and may have decreased again in the 1990s.

Chart 10 Total fertility rates for urban and rural areas by component age groups 1978–95

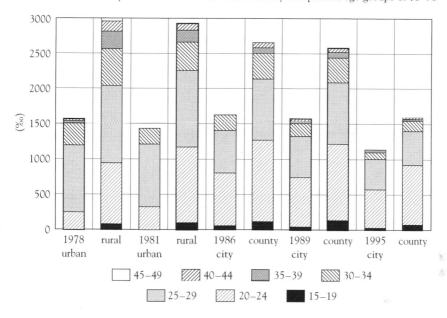

	1978		1981		1986		1989		1995	
	urban	rural	urban	rural	city	county	city	county	city	county
TFR	1565	2976	1409	2924	1686	2619	1517	2539	1090	1556
15–19	1.8	15.6	2.4	17.6	8.2	22.4	9.4	25.9	4.6	13.1
20–24	48.4	173.8	62.0	213.0	147.9	230.0	139.6	218.7	108.9	170.3
25–29	188.4	220.4	179.2	221.0	123.7	174.1	118.1	173.1	86.5	94.2
30–34	61.8	102.4	32.0	78.2	39.8	72.4	32.0	65.7	20.4	29.6
35–39	1.8	52.6	5.2	35.8	0.9	23.3	9.8	23.2	4.4	6.4
40–44	2.8	25.4	0.4	15.8	1.9	8.3	2.0	7.0	0.9	1.9
45–49	1.0	5.0	0.6	2.8	0.4	1.6	0.6	2.0	0.3	0.8

Note: total fertility rate in ‰ by summation of age-specific rates; 1995 figures are unadjusted

Sources: fertility survey 1982 in ZJSN 1986; microcensus 1987 in ZRTN 1988; census 1990 in Zhongguo 1990 nian renkou pucha ziliao, Vol. 3; microcensus 1995 in: 1995 nian quanguo 1% renkou chouyang diaocha ziliao

Parity progression ratios for the cities from the period 1955 to 1981 period put these figures into historical perspective. In the mid-1950s the ratios up to progression from fourth to fifth child were uniformly above 90 per cent. The share of urban women having four or more births began to fall sharply from 1963 to 1967 and then again after 1969. However, in 1975 the ratio of urban women with one child who progressed to having a second child still amounted to nearly 90 per cent; and the ratio for progression from a second to a third child continued to stand at almost 50 per cent. In the rural areas, where the fertility decline started later, these figures for 1975 even amounted to 98 per cent and 88 per cent, respectively.[24] The birth order components of rural TFRs therefore look different

Chart 11 Total fertility rate urban and rural areas by component birth orders 1978–95

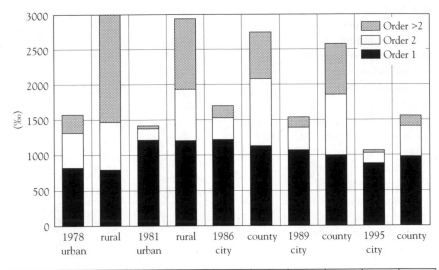

	1978		1981		1986		1989		1995	
	urban	*rural*	*urban*	*rural*	*city*	*county*	*city*	*county*	*city*	*county*
TFR	1565	2976	1409	2924	1686	2619	1517	2539	1090	1556
Order 1	808	784	1194	1176	1188	1107	1055	980	846	956
Order 2	498	671	182	740	332	954	330	867	166	435
Order >2	259	1519	34	1007	165	657	133	690	30	135

Note: total fertility rate in ‰ by summation of age-specific rates; 1995 figures are unadjusted

Sources: fertility survey 1982 in ZJSN 1986; microcensus 1987 in ZRTN 1988; census 1990 in Zhongguo 1990 nian renkou pucha ziliao, Vol. 3; microcensus 1995 in 1995 nian quanguo 1% renkou chouyang diaocha ziliao

by necessity. The 1978 fertility rate for third and higher-order births, for instance, continued to be larger than either the one for first or the one for second births.

Chart 11 shows a continuous downward trend for the combined total fertility rate in rural areas. However, this trend is disrupted once data for 1982 and 1987 are added. In contrast to the cities, there was no real decline of rural fertility rates for second births in the 1980s. Massive changes, though, are recorded in respect of fertility rates for higher-order births, which in 1989 were down to almost one-third of their level in 1978. Nevertheless, higher-order births continue to be anything but negligible. A large drop is claimed only in the 1995 micro-census results.

12.7 Fertility by social characteristics

By virtue of their better educational and health institutions, their tighter housing conditions, their higher standard of living and their better job opportunities, the cities boast many conditions conducive to birth control.

Apart from the easier-to-measure factors on the economic and social plane, cultural aspects such as gender roles, family structure or changes in values and needs also play a part. Political differences in comparison to the villages such as stricter birth-planning regulations and greater governmental capacity stand out. In this sense, the difference between urban and rural birth levels already provides some clues to the mechanisms involved in Chinese fertility dynamics. Data available from the fertility surveys of 1982, 1988 and 1992, the 1987 micro-census and the fourth national census in 1990 permit further study of some of these factors.[25] With due regard to the conceptual difference between childbearing ideals and actual fertility levels, this information may be combined with the discussion of family size and sex preferences in section 7 above.

In order to measure the social characteristics of women of reproductive age, the 1990 census figures are clearly the most exhaustive source. They tally with most of the 1987 microcensus data and are the preferred point of reference in the following discussion. Unfortunately, the cruder tabulations from the 1982 census do not lend themselves to easy comparison. The 1992 fertility survey data are very extensive, too, but they suffer from a general lack of reliability. Moreover, the various datasets are not always compatible in terms of methodology. Nevertheless, they provide basic knowledge on fertility levels by educational standard, occupational group and industrial sector. The analysis of the census figures may be further refined by differentiating age groups and birth orders within social strata. Some historical perspective is provided by internally consistent data for the 1980s from the 1988 fertility survey and by a retrospective analysis of the preceding 1982 fertility survey results. Directly enumerated material from earlier decades or representative information on developments in the 1990s is sparse, however.

Chart 12 presents some of the census data for checking the influence of education on the fertility record. It shows a stringent relationship between the years spent in school by women of reproductive age and the hypothetical number of children born to these women. The different categories for educational attainment, however, include those with unfinished school attendance at the specified level. Moreover, school systems have be varyied over the decades. The various types of institutions listed in the chart may therefore be taken to mean the following total years of school: four to six (elementary), seven to nine (junior high), ten to twelve (senior high, technical), and thirteen to sixteen (college, university). Calculated for a maximum of sixteen years of school attendance from the primary to tertiary level, the data show that each additional year in school reduces the TFR by a statistical average of more than 0.1. The effect of education is greatest when those with a completed elementary and a completed senior high school education are compared. It then amounts to an overall difference of nearly one child for four to six additional years of education.

Disaggregating the figures by age group and birth order highlights the following trends: Persons with a low educational standard (illiterates, elementary or junior high school level) show a strong concentration of early childbearing within the age group 20–24. Their age-specific fertility rates for the

Chart 12 Total fertility rates for educational levels by birth order 1989

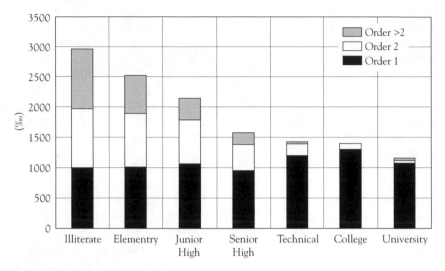

1989	Illiterate	Elementary	Junior High	Senior High	Technical	College	University
TFR	2959	2519	2143	1581	1440	1412	1161
Order 1	1007	1009	1065	964	1213	1314	1090
Order 2	974	894	726	420	195	90	63
Order >2	979	617	352	196	32	8	7

Note: total fertility rate in ‰ by summation of age-specific rates

Source: Census 1990 in Zhongguo 1990 nian renkou pucha ziliao, Vol. 3

following age group 25 to 29 get depleted, while childbearing beyond age 30 makes up under 17 per cent of the TFR. First births are even more concentrated in the young age groups. Among illiterates and women with only an elementary school education, very early childbearing in the age group 15 to 19 still contributes 21 per cent and 13 per cent to the TFR, respectively. These women also produce their second children rather early, usually between 23 and 25 years of age. The TFRs for higher-order births among less educated persons are raised, too. These births usually occur in the age brackets 25 to 34.

In contrast to this group, the fertility rates of persons with senior high school education are spread more evenly within the age group 20 to 29. While the majority of first children are still produced between by women between 20 and 24 years of age, the relative decline in the age group 25 and 29 is not as steep as among people with only a few years of education. Second children are mostly born to women of between 25 and 29 years of age; some are produced until age 34, after which the numbers dwindle fast. The greatly reduced number of higher-order births is distributed more or less evenly in the age groups 25 to 34. For the three following groups of persons, who have been attending either technical school, college or university, a very regular pattern may be discerned.

At each of these levels a progressively steeper decline of fertility rates sets in. It not only involves a drop in overall fertility but also a progressively larger decrease of second and higher-order births. At the same time, childbearing is increasingly delayed, so that the highest fertility rates for these women are recorded in the age group 25 to 29. It is here that most first children are born. The few second and higher-order children are mostly produced at ages 30 to 34 or still later in life.

Scrutinizing the retrospective data shows that between 1955 and 1967 urban areas have consistently displayed a negative relationship between education and fertility levels, the latter decreasing with additional years of schooling. Rates for city women with high school education began to fall in the mid-1950s, at a time when contraceptive counselling and the provision of contraceptive devices started during the first birth-planning campaign. The fertility decline for other strata was slower, so that both intra-urban variation and rural–urban differences increased. The greatest impact of education on fertility levels was recorded in the period 1964 to 1967. This changed in the 1970s, when differentials became reduced.[26]

Information from the 1988 fertility survey reveals that with the advent of the one-child policy fertility variation among women with different educational levels resurged during the period 1979 to 1984, before it fell back again at the end of the decade. The largest TFR reductions during the 1980s were recorded for women with higher education. Combining these data with attitudinal surveys among young and well-educated city girls points to far-reaching changes among this segment of the population. Between 1981 and 1987 fertility of less educated persons diminished, too, while that of women with high-school education increased. In the suspect figures of the 1992 survey, fertility variation by educational level decreased markedly. This was caused by sharply falling birth levels among undereducated peasants and seems to be exaggerated.

The continuous rise of female school enrolment since the 1950s has certainly bolstered the role of education in reducing fertility levels. The force of the drive for raising mass education may be gleaned from the fact that the third population census in 1982 still recorded 92 per cent of all women at and above 50 years of age as illiterates. For women in the age groups 15 to 49, who all entered their reproductive period after the founding of the People's Republic, that percentage dropped to 36 per cent; in the fourth census eight years later it was down to 15 per cent. While in 1982 the average woman of childbearing age had completed about five years of education, in 1990 this figure was up to about 5.5 years.[27]

Such data may be combined with corresponding information for the advancement of women along the ladder of academic success. On closer look, however, the numbers conceal just as much as they reveal. For once, fertility by educational attainment displays strong interaction with the rural–urban dichotomy. Table 30, which shows the 1990 census data on fertility and education by place of residence, demonstrates that within educational strata fertility falls along the categories of city, town and county population. The drop for junior and senior high school levels is particularly steep. It affects nearly half of the women of reproductive age, where urban residence rather than

Table 30 Total fertility rate for educational level by place of residence 1989

	Illiterate	Elementary	Junior High	Senior High	Technical	College	University
TFR	2959	2519	2143	1581	1440	1412	1161
Cities	2556	2080	1545	1288	1303	1332	1113
Towns	2547	2081	1656	1429	1607	1653	1569
Counties	2998	2589	2505	2055	1603	1592	1625

Note: total fertility rate in ‰ by summation of age-specific rates

Source: Census 1990 in Zhongguo 1990 nian renkou pucha ziliao, Vol. 3

educational standard is the dominant factor. Urban-rural fertility variation for the other types of education is less. Neither does it have a major effect, as most illiterates and women with only elementary school education live in the countryside (86 per cent), while most women who have attended higher institutions of learning reside in the cities (82 per cent). This is why in these cases the national averages closely resemble either the county or city figures. Similar conclusions on the fertility effects of residence and educational attainment have been reached on the basis of the 1982, 1987 and 1992 datasets. Furthermore, all studies demonstrate strong variation from one province to another. An earlier analysis of the 1982 fertility survey resulted in the discovery that with the rising age of women the effect of education on fertility levels decreased, while that of rural–urban and provincial differences increased.[28] Unfortunately, the materials at hand do not permit a repeat of such calculations for later years.

An even more fundamental problem arises in the interpretation of data, as the crude census figures are insufficient to discuss how higher educational levels lower fertility rates. Causal relationships become increasingly complicated if the interplay with other factors is examined. The only clear point seems to be evidence that longer schooling delays marriage and thereby leads to a shortening of the period for childbearing. Beyond this observation, however, only hypotheses may be formulated. It is likely that higher education changes needs and values, as it has done in the West. Under this premise, striving for personal liberties and self-fulfilment, career goals and higher consumption would be key factors in lowering child numbers. The latter point may be reinforced by rising costs for the upbringing of children through longer periods of schooling and less income from child work. Education that is raising the status of women and giving them more say in family planning matters *vis-à-vis* husbands or relatives may also be included in the bracket of changing values and needs. Greater contraceptive knowledge would be another mechanism by which education lowers fertility.

But there are also hypotheses conflicting with the thrust of these arguments. In most cases, marriage and childbearing still furnish sufficient reason for being expelled from Chinese schools. Access to more education thus signifies more freedom of choice and loss of individual liberty at the same time. Even more important is the fact that most better educated persons are employed in the urban state sector, where they are more susceptible to government pressures for birth control later on. The picture becomes still more blurred when village and county-level case studies are taken into account that show how other local differences can largely mute or even cancel the influence of education on fertility behaviour. Instead of individual traits, a combination of political, economic and social factors at community level thus play a decisive role. Variance of fertility levels among different localities is therefore often greater than differences between social strata crossing community lines. This holds true for education as well as for other individual characteristics commonly cited as determining factors of childbearing.[29]

The same caveats also hold true for the analysis of fertility figures arranged according to occupational groups. They, too, are subject to the influence of residential factors, provincial and local differences. Not surprisingly, the figures in Chart 13 once again confirm the overriding importance of the rural–urban fertility gap. Classifying persons by occupation rather than residence even exacerbates the difference, since only rural inhabitants who largely work in

Chart 13 Total fertility rates for occupational groups by birth order 1989

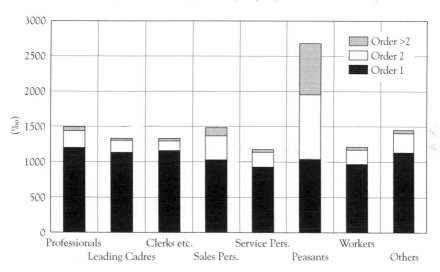

1989	Profess.	Lead. Cadres	Clerks etc.	Sales Pers.	Service Pers.	Peasants	Workers	Others
TFR	1474	1333	1313	1476	1186	2679	1228	1466
Order 1	1194	1129	1153	1041	929	1038	975	1115
Order 2	237	179	152	335	207	934	204	267
Order >2	43	26	17	100	50	707	49	48

Note: total fertility rate in ‰ by summation of age-specific rates; all data excluding the military

Source: Census 1990 in Zhongguo 1990 nian renkou pucha ziliao, Vol. 3

farming, forestry, husbandry, fishing or hunting are covered under the rubric peasant, while villagers in non-agricultural pursuits are excluded. Vice versa, persons with urban registration but predominantly agricultural activity would also be subsumed under the peasant group. The census data show that this categorization creates overall differences of more than one child in the TFR. They are smallest for first birth and invariably increase with birth order. In 1990 nearly 75 per cent of all women of reproductive age were counted as peasants.

More interesting are the differentials between the various non-agricultural occupations. Generally, they remain small. Slightly higher TFRs with concomitantly larger shares of second and higher-order births are observed for sales personnel. This is probably caused by the fact that this occupational group also includes rural peddlers, retailers, wholesalers, or those working for government procurement. Educational levels in this group are low. The most depressed fertility rates are recorded for workers and service personnel, who tend to be urban inhabitants but may include some villagers with full-time jobs in private, town or township enterprises. Most members of this group are wage-earners and vulnerable to pressures for birth control. This also holds true for other mostly urban groups such as professionals, leading cadres and clerks. In 1989, their TFRs were artificially raised by the heaping of age-specific rates for first births. This indicates that these groups have been most affected by changes in the marriage age. Cadres, incidentally, were also conspicuous for having more early births during 15 to 19 years of age than all other groups, apart from peasants and sales personnel.

The occupation-specific fertility figures accord with further data on births by economic branches in which women were employed. These statistics offer few additional insights and therefore are not reproduced here. They may be simplified further by bracketing the various branches under the three industrial sectors. This was also how the 1988 fertility survey handled the data. It also supplied information for non-employed women, namely housewives, laid-off women, students and others. Non-employed women trailed behind peasant women but always had more children than women employed in the secondary or tertiary sector. A comparison of the figures for 1980 and 1987 was striking for the lack of change it revealed. Only the TFR for women employed in the secondary sector (industry, mining and construction) had decreased slightly; TFRs for unemployed women or those with jobs in the tertiary sector had increased slightly; those for peasant women had even gone up by 13 per cent. This was a vivid expression of the situation at the height of the 1987 fertility peak. No representative data exist from the more recent period.

Nor are there sufficiently representative data at national level that allow us to examine the relationship between income and fertility. This is a subject of crucial importance in the course of China's economic reforms. It is also an area where continuity or break with older patterns of Chinese culture is at issue. Fieldwork in China from the first half of the twentieth century and historical data point to a positive association between wealth, power and large numbers of children. It seems that in contrast to nineteenth-century Europe, it was the rich rather than the poor who had many children.[30]

Weak evidence exists from the 1986 migration survey in seventy-four cities and towns, which, as a side product, also supplied approximate data on the urban population's monthly income at that time and the number of children ever born to various age groups of women. It invariably produced the highest number of children for non-earning women. In all other cases, it resulted in a strongly negative relationship between both variables for the cohorts of women born before the founding of the People's Republic. For the younger generations the relationship was beginning to weaken.[31] For women born after the early 1950s and who became marriageable after 1972, the income group made little difference. This could hint at the impact of the birth-planning campaign, which may have cancelled the family economics of childbearing. It is, however, open to debate whether the earlier circumstances may be interpreted as rising wealth having led to fewer children in the urban population. Personal monthly income in 1986 is a rather feeble indicator for illuminating the economic situation of older women at their time of childbearing decades before.

Information for the rural areas is also limited and largely localized. This is unfortunate, because the relative weakness of occupational differentiation in the countryside, the lack of social provisions from the state and the significance of the household economy turn income into an even more important indicator there. The few village samples indicate a wide variety of circumstances prevailing in the countryside. A number of rural surveys, all conducted during 1992, may serve as an example.

A larger survey in Shaanxi province produced a positive relationship between income and fertility in the lower income brackets; in the higher income groups, though, the number of children levelled off. Parallel village surveys in Jilin and Heilongjiang resulted in a consistently positive relationship apart from the second highest income group, where the average number of children fell, while a study conducted in two counties of Shandong and Hebei provinces respectively resulted in a negative relationship. In these areas, increases in wealth generally were associated with reduced fertility. In one of the four counties under investigation, however, the rich had more births than the poor, because fine collection had effectively turned into a mechanism for buying off further molestation from state-promoted birth control.[32]

Similarly inconclusive are the empirical studies on migrant fertility, another hotly debated topic ever since the numbers of migrants and floating population spectacularly increased in the course of economic reforms during the 1980s. In contrast to the host of articles and regulations on migrant childbearing, reliable fertility data for this stratum are scarce and many pertinent studies rather superficial. This has to do with the intrinsic disparateness of the migrant population and the difficulties of conducting survey work among them. According to the definitions of the 1990 census, approximately half of this population group are rural–urban migrants; one-third move between different urban places; the rest either change from one rural residence to another or relocate from urban areas to the countryside. Real migrant numbers are larger than in the census results, though. In the mid-1990s they amounted to an estimated 50 million persons with more sustained types of movement. Migrants and floating population include those with a permanent change of abode, seasonal workers, commuters, transferred personnel, job-hunters, dependants and a multitude of other subgroups. Often, travellers and other short-term transients are also included.

Usually, the floating population of young rural–urban migrants in search of work receives most public attention. It is this group which poses the worst social problems for urban administrations and the highest threat in terms of breaching the one-child policy. This applies not so much to unmarried migrant wage-earners in more or less regular employment, who usually live in crammed dormitories, have a long workday and are geared to income–maximizing activities, but rather self-employed migrant couples in economic sectors and living conditions that are hard to control and that offer incentives for increasing family manpower.[33]

Relevant reports continue to estimate that the majority of migrants have two or more children and that more than half – in some areas even 80 to 90 per cent – of all unauthorized births are produced by them. The reports emanate mostly from the coastal boom regions, which serve as the preferred areas of attraction, or some densely settled hinterland provinces such as Sichuan, Hunan or Anhui, which function as major exporters of excess manpower. The difficulties accumulate in large cities, where tight birth control for registered residents conflicts with implementation problems among in-migrants. Quantifying this gap, however, poses almost insurmountable problems. All empirical investiga-tions of migrant fertility suffer from a diverse handling of definitional questions, sampling problems and the non-cooperation of respondents, who do their best to obscure the real situation.

A Shanghai survey of 1988 claimed only 0.6 per cent unauthorized births among women with permanent household registration in the city, contrasting with 15.3 per cent for migrant women. The latter group included all types of short-term transients with no permanent registration in the city. In other surveys conducted in the cities of Chongqing and Xi'an two years later, the figures amounted to 6.6 per cent and 11.8 per cent, or 0.7 per cent and 14 per cent, respectively. The ongoing acute nature of the issue is indicated by the fact that in 1995 the Birth-Planning Commission continued to point to provinces with two-thirds of all unauthorized births in the migrant group. A 1996 migrant survey in Beijing resulted in about 30 per cent unauthorized births among migrant women since 1991. Guangdong data from the 1995 micro-census, however, yielded a disproportionally low fertility of the migrant population.[34]

Although none of the figures cited above are very reliable, the existence of a disproportional number of unauthorized births among certain segments of the migrant population is not in doubt. But there is a further way of looking at the issue. Experience in many developing countries shows that rural-urban migration ultimately lowers fertility by adaptation to city life. The time horizon for this process varies, though, and depends on such factors as migrant selectivity, employment patterns, finding a marriage partner, the permanency of migration, and the links entertained with the places of origin. In most cases, fertility rates of rural–urban migrants tend to hover somewhere between rural and urban levels.

Some Chinese research suggests that this pattern exists in China, too. It also corroborates the plausible thesis that migrant fertility in major cities is generally lower than the corresponding rates for small cities or towns. But the figures from the 1986 migration survey in seventy-four cities and towns and the 1988 national fertility survey, which are cited in support of these arguments, are heavily biased and do not suffice for verification.[35] A small study of a group of migrant women in Beijing highlights the problems. It notes the persistence of strong expectations for swift childbirth after marriage and finds little evidence of migration prolonging that interval. Noting abnormally high sex ratios for children born prior to migration, it speculates on a selection process that releases young women for migration once they have fulfilled their obligation to produce a son.[36] This indicates the complex nature of the social processes involved and should serve as a warning against premature generalizations.

12.8 Fertility by ethnic group

National minorities constitute another important subgroup for the population dynamics of China. With a combined share of only 6 to 8 per cent of the total population, their impact on national fertility levels remains limited. The picture changes, however, once a regional perspective is adopted. Most areas of West China are characterized by large minority shares, ranging from still solid majorities in Tibet (more than 90 per cent in 1990) and Xinjiang (more than 60 per cent) to other parts of the Northwest (Qinghai, Ningxia) and Southwest (Guangxi, Guizhou, Yunnan), where ethnic groups constitute between 30 and 40 per cent of regional population totals. Shares in Inner Mongolia (about 20 per cent) and parts of the Northeast, the former Manchuria, are above average, too (10 to 15 per cent in Liaoning and Jilin).

The ethnic mix of the provinces has been subject to diverse political, social and economic influences. The greatest role has been played by factors such as low standards of living with extremely high mortality levels among many ethnic groups, heavy Chinese in-migration for both political and economic reasons, mixed marriages with Han-Chinese, reshuffling of territorial organization, the strength of historical identities, and changes of ethnic self-designation due to either assimilationist pressures or restorative incentives. Despite official recognition of minority status in the 1950s, the forces provoking minority decline prevailed until the end of the 1960s. Since the tightening of birth control in the 1970s, however, birth-planning privileges for the national minorities have reversed this situation, so that minority shares are growing. The end of the Cultural Revolution, the re-extension of minority privileges and the start of the one-child campaign in the late 1970s boosted incentives for minority growth even more. The most spectacular rates of increase were recorded in Liaoning, Inner Mongolia, Hunan and Guizhou, where massive reclassification of nationality status took place. Yet, without exception, all other provinces have also witnessed minority growth outpacing rates of increase for the Han majority. Since the mid-1980s, the gradual introduction of birth planning for the minorities has reduced, though not levelled, the fertility gap.[37]

Demographic data on minority populations from earlier decades are very limited. As a rule, they are restricted to birth and death rates defined by territorial units with a large Han-Chinese component. Even more problematic are simple population totals for individual minorities, since their changes may be caused by either natural increase or reclassification. It is only with the third population census of 1982 and the national fertility survey of the same year that more rigorously defined fertility data for the minorities become available. The fourth census of 1990 then extended this database to all separate ethnic groups. Retrospective data document that in 1964 the TFR for the combined minority total (6.72) surpassed the TFR for the Han-Chinese (6.03) by more than 10 per cent. By 1981 the differential had grown to almost 80 per cent (4.49 versus 2.52). This was almost entirely caused by the widening fertility gap in the rural areas, where Han-Chinese birth numbers shrank much more rapidly than minority ones. In contrast, the fertility of minority women in urban areas more or less equalled that of the Han-Chinese majority. These trends, of course, were the products of the second birth-planning campaign among the Han-Chinese. Whereas their fertility rates declined due to political intervention, population developments among the minorities in rural areas were characterized by a greater degree of spontaneity. [38]

Census results for the fertility rates of individual minorities are collected in Table 31. Viewed together with figures from the 1988 fertility survey and some earlier local investigations,[39] they indicate that in the second half of the 1980s the fertility decline among the minorities accelerated. In 1989, the differential between total fertility rates for the Han-Chinese and all national minorities had shrunk. The latter surpassed the former by only 27 per cent. However, the aggregate total for all ethnic groups also hides a wide variety of circumstances. Minorities with fertility rates below replacement level (Koreans, Manchu, Russians, Xibe) contrast with other ethnic communities among whom birth numbers remain excessively high (most Turkic groups from Xinjiang and some Southwestern border tribes). Mongols, Hui and small Northeastern minorities evince fertility levels close to the Han-Chinese majority. For most South-western groups, however, the total fertility rate ranges between 2.3 and 3.6 – clearly lower than in 1981 but still noticeably above the national average. Larger minorities with high birth numbers include the Uygur, the titular nation and most important group of Xinjiang Autonomous Region, the Tibetans, as well as the Zhuang, Miao and Yi of the Southwest. While elevated fertility is largely due to higher-order births during later stages of life, some Southwestern and Northwestern minorities are also noted for early marriages and childbearing below 20 years of age. Prominent examples are the Uygur and Kirgiz of Xinjiang, as well as the Yi, Thai, Hani and other nationalities settling in Yunnan.[40]

Among the national minorities both different urbanization rates and education levels lead to greater fertility variation than among the Han-Chinese. This mechanism also works if various minorities are compared. Highly

Table 31 Minority population and total fertility rate by ethnic group 1981/82, 1989/90

	Million 1982	TFR 1981	Million 1990	TFR 1989
Han	936.675	2.51	1039.188	2.30
All Minorities	67.239	4.24	91.323	2.91
North:				
Mongol	3.411	3.16	4.802	2.24
Northeast				
Manchu	4.305	2.10	9.847	1.86
Koreans	1.765	1.91	1.923	1.56
Xibe	0.084		0.173	1.88
Dagur	0.094		0.121	2.25
Evenki	0.019		0.026	2.56
Oroqen	0.004		0.007	2.35
Hezhe	0.001		0.004	2.39
Central-South:				
Zhuang	13.383	4.67	15.556	2.91
Tujia	2.837	3.26	5.725	2.55
Li	0.887	7.55	1.112	3.51
She	0.372		0.635	2.32
Shui	0.287		0.347	3.57
Mulam	0.090		0.161	2.71
Maonan	0.038		0.072	2.44
Jing	0.013		0.019	2.73
Southwest:				
Miao	5.021	5.34	7.384	3.16
Yi	5.454	5.21	6.579	3.08
Tibetans	3.848	5.84	4.593	3.81
Buyi	2.119	5.15	2.548	3.53
Dong	1.426	4.45	2.509	2.67
Yao	1.412	5.39	2.137	2.94
Bai	1.132	3.26	1.598	2.81
Hani	1.059	5.66	1.255	3.40
Thai	0.839	3.65	1.025	2.68
Lisu	0.482	5.60	0.575	3.60
Gelao	0.054		0.438	2.83
Lahu	0.304		0.412	3.73
Va	0.299		0.352	3.98
Naxi	0.252		0.278	2.44
Qiang	0.103		0.198	2.92
Jingpo	0.093		0.119	4.22
Blang	0.058	6.38	0.082	4.24
Pumi	0.024		0.030	3.38
Achang	0.020		0.028	3.72
Nu	0.023		0.027	4.24
Jinuo	0.012		0.018	2.98
Deang	0.012	5.82	0.015	5.04
Monba	0.001		0.007	4.19

	Million 1982	TFR 1981	Million 1990	TFR 1989
Dulong	0.005	6.10	0.006	5.41
Lhoba	0.001		0.002	3.99
Others	0.800		0.752	3.51
Northwest:				
Hui	7.228	3.13	8.612	2.62
Uygur	5.963	5.59	7.207	4.66
Kazakh	0.908	6.85	1.111	4.76
Dongxiang	0.280		0.374	3.44
Kirgiz	0.113		0.144	6.16
Tu	0.160		0.193	2.81
Salar	0.069		0.088	4.15
Tajik	0.027		0.033	6.16
Uzbek	0.012		0.015	2.77
Russians	0.003		0.014	1.62
Baoan	0.009		0.012	2.66
Yugur	0.011		0.012	2.13
Tatar	0.004		0.005	3.37

Note: total fertility rate by summation of age-specific rates

Sources: calculated from data in ZRTN 1988, 1992, 1996; Yang Kuifu 1995; Yuan Yongxi 1996, 52; Zhang Tianlu and Huang Rongqing 1996, 328; *Minzu gongzuo*, 20 December 1996

urbanized groups with above-average education and long life-expectancy generally display reduced fertility. Vice versa, most high-fertility groups tend to be characterized by a predominantly rural character, a high incidence of illiteracy and raised mortality levels, especially among infants. But there are exceptions to these rules. Most Xinjiang minorities, for example, show high fertility rates despite low rates of illiteracy; sometimes even urban residence barely reduces their birth numbers. Parallels with Muslim populations in other parts of the world are striking. Cases as such weaken the relationship between the TFR and the social indicators for the various ethnic groups. For life-expectancy the correlation coefficient stands at -0.64, for urbanization rate -0.50, for illiteracy 0.47.[41]

The moderate strength of these associations points to the existence of other causal factors in fertility dynamics, most important among them being the more lenient policies for higher-order births, the dissimilar degree of enforcement capacity, and the divergent contraceptive rates. The level and composition of the latter vary greatly between different nationalities.[42] A recent macro-analysis of 1990 county-level birth data, which includes the titular nationality of autonomous areas as one variable among others, reaches similar conclusions. To a large degree, ethnic fertility differentials arise from differences in other socioeconomic factors such as educational levels, urbanization rates and social products. Divergent birth-control policies play an overriding role. Once these factors are controlled for, the role of the ethnic element becomes reduced in most cases. Yet it still remains, and it can sometimes even outrank other socioeconomic factors to become the most important determinant of fertility. This might have been the case for Uygur and Tibetan autonomous areas, where it pushed up fertility levels, while it reduced them in Mongolian, Hui, Manchu, Tujia and Yi autonomous areas. Although methodical considerations may invalidate some of these results, the differentials serve as a reminder of other factors transcending the standard fare of development indicators.[43]

As a subgroup of the total population, China's national minorities are often treated as one entity. This is also the dominant approach in demographic analysis, where most ethnic groups are considered too small to deserve separate treatment. But focusing on the role of ethnicity draws a host of social and cultural items into the picture, among them religious beliefs, marriage and matchmaking customs, family structures, gender roles or child-feeding practices. They underline the importance of factors that are usually neglected in formal analyses and lead to the realization that the ethnic groups of China are not a homogenous mass but rather an extremely rich and diversified universe.

13 Changes in sex and age structure

13.1 Sex at birth and in age groups 0–4

One of the most heatedly debated topics raised by Chinese population policies is the distorted sex ratio at birth. In contrast to the normal situation, where this indicator amounts to between 1050 and 1070 new-born boys per 1000 new-born girls, indicators for China have risen way beyond this margin. Simply put, some 120,000 infant girls were missing in the third census of 1982. Seven years later, this number climbed to nearly 600,000 in the adjusted census figures for 1989. Without the adjustments it would have reached more than 1 million. As the distorted sex ratio extends beyond infancy, and mortality for young girls between 1 and 5 years of age is abnormally high, too, the dimensions of the problem are still greater, and they continue to grow. During recent years the sex ratio for age group 0 has continued to rise, and the annual number of missing infant girls amounts to almost 1 million.[1]

The issue has at last been recognized within China. When evidence for the distortion together with reports on infanticide or child abandonment accumulated in the mid-1980s, politicians and population specialists reacted defensively at first. While treating infanticide or abandonment as isolated cases, they doubted that international standards for the sex ratio were applicable in the Chinese case. Instead of the standard value, it was claimed that a range up to 1100 was normal for the country. Speculations linked it to unknown racial characteristics of the Chinese.[2]

It was only after the 1990 census with its even more biased sex ratio at birth that concern grew. Since then, sensational reports on the missing girls and their long-term effects have appeared in China too, and a new series of national conferences has been devoted to the issue. They have called the distortion 'ominous', acknowledged the increasing severity of the problem since the early 1980s and discarded the idea that the imbalances can be traced to biological specifics of the Chinese race. Quite the opposite: human intervention has been unequivocally blamed for the situation. Meanwhile, measures have been taken. Regulations and controls for checking infant deaths and sex-specific abortions have multiplied, and the sex ratio at birth is increasingly used as an integral part of regular birth-control evaluations.[3] However, different reasons are advanced for explaining the number of missing girls, and the link to the one-child policy remains a sensitive issue.

The population figures at hand elucidate major aspects of the problem. They offer yet another example of the possibilities and limits of demographic analysis in the evaluation of birth-control performance. They also permit intimate glimpses into patterns of gender preferences among different strata of the population, and the social dynamics produced by the interplay of cultural and political forces. Census materials and survey results can be compared, and detailed items on births and infant deaths during the preceding years, the total of children ever born, and the number of survivors can be used for exploring internal data consistency. Furthermore, the figures can be disaggregated for the provinces and for various social strata or combined with other relevant data. Finally, they can be used for a retrospective calculation of past trends, which can then be related to contemporaneous developments in other areas.

But although such exercises expose revealing patterns, they cannot correct really determined falsification. All calculations and adjustments employ certain standard indicators, biological rules, and methods gained from historical materials and international experience. They also exploit disagreements between various datasets. Ultimately, however, they have to assume the accuracy of at least some of these figures and thus can be discounted, once all figures are falsified in a systematic way over a long period. This can be demonstrated most easily for infant mortality. There exists no sophisticated formula for resurrecting dead infants whose births were never recorded, whose deaths never entered the registers, who are consistently omitted from all later tabulations of children ever born, and who cannot emerge as survivors afterwards. Keeping these caveats in mind, the available information results in the following picture.

As shown in Table 32, the first two censuses of 1953 and 1964 resulted in sex ratios that moved within the normal range. Although no precise figures for sex at birth are available from these counts, the data for age group 0 approximate them. This age group comprises infants from the day of their birth up to their completed first year of life. Due to usually higher male than female mortality, the sex ratio of this age group should normally be a little lower than the sex ratio at birth. The same effect should show up for the following age groups. Chinese sex ratios for infants and young children as determined by the first and second census stay within the normal range for the first three years of life, but, contrary to the general rule of slow decline over the following years of life, they gradually increase, thus hinting at higher female mortality caused by neglect. With the third census of 1982 the sex ratios become distorted. Girls are missing at birth as well as in the age groups 0–2. With each new population count the imbalance becomes more severe. The latest figures for the period 1997 to 1998 show a sex ratio of 1170 for the age group 0. While the bias is clearly more serious in the countryside, the figures for the cities are also skewed.

The census and micro-census data thus suggest that the problem has newly arisen and become aggravated in the course of the one-child campaign. Retrospective time series from the 1982 and 1988 fertility surveys may be used for checking this hypothesis. They show that infant girls have also been missing among the cohorts born between 1936 and 1950. For these generations, sex

Table 32 Sex ratio of births and cohorts ages 0–4: national totals 1953–95 (males per 1000 females)

	Births	Age group				
		0	1	2	3	4
1953		1049	1056	1066	1086	1049
1964		1038	1053	1064	1070	1087
1981	1085					
1982		1076	1078	1074	1067	1062
–, cities		1069	1072	1075	1068	1068
–, counties		1077	1079	1073	1066	1060
1986	1109					
1987		1096	1116	1100	1099	1087
–, cities		1084	1076	1093	1097	1091
–, counties		1100	1121	1105	1103	1087
1989	1113					
1990		1118	1116	1101	1091	1085
–, cities		1089	1088	1080	1074	1073
–, counties		1122	1120	1104	1094	1086
1992	1159	1157				
–, non-agricult.	1074					
–, agricultural	1172					
1995	1156					
1995		1166	1211	1213	1192	1150
–, cities		1119	1153	1128	1099	1109
–, counties		1177	1231	1237	1209	1163

Sources: Calculations from census and microcensus materials. For 1953: Zhongguo renkou congshu 1987–93. For 1964,82: Zhongguo 1982 nian renkou pucha ziliao; own calculations from data in ZRTN 1988. For 1987: Zhongguo 1987 nian 1% renkou chouyang diaocha ziliao. For 1990: Zhongguo 1990 nian renkou pucha ziliao. For 1992: State Family Planning Commission 1997, 70. For 1995: 1995 Quanguo 1% renkou chouyang diaocha ziliao; ZRTN 1997

ratios at birth between 1138 (average for 1936–40) and 1083 (average for 1946–50) result from the *ex post* tabulations. The ratios stay at an average level of 1090 in the first decade of the People's Republic and fall to less than 1070 during the Great Leap Forward. For the 1960s and 1970s, data from both fertility surveys overlap. However, whereas in the 1982 survey biased sex ratios between 1070 and 1080 start to reappear in 1964, the imbalances level out in the 1988 survey, only to re-emerge in 1980.[4] The record for the second and third birth-planning campaigns is therefore inconclusive. It may be that faulty memory and problems of survey design are at work. This would seem to apply mostly to the 1988 survey, whose retrospective data for the 1960s and 1970s are considered to be weak.

Chart 14 forcefully demonstrates that the biased sex ratio is caused exclusively by second and higher-order births. There is a tendency for it to become exacerbated with each successive delivery. In contrast, the distribution of first births between the two sexes remains normal. This has also been the rule for all other large-scale enumerations. The same situation prevails if authorized and unauthorized births are compared with each other. The sex ratios for births within plan then tend to stay inside the normal range, while those for births outside plan are abnormally high (rising from 1092 in 1981 to a maximum of 1194 in 1986). This indicates a strong connection between sex ratio and birth-control policy.[5] Somewhat surprisingly, the proportion of missing girls among the non-agricultural population in urban areas is even greater than among peasants, rural–urban migrant workers, and other parts of the population classified under agricultural registration status.

Chart 14 provides further evidence of the prevalent son preference. It points to a situation where the sex of the first child is left to providence, but male offspring are favoured by human intervention afterwards. The urge to secure the birth of a son grows if it has not been satisfied during preceding births, thereby driving up the sex ratio for following births. Even in the cities there has been no value change on a mass scale for countering this impulse. As infanticide or large-scale concealment can be ruled out under the urban conditions of tight control, sex-specific abortion seems to be the most plausible explanation for the high sex ratios there. It seems that the better educational standards and the more sophisticated medical amenities of the cities facilitate rather than hinder sex screening. Of course, such linkages apply only to the small percentage of second and higher-order children born in the urban areas. Because the overwhelming number of second and higher-order births is produced in the countryside, the rural sex ratio for the total number of births still surpasses the urban one.

The census data for the countryside in Chart 15 corroborate the thesis of progressively greater son preference, and they illustrate the importance of

Chart 14 Sex ratio by birth order and registration status 1989 (M/F × 1000)

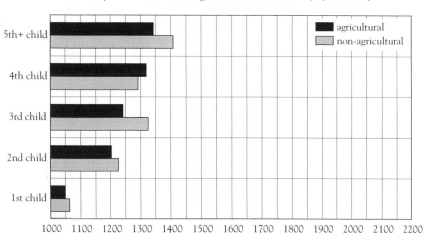

Source: 1990 census data from Kua shiji de zhongguo renkou (zonghe juan) 1994, 45

Chart 15 Sex ratio by birth order and existence of son, agricultural population 1989 (M/F × 1000)

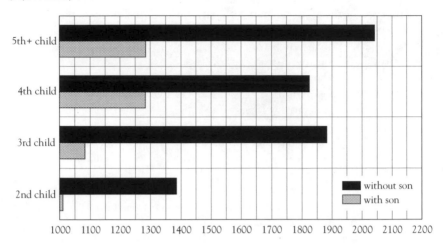

Source: 1990 census data from Wu Cangping 1996, 202

gender roles and the social mechanics at work even more graphically.[6] If no son has been born before, the proportion of missing girls among second, third, fourth and fifth births assumes huge proportions. The same trend shows up in a retrospective analysis of 1990 census data for the period 1971 to 1980. While infant girls are tolerated, maybe even desired, if the first or second child is a boy, they are once again conspicuously lacking among fourth and fifth children. Numbers of such higher-order births have fallen sharply in the villages, too. In the census figures for 1989 they comprised little more than 10 per cent of the birth total. But if they do occur, a son is clearly preferred, even if another boy has already been born before.

The data discussed so far are national figures. Table 33 provides figures to show the situation in the provinces. It documents that regional differences of the sex ratios at birth have been small during earlier decades but have increased sharply in the 1980s. The greatest gaps developed between the censuses of 1982 and 1990. In most cases, differentials for the rural county population are responsible for this state of affairs. Some regions have always evinced sex ratios below the national average. This applies to all provinces of the Southwest and Northwest with their high shares of minority populations. Son preference among these ethnic groups is markedly less than among the Han-Chinese majority; some of the minorities give women a much better deal than in traditional Chinese culture. Only Zhuang and Manchu display sex ratios at birth that rival the Han-Chinese figures. Raised levels above the national average, albeit to a lesser degree, are also recorded for the Yao, Tujia, Hani, Mulam, Blang and Pumi nationalities of the Southwest. For all other ethnic groups, most notably all Muslim groups of the Northwest, the proportions are more or less normal. Among some of them, sex ratios in the age group 0 also document a preponderance of infant girls. Tibetans are the most prominent

Table 33 Sex ratio of cohorts age 0 by provinces, 1953–90 (males per 1000 females)

	1953	1964	1982	1990	cities	counties
Beijing		1055	1067	1080	1070	1097
Tianjin	950		1059	1103	1050	1171
Hebei	1052	1040	1072	1126		1132
Shanxi	1107	1059	1086	1092	1087	1090
Inner Mongolia	1068	1052	1062	1088	1085	1088
Liaoning	1036	1038	1064	1104	1060	1138
Jilin	1018	1027	1074	1078	1049	1087
Heilongjiang		1025	1056	1067	1055	1075
Shanghai		1063	1067	1048	1056	1032
Jiangsu		1048	1077	1149	1122	1155
Zhejiang	1074	1062	1076	1180	1063	1204
Anhui	1069	1054	1113	1107	1087	1108
Fujian	1077	1056	1060	1107	1121	1099
Jiangxi	1034	1046	1069	1117	1113	1118
Shandong	1040	1030	1092	1163	1146	1167
Henan	1052	1022	1099	1171	1131	1174
Hubei	1037	1040	1067	1094	1089	1093
Hunan		1045	1064	1104	1074	1109
Guangdong	1067	1063	1104	1120	1129	1107
Guangxi	1056	1041	1107	1223	1146	1231
Hainan				1148	1098	1134
Sichuan	1039	1026	1072	1117	1077	1126
Guizhou	1032	1017	1055	1003	1000	1000
Yunnan	1018	1009	1041	1072	1047	1074
Tibet			994	1003	1001	1002
Shaanxi	1046	1047	1091	1121	1112	1122
Gansu		1015	1055	1117	1095	1119
Qinghai	1023	1020	1022	1039	1060	1036
Ningxia	1035	1017	1051	1064	1074	1064
Xinjiang	997	1026	1039	1035	1051	1033
China	1049	1038	1076	1118	1089	1122

Sources: own calculations according to sex- and age-specific provincial population figures of the 1953, 1964, 1982 and 1990 censuses in Zhongguo renkou congshu 1987–93, 32 vol.; Zhongguo 1982 nian renkou pucha ziliao; ZRTN 1988; Zhongguo 1990 nian renkou pucha ziliao; Sheng renkou pucha bangongshi 1992–93, 85 vol.

example. Cultural factors as well as different environmental conditions are at the root of these differences.[7]

While the minority regions of West China are underdeveloped, other areas with low sex ratios are located in the more modernized parts of the country. Predominantly, these are provinces and municipal regions of the North and Northeast featuring high urbanization rates and an elevated social product. Beijing, Tianjin and Shanghai, as well as the three Manchurian provinces, belong to this group, but strangely enough, hinterland provinces such as Shanxi,

Inner Mongolia and Hubei are also included. At the other end of the spectrum, some affluent provinces, such as Zhejiang and Guangdong, have always displayed an above-average sex ratio. In the last two censuses they have been joined by densely settled, agrarian provinces such as Shandong, Henan and Guangxi. At present, the latter region displays the highest sex ratios of China; peak values have been reached in its better-off areas.[8] Jiangsu, Hainan and Anhui have figured among the cases with very high sex ratios, too. It is conspicuous that many of these provinces figure among areas with a high incidence of infanticide or child abandonment in the past. This group includes both modernized and backward regions.

Apart from the ethnic mix, there is no clear-cut rule for predicting the provincial ratios from social, economic or political characteristics, such as fertility and development levels or differences in birth-control policies. The province-level data do not support the hypothesis that different kinds of policies for second births, among them second-birth permits for couples with one daughter only, function as an underlying cause for the divergences. The varying extent of urban-rural differences in the provinces also does not lend itself to easy generalization. In most cases, the sex ratio for the cities is lower than in the countryside, and this difference increased between 1982 and 1995. Ratios for the county population in age group 0 exceeded those for the cities by 0.7 per cent in 1982, 1.5 per cent in 1987, 3.0 per cent in 1990 and 5.2 per cent in 1995. In the 1990 census, differences in Tianjin, Liaoning, Zhejiang and Guangxi were particularly large, but there were also adverse examples, where the urban sex ratio at birth exceeded that for the countryside. Such instances could be found in the well-developed coastal regions of Shanghai, Fujian and Guangdong as well as in the Northwestern regions of Qinghai, Ningxia and Xinjiang.[9] The irregular nature of such differentials is one of the facts on which Chinese authors base their refutation of a link between the one-child policy and the issue of missing infant girls.

Better clues for explaining the distorted sex ratio are provided by education- and occupation-specific data, which are available from the 1990 census. For the rural areas, they point to a linear relationship between a higher number of years in school and a rising proportion of missing girls. In the cities, the sex ratios for births by persons with junior or senior high school education fall behind those for illiterates or women who have attended elementary school, but they increase again for academics. These results confirm a conclusion that has already been reached: apparently, better schooling is used for more effective sex screening. Since more years of education reduce the number of childbirths, high sex ratios caused by a large number of unreported infant girls are unlikely for the better educated segment of the population. Infanticide can largely be ruled out, too. The only remaining explanatory factor is sex-specific abortion.

Equally revealing are the relationships that show up if sex ratios are analysed for the influence of the occupation factor. Such analysis reveals that in the countryside, births among peasants, cadres and other white-collar personnel are most heavily slanted in favour of sons. These social groups are either hard to control or enjoy disproportionate access to knowledge and power. Sex ratios at birth for children of workers in the non-agricultural branches of the rural economy are significantly lower. Similarly low are sex ratios at birth among urban workers and cadres, who seem to be subject to tighter control. In the cities, specialists and technical personnel, as well as employees of the trade and service sector, are most successful in securing male offspring. Many members of these groups either work in deregulated sectors of the economy or again possess high educational qualifications.[10]

While disaggregation of data may identify regional or social patterns in the distribution of infant girls and boys, it does not answer the question as to the means by which the bias is created. Four major mechanisms are usually cited that may complement each other or compete as rival explanations. The factor with the seemingly highest explanatory value is under-registration of births. Its lower margin is indicated by cross-checking census figures for births, infant deaths, children ever born and survivors. These figures allow testing of the assumption that not all infants who died soon after delivery are later reported as births, and that figures for all children ever born and survivors may indicate a larger number of births than is directly enumerated.

The census results show that excess survivors and infant deaths omitted in the direct enumeration of births amount to altogether 4.3 per cent of infant girls and 2.1 per cent of infant boys born in 1989. By adding these children to the directly recorded birth figures, the sex ratio at birth is reduced from 1139 to 1113. It may be lowered further to 1090 if 1986–91 survey data on hospital deliveries are accepted as representative. The hospital conditions rule out infanticide or under-reporting, leaving only prior sex-specific abortion as a plausible explanation for the still remaining difference to a normal sex ratio of 1050 to 1070. Depending on where the standard value for the sex ratio is precisely set and whether calculated or directly enumerated births are used for comparison, these various figures mean that in 1989 between 40 and 70 per cent of the excess value in the sex ratio was caused by under-registration.[11] Under-registration may be even greater if allowance is made for the possibility that the survival rates used in the calculations are based on inaccurate figures. Conventional wisdom would have it that most concealed births re-emerge at some later date, when vaccinations, school enrolment, housing or employment formalities are required. But this may take years and would become visible only in later population counts.

Closely linked with the problem of under-registration is the increasing number of adoptions, which were covered in the 1988 fertility survey. As already discussed in section 8, the number of children given away for adoption greatly increased in the 1980s, and about 75 per cent of these were infant girls. It is not clear how these adoptions influence census results. As registration is a prerequisite for obtaining benefits, adopted children would tend to be listed under household members, but in the majority of cases they are not included among the births of their foster-mothers. If concealment is practised and children who are given away are also omitted from the births of their own mothers, an undercount ensues. Adoptions thus contribute to the pervasive under-registration of births. It has been calculated that adding their number to the birth totals for the period 1980 to 1984 brings the sex ratio down to a normal level. Repeating the same procedure for the period 1985 to 1987 would reduce it to a value of around 1090 – the same level as that recorded for the hospital deliveries mentioned above.[12] Of course, adoption numbers are vulnerable to the same kind of falsification as other figures. Children may be given away for short periods and reclaimed later on in order to evade detection. Moreover, the analysis of adoption numbers cannot be carried on beyond 1987, as no other nationwide survey has included adoption topics in the questionnaire.

Although adoption and large-scale under-registration may explain a great part of the biased sex ratio at birth, these factors do not tell the whole story. Prenatal sex determination with consecutive abortion of female foetuses has already been mentioned as a further cause for distortion. Sex screening became possible when ultrasound B machines were first introduced into China in 1979. Since the mid-1980s they have spread rapidly to all counties and to the majority of towns and townships. This has turned China into a parallel case of South Korea, Taiwan and other parts of the Chinese culture area, where the new technology has likewise led to a dramatic rise of sex-specific abortions.[13]

Chinese analyses of the 1990 census blame sex screening for some 30 per cent of the distortion in the sex ratio. Applying different methods of calculation can raise this share to more than 40 per cent. However, all these methods rely on indirect evidence. They assign the unexplained residual of missing girls to sex-specific abortion, once every other conceivable reason for lowering the number of infant girls has been taken into account. It may well be that despite strong legislation against it, sex-specific abortion is increasing. This is the message of a 1993 survey on terminated pregnancies in South Zhejiang, another area notorious for its extremely high proportion of missing girls. Instead of relying on circumstantial evidence, the survey was able to directly record the sex discrimination surrounding abortions. The figures collected showed that the number of aborted female foetuses was twice that of aborted male foetuses if there was no son among the one or two children born before. For women who had borne three daughters but no son, the number of aborted female foetuses was three times higher than the number of male foetuses.[14]

Among the various reasons advanced for explaining the biased sex ratio, increased female infant mortality caused by infanticide, abandonment or neglect is the hardest to track down. After a flurry of press reports on the subject, it was investigated in the 1988 fertility survey. The questionnaire contained questions on the number of infanticide or abandonment cases in the sample localities. The results in the 13,000 or so grass-roots units covered were never published, though, and it is doubtful they yielded reliable figures. Assessments of the situation vary in the literature. While some Chinese specialists dismiss the problem as being of only minor importance, others discern an increasing trend.

Viewed from a historical perspective, infanticide is no newcomer to the Chinese scene and has been practised for centuries. Together with fatal neglect and raised mortality due to earlier weaning of girls, it was most likely responsible for the skewed sex ratios at birth that were recorded in the republican period, when no technology for prenatal sex determination was available. Anhui, Henan, Guangdong and Guangxi were notorious for the practice, and even urban areas were not free from it. The few more reliable population surveys conducted in some rural areas during the 1930s and 1940s produced sex ratios of between 1100 and 1266.[15] The retrospective data for the late 1930s and 1940s from the 1982 fertility survey that have been cited above also fall within this range. They hint at excess female infant mortality in the order of 10 to 15 per cent.

These percentages dropped sharply in the course of the 1940s, and fell even further through the forceful social policies of the People's Republic. In contrast to the cruder census results for 1953 and 1964, however, the retrospective survey data document that a residual of approximately 2 per cent missing girls continued to be present throughout the 1960s and early 1970s. Between the mid-1970s and mid-1980s, before ultrasound technology became available on a mass scale, it increased again to nearly 5 per cent. A retrospective analysis of the 1990 census raises the figure of missing girls during the period from 1971 to 1980 to as high as 8 per cent. Interestingly enough, it also finds some 4 to 5 per cent missing boys at parity 3 or higher. It is open to interpretation whether these were signs of increasing infanticide, abandonment, neglect or adoption. The latter factor probably worked to the benefit of missing boys.[16]

The 1990 census data and figures from the 1988 fertility survey permit further examination of female infant mortality. They establish an overall trend of stagnating infant mortality during the late 1970s and 1980s. The figures further show that the normal situation of an excess of male over female infant mortality was reversed at the end of the 1980s. If the sex distribution of infant deaths enumerated by the 1990 census is compared with the normal proportion of female relative to male infant mortality, the outcome is a greater number of dead infant girls than expected. These could be interpreted as unnatural deaths due to infanticide, abandonment or neglect. Surveys from the 1990s exacerbate the phenomenon and even suggest newly rising infant mortality.[17]

Of course, the calculation of excess numbers depends on the reliability of census data, and here the problems start again. As everywhere in the world, infant deaths and the infant mortality rate calculated from them belong to the kind of demographic information that is most difficult to collect. In developing countries the complications are particularly great. This is caused by cultural taboos, deficiencies of the health system, difficulties of distinguishing stillbirths from postnatal deaths and the opportunities for manipulation arising under such circumstances. Under current conditions in China, such manipulation could involve both parents and doctors. A rule of thumb states that figures for deaths occurring recently are more reliable than those for more distant periods. The Chinese infant mortality rates obtained from the latest census figures demonstrate the effect of such problems. They vary to a large extent depending on the question of whether they are measured for the past six, twelve or eighteen months before the population count. The closer the reference period to the census date, the higher the general level of infant mortality as well as the excess of dead infant girls.

Applying the infant mortality rates obtained for January to June 1990 to the number of births in 1989, and adjusting the result by the standard proportion of female relative to male infant mortality, produces an excess number of approximately 140,000 dead infant girls. Including this figure in the unadjusted total of missing girls for 1989 would result in 13 per cent of these children being eliminated by unnatural death, 41 per cent aborted after prenatal sex determination, and 46 per cent concealed by non-reporting of births. Applying the even more skewed infant mortality rates obtained from the 1992 fertility survey would change the absolute number to more than 200,000 and the percentages to 20 per cent, 34 per cent and 46 per cent, respectively. The lower figure for the number of unnatural deaths would be equal to 1.2 per cent of all infant girls born in 1989, and would contrast with an estimate for female infanticide in the range of 5 per cent between 1851 and 1948.[18]

It cannot be ruled out, however, that some of the missing girls are reported as dead even though they are living. Misreporting may therefore contribute to the highly untypical preponderance of female versus male infant deaths and to the recent survey figures indicating a resurgence of infant mortality. As the birth numbers used in the calculation of percentage shares may still be under-estimated, the relative weight of excess deaths and prenatal sex determination could also be lower than indicated by the percentages cited above. As with the situation for fertility data, the discussion of infant mortality and sex ratio at birth thus leads into a data maze and exposes many opportunities for falsification. Nevertheless, the demographic exercises can establish dimensions and proportions for the factors involved. They suggest that infanticide is not the main reason for the distorted sex ratio and that under-registration of infant girls or sex-specific abortion play a greater role.

As far as the underlying causes are concerned, cultural traditions of long standing, scientific breakthroughs, and policy elements enter a complex symbiosis. While birth control cannot be blamed for the overriding influence of the son preference as such, it denies couples the chance to realize their wishes by producing more children. The response is a mixture of evasion, technology and violence that discriminates against infant girls and drives up sex ratios. As shown by the strong variation of regional data, many intervening factors can modify this general trend. In the same vein, the examples of Taiwan and South Korea, where sex ratios at birth are also rising incessantly, caution against simplified conclusions. It is a fair guess that China would face a large number of missing girls under conditions of spontaneous fertility decline, too.

13.2 Age structure

Fertility, mortality and migration are the three aspects of demographic behaviour which influence population structure. The latter two elements will be largely ignored in the following discussion, which concentrates on the influence of fertility levels and birth control. Also not covered are the widely varying conditions in China's provinces. Regional population structures differ markedly, depending on their specific mortality and fertility pattern, the varying impact of birth control, the extent of migration and other factors. Very young populations in the Southwest and the Northwest or elderly populations in the highly urbanized coastal regions mark the two ends of the spectrum. Shanghai is in the forefront of this development. As the region with the earliest beginnings of both voluntary and state-induced fertility decline, it is starting to share all the problems of Western societies with a heavy load of supporting old people.

The age pyramids from the 1982 and 1990 censuses in Chart 16 show glaring projections and indentations, sharp oscillations even among neighbouring cohorts and repeated changes of overall shape. These produce an irregular form in the pyramids, differing from the usual smooth shapes. The sometimes abrupt differences in cohort size make planning and policy implementation in the social sphere extremely difficult.

Chart 16 displays a highly regular pyramid form for all cohorts born prior to 1930 (age groups above 52 in 1982, above 60 in 1990). It serves as a reminder of the difference between historic and demographic reasoning that the incessant warlord battles and natural catastrophes of the first decades of the twentieth century left only relatively small legacies. This is caused by the prolonged and increased mortality risk to which older generations have been submitted. It planes former irregularities. Levelling may be reinforced if, due to slight population increase in the past, the cohorts have been small anyway, or if the differences between them have not been spectacular.

The pyramid takes on an almost rectangular shape for cohorts born between 1933 and 1943 (age groups 39 to 49 in 1982, 47 to 57 in 1990). This can be created by the double effect of extended mortality plus decreasing births. While larger cohorts at the beginning of this period melt away under prolonged mortality risk, the following years see falling birth numbers. This is exactly the scenario for the heyday of the Guomindang era and the following period of the Sino–Japanese war. Birth cohorts increased again in 1944, and this development accelerated rapidly with the new-found stability after 1949. Indicative for periods of high natural increase, the pyramid slopes flatten as yearly increases of base size outpace the former pattern of growth, and cohorts are not yet diminished by prolonged mortality.

However, 1949 also acts as a dividing line in another sense. After the founding of the People's Republic the pyramid loses all regularity. A major factor behind the irregularities are the three peak periods of births between 1950 and 1958 (age groups 24 to 32 in 1982, 32 to 40 in 1990), 1963 and 1971 (age groups 11 to 19 in 1982, 19 to 27 in 1990), and 1986 to 1990 (age group 0 to 4 in 1990), as well as the ruptures between them. During each peak period the average birth number per year exceeded 20 million. There is a deep trough between the first and second period caused by the catastrophe of the Great Leap Forward, when the total fertility rate plunged from its former level of 6.4 (1957) to 4.0 (1960), while the mortality rate rocketed. The trough is partly compensated by the extremely large number of births and the rapidly falling mortality in 1962/63, which cause the pyramid to protrude again. Birth reductions effected by the start of birth control are clearly visible thereafter, as is the upheaval of the Cultural Revolution, which creates new notches and

Chart 16 Age pyramids

1982

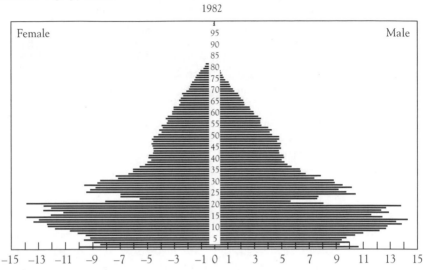

1990

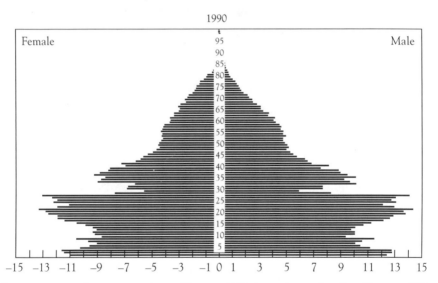

Sources: census and microcensus data in Zhongguo 1982 nian renkou pucha ziliao; Zhongguo 1990 nian renkou pucha ziliao

another protrusion. In terms of size, the cohort born in 1969 (age group 13 in 1982, 21 in 1990) rivals that born in 1963.

The restoration of state administration and the beginning of the third birth-planning campaign lead to a regular reduction of cohorts born in the 1970s (age groups 3 to 12 in 1982, 11 to 20 in 1990). However, since the break with the preceding period is not nearly as abrupt as in the Great Leap Forward, the pyramid is transformed into an urn that is progressively hollowed out. The beginning of the one-child policy produces another large reduction of cohort size during 1981. In the earlier pyramid it had already begun with the cohort of 1980 – a deceptive impression due to faulty data. The strong cohort of 1982 (age group 8 in 1990) emerges in both pyramids and signals another change in the pattern. Mirroring the changing fortunes of the one-child campaign, a pyramid form re-emerges with the cohorts born after 1983. Its base is cut back by the tightening up beginning after 1988. On closer examination the youngest cohorts of the 1990 pyramid also show initial deformation due to the biased sex ratio at birth. In comparison to the 1982 census, sex ratios for the age groups 1 to 19 have deteriorated, too. In both pyramids this is paralleled by even larger bias for cohorts born in the 1930s and 1940s. It is only beyond 60 years of age that greater male mortality finally eliminates the excess of men.

Besides the short-term influences discussed above, the irregular shapes of the age pyramid are also formed by the long-term effects of large and small cohorts passing through different stages of life. As the number of births in a given year is determined both by the number of children per woman and the total number of women of reproductive age, these two effects are superimposed upon each other, enhancing or muting the direction of their individual changes.

This is illustrated in Chart 17, which also contains manifestly defective data from the 1995 micro-census. The chart sketches the process by which the widely differing sizes of cohorts of reproductive age has been influencing the Chinese birth record.[19] In the 1980s, the total number of women in the age bracket 15 to 49 consistently increased. Even more revealing were changes for the age group 20 to 29, which contributed between 75 per cent and 85 per cent to total fertility. In 1982, this age group consisted of the depleted cohorts of the

Chart 17 Women of reproductive age 1982, 1990, 1995

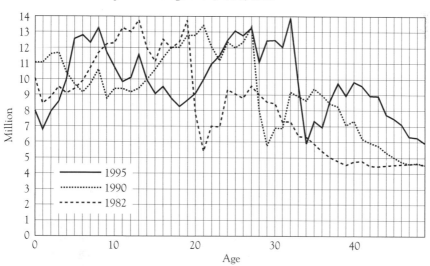

Sources: census and unadjusted microcensus data in Zhongguo 1982 nian renkou pucha ziliao; Zhongguo 1990 nian renkou pucha ziliao; 1995 nian quanguo 1% renkou chouyang diaocha ziliao

Great Leap and of women born in the 1950s, who were clearly more numerous than those born before the founding of the People's Republic. Waiting to move into the high-fertility age group were the extremely large cohorts of the second peak period of births between 1963 and 1971. By 1990 they had entered the scene, and by 1995 they dominated it. The size of subsequent cohorts signalled an easing of pressure in the second half of the 1990s, to be followed by yet another wave of births in the future.

Similar graphs can also be plotted for other critical segments of the population. Basic among these are three large age groups defined by their potential participation in economic life. For comparative purposes, here they are given in percentages and in the internationally accepted standard brackets of children aged 0 to 14, working-age population 15 to 64, and elderly people aged 65 and above. Although Chinese law stipulates different ages for entry into the labour market (16 years) or retirement (55 for women, 60 for men), these rules do not apply to the peasant majority of the population.[20] In the cities they are often also breached by delayed retirement of cadres, advanced retirement of surplus employees and widespread sideline employment of pensioners. Besides, real numbers of gainfully employed people are always smaller than potential figures, since housewives, students, soldiers, unemployed persons and other non-active groups have to be deducted from the working-age population. Chart 18 therefore mirrors the demographic constraints on Chinese economic life rather than the actual employment situation as such.

Chart 18 shows the initial growth and subsequent shrinking of the young population due to the waves of births in the 1950s and after the Great Leap, followed by fertility decline in the ensuing decades. It also illustrates the extent of the rural–urban divide. As a result of the wide fertility differentials of the 1970s, the percentages of children in 1982 differed considerably. The same might be said of the share of active persons, where more than ten percentage points separate cities and villages. Since then, fertility decline in the rural areas has diminished the overall percentage of children and brought the county figures closer to the city level. In many Chinese regions, the scarcity of children has become a fact of life catching the eye. Figures for the share of children among the total population have come down considerably from the formerly high levels of 36 per cent and 41 per cent recorded by the censuses of 1953 and 1964, respectively. The 1990 levels signify that as a whole the country's population is no longer young. It comes closer to averages for developed countries (22 per cent in 1990) than to those for developing countries (36 per cent). The falling numbers of children have had palpable consequences for the educational sector. Whereas the first three decades of the People's Republic were characterized by large bottle-necks in school enrolment, the 1980s and 1990s have seen growing instances of redundant school facilities for young children. This situation has arisen because even the absolute size of the school-age population has dropped. Between 1982 and 1990, the number of persons in elementary and junior high school age diminished by 20 per cent, although in the 1990s, it increased again by about 10 per cent.[21]

Chart 18 Age structure of total population 1953, 1964, 1982, 1990, 1995 (million)

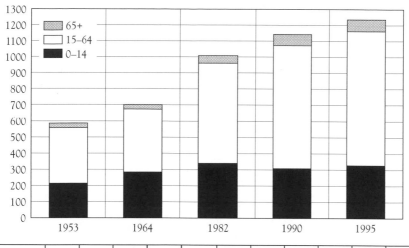

	1953	1964	1982			1990			1995		
	total	total	total	city	county	total	city	county	total	city	county
0–14, %	36.3	40.7	33.6	26.0	35.4	27.7	21.8	29.6	26.7	21.1	28.7
15–64, %	59.9	55.7	61.5	69.3	59.6	66.7	72.8	64.7	66.6	71.9	64.6
65+, %	4.4	3.6	4.9	4.7	5.0	5.6	5.7	5.7	6.7	7.0	6.7

Note: all data including the military; data for 1953 and 1964 with adjustments by A. Coale

Sources: census and unadjusted microcensus data in Zhongguo 1982 nian renkou pucha ziliao; Zhongguo 1990 nian renkou pucha ziliao; 1995 nian quanguo 1% renkou chouyang diaocha ziliao; adjustments for 1953 and 1964 in Coale 1984, 78–79

The depletion of the child population has been accompanied by an increase in adult age groups. During the periods 1967 to 1972 and 1978 to 1986, the large cohorts of youngsters born in the 1950s and 1960s had moved into the bracket of the working-age population. With a further delay of five to ten years they became marriageable, too. This pushed up the percentage of persons aged 15 to 64 from the 56 per cent recorded in 1964 to the current 67 per cent. It also led to constant rejuvenation within this group. While the share of youth and young adults aged 15 to 29 grew constantly, that of older persons aged 45 to 59 fell on a corresponding scale.

Because the additions created by high fertility were not balanced by similarly large cohorts retiring, the overall increase of the active population has been particularly large. Between 1964 and 1990, the increase amounted to the astonishing numbers of 369 million for the age range 15 to 64 and 337 million for persons within the legally defined period of active life (men aged 16 to 59 and women aged 16 to 54). For the period 1990 to 2000, these figures amounted to 100 million and 93 million, respectively. Until 1990 the net increments to the working-age population (new entrants aged 15 minus retiring persons aged 65) averaged more than 16 million per year, with particularly high additional numbers from 1978 to 1988. At the same time, percentage figures for the old population have stayed small with barely any difference between city and countryside. The change in comparison to 1953 (4.4 per cent) and 1964 (3.6 per cent) has been limited, too. In absolute terms, it amounted to little more than 38 million between 1964 and 1990. Although the social changes of the reform period have produced initial signs of approaching problems of an ageing population, these have still been cushioned by the small overall percentage of the elderly population.

The net effect of these shifts in age structure has been a change in the dependency ratio, which indicates the number of children and old people as a percentage of the active population aged 15 to 64. Used for weighing the social burden of earners, this basic indicator stood at 67 per cent in the first census of 1953. The large birth cohorts of the mid-1950s and of 1962/63 raised this figure to 79 per cent in the second census of 1964. Since then, the structural changes outlined above have reduced it to 62 per cent in 1982 and 50 per cent in both 1990 and 1995.

The current characteristics of Chinese age structure – large percentage reductions of the young population without a corresponding increase in the old population – have led the country's politicians and demographers to speak of a 'golden age'. This term may be true as far as the general proportions and the burden posed by dependants are concerned. However, the favourable percentage figures conceal the fact that population growth has translated into a tremendous increase in the potential labour force. Annual rates of increase for the working-age population continue to outstrip those of the total population by large margins. This has contributed to serious employment problems and dampened the increase of economic productivity. The asset of a favourable demographic structure during the last decades thus has to be balanced against the perennial problems of excessive population growth.

Part VI

Conclusions and future perspectives

14 Looking back: causal structures and policy impact

The review of Chinese population policy and the country's demographic record over the past fifty years testifies to the violent ruptures in modern Chinese history: political and legal birth-planning norms, the social response evoked by them and their problems of implementation document the sharp volte-face of the Mao era, the policy cycles and recurrent upheavals shaping Chinese society during that period. Moreover, they continue to reverberate with the disasters shaking the country in the preceding epoch. Finally, they document the impact of two recent decades of reform policies with the profound transformations produced by them. The fertility indicators resulting from such a complex interplay of divergent forces tell the same story in another way.

Secular changes have left their mark in the jagged contours of recent Chinese population history, too. Most important is the cluster of socioeconomic developments associated with modern society and extending into China on a similarly tortuous course: urbanization, industrialization and rising mobility, improving standards for health, education and private income, changing occupational patterns with resulting social differentiation and individual emancipation, the disintegration of traditional world orders and the accompanying mental changes. They all show highly significant Chinese characteristics produced by the far-reaching, manifest interventions of politics and the more elusive influences of history and culture.

Among the cultural factors in the setting of birth control, the ethics flowing from ancestral cult and the Chinese family system have played the most visible role. Defining standards for human obligations in marriage, sexual conduct, childbearing and rearing of offspring, they have furthered early marriage, constrained sexuality and prevented extra-marital childbirths. Even more important, they have promoted a marked son preference and helped to push up recent fertility rates beyond the prescribed limits. The data at hand clearly demonstrate that the lower birth numbers have been, the more prominent this issue has become. Secularism of the elite and folk traditions of regulating excess births by way of infanticide seem to have furthered the acceptance of abortion and the principle of birth control – even if countervailing forces have been part of the national heritage, too. Furthermore, strong traditions of collectivism with few individual rights have turned birth control into a field of contention between family interests and government wishes rather than into a human rights issue in the Western sense.

Certainly, the list of cultural factors influencing birth control is not confined to traditional elements. In recent times, the increasing role of international contacts and outside influences via the media would be a subject worthy of further study. As a whole, the pace of change in the cultural realm lags far behind the transformations in other areas and may sometimes even run against them. This is demonstrated by the tenacity with which traditional gender roles and family institutions are preserved or even revived against the combined onslaught of political interventions and modernization forces in the social and economic sphere. Present family-size preferences have certainly come down from the former standards for the number of children per couple. In the cities, they indicate that profound changes of outlook have taken place. At the same time, the majority of the population stubbornly clings to an ideal of at least two children per couple and shows little evidence of internalizing the one-child norm.

Historical consciousness has been another force in moulding attitudes. Above all, this applies to the memory of population issues figuring prominently in the context of national greatness, social order and economic subsistence. The deeply ingrained notion of dynastic cycles has turned a large population into a symbol of prosperity, power and the ability to cope with outside threat; at the same time, historical memory has also interpreted a large population as an omen of approaching crisis and downfall. Both strains have influenced attitudes in the twentieth century, when population issues were linked to the politics of national survival. Over the entire century, the desire to use large population numbers to deter foreign aggression has permeated Chinese political thinking. It has receded only slowly, to be replaced by the fear of overpopulation spelling ruin for the country.

History has also worked in more subtle ways. It has left enduring structural problems and long-lasting patterns of behaviour influencing the implementation of political measures. The legacy of autocratic rule in a centralized, bureaucratic state with strong normative powers and coercive registration of the population, limited capacity for rule enforcement, continuous delegation of powers and mutual surveillance in grass-roots units shows up time and again. This has been balanced by a highly sophisticated verbal culture and time-honoured ways of evading governmental interference. Bending the law has been facilitated by the high esteem of personal relations and the prevalence of clientelism overriding legal provisions. Current techniques for data manipulation strikingly resemble the subterfuges used by the imperial bureaucracy for producing wrong population numbers and covering up defective or non-existent registration. The traditional policy cycle of vigorous household registration, ensuing data corruption, imperial wrath, bureaucratic rectification and renewed lapse into manipulation thus seems strangely familiar.

Most cultural and historical elements cannot be readily measured. While this does not cancel out their influence, it precludes precise judgements as to their role in relation to other factors and the extent of continuity or change. This is different for the more easily quantifiable trends in the socioeconomic sphere. A number of specialized studies have tried to test the association between annual fertility rates and regularly available per capita indicators of development by way of macro-level statistical analysis.[1] Such approaches supplement survey and census materials, which have the advantage of direct enumeration but are only intermittently available and cover merely some of the dimensions involved.

The relevant studies assume that objective factors influence the subjective wishes of the population and serve to reduce birth numbers on the basis of self-interest and voluntary family decisions. There can be no doubt that such mechanisms play a role in China, too. By conventional reasoning, rises in private consumption and social product, urbanization and non-agricultural employment, female education, occupation and life-expectancy tend to show particularly high associations with reduced childbearing. However, the crux of the matter is how to assess their weight in relation to cultural factors and political intervention in fertility matters. While some of the studies neglect the political aspects completely, others have paid attention to the issue. However, measuring the influence of birth control is extremely hard. Usually, the few available indicators are neither fully reliable nor sufficiently valid, so that many conclusions remain open to debate.

Even within the confines of purely economic treatment, the problem of political campaigns causing wild fluctuations in the statistical record creates almost insurmountable problems for modelling longer periods of time. Moreover, interdependencies of many important indicators with consequent statistical collinearities are prevalent, and a number of these remain highly problematic in terms of causal reasoning. Strong associations between low fertility and high educational attainment, for instance, remain essentially ambivalent. They are usually interpreted as socioeconomic development furthering spontaneous fertility decline. But, in the Chinese context, increased governmental capacity for birth control among students and graduates in state-sector positions also plays a role. Ethno-specific differentiation in turn may indicate both different fertility behaviour of China's minorities and varying nationality policies of the Party. In comparative analyses of regional development, the situation for factors such as urbanization, personal consumption or social product is similar. A conundrum is created by the fact that the wealthy and highly urbanized regions of China tend to be the same areas where stern one-child policies with few exemptions and tight enforcement prevail. In other cases, the assumed association between economic progress and successful birth planning remains tenuous. The example of the rich Guangdong province with its comparatively high, though falling, fertility is thought-provoking in this regard.

Against this background, inferential statistical analysis poses a number of intricate problems. It is not pursued further here. Instead, a less rigorous discussion of the changing role of socioeconomic and political elements for fertility dynamics within a periodization scheme is the favoured approach. It is augmented by some general conclusions as to the role of marriage age, contraception and abortion in the respective periods. Summarizing the findings in the various chapters of this book, own calculations from the statistical record and results from the relevant analyses mentioned above, the following conclusions may be drawn for the sequence of phases since 1949.

In the first phase from 1949 to 1957, a largely compensatory movement towards restoration of pre-war fertility levels may be discerned. Coinciding with the rise in fertility, health standards improve, social product and consumption levels increase and mortality plummets. This produces an upsurge of population growth and a positive instead of the expected negative correlation with economic indicators. Although urbanization rates climbed markedly in the early 1950s, no clear rural–urban fertility divide has yet evolved. Interregional differentiation is small, too. Retarded childbearing produced by a gradual increase in marriage age is offset by greater marital fertility. Even if negative relationships between educational attainment and fertility have shown up since the mid-1950s, the spread of female education remains far too limited to allow for a greater role of this factor. The same applies to occupational differentiation. There is some back-stage lobbying of women cadres and labour representatives in favour of voluntary contraception and abortion, but it does not yet suffice to leave a permanent mark on the patchy demographic record. On the whole, the evidence for spontaneous fertility reduction leading state-run birth control remains weak. Essentially, Chinese fertility dynamics remain within their traditional framework with no modern types of human intervention.

No data can be cited that would substantiate any major demographic impact of the first, half-hearted birth-planning campaign from 1954 to 1958. This campaign is severely constrained by historically grounded and ideologically reinforced demographic perceptions of the Party leadership, above all by the convictions of Mao Zedong. For a number of years, the Party stresses the positive role of high population numbers and denies the option of voluntary birth planning to the Chinese public. Later on, it grants access to contraceptives, abortions and sterilizations only hesitatingly. On the whole, their use remains minimal during the 1950s. Ideological dogmatism, political nationalism and cultural conservatism act as the main barriers against state-controlled birth planning, even if they begin to struggle with concerns for the viability of the country's economic base among a group of academics and Party leaders. It is this very same group which instigates the first birth-planning initiatives and which is responsible for enlarging them to a grand national enterprise three decades later.

Early campaigns such as land reform in 1953 and the collectivization drive in 1956 have left only slight traces in the demographic record. Their impact has been small in comparison to the Great Leap Forward of 1958 to 1960 and its aftermath in the two following years. Triggering a steep drop in private consumption and the greatest famine of the nineteenth century, it drives mortality up to unprecedented levels and allows fertility to fall to a record low. In a perverse way, this happens while achievement reports exalt the well-being of the nation, political pronouncements praise the salutary effect of high birth numbers and the first birth-planning campaign grinds to a halt. In addition to the famine, large-scale rural–urban migrations with subsequent return movements may have also contributed to the sharp oscillations of fertility. There is a rather strong inverse relationship between galloping urbanization rates and falling fertility in 1958 to 1960, followed by opposite circumstances in the next two years. But the mayhem of the period, the repeated reversals of policy and the beginning recovery in 1962 make the overall relationship between population trends and other socioeconomic indicators tenuous between 1958 and 1962. Only Shanghai is launched on the road to permanent fertility decline, turning the metropolitan region into the first such area nationwide. In the rest of the country a new wave of births arrives. High fertility corresponds with low mortality and vice versa.

It is only after 1963 that a simultaneous decline of all vitality rates sets in. In the process, mortality quickly falls to its old level before the Great Leap, whence it starts a slow but sustained decline to standards resembling the situation in industrialized countries. It has stabilized at this low level since the late 1970s. Even if today the death of the first child continues to rank as the most important predictor for having a second birth, such circumstances affect only few people – local deviations apart. Mortality therefore no longer plays a direct role in determining population dynamics. Indirectly, however, low infant mortality rates promote fertility decline by removing the need to bear many children in order to make up for death in young age.

The fertility record of the 1960s is less than clear-cut. Sharp oscillations may be seen between the record height of 1963, the conspicuous drop of 1967 and the remainder of the 1960s, when birth indicators hover on the level of the preceding decade. These fluctuations make it hard to frame a pronouncement as to the effects of socioeconomic versus political factors. Obviously, economic recovery and the normalization of life after the Great Leap lead to compensatory behaviour and drive up fertility again. The second birth-planning campaign from 1962 to 1966 works in the other direction. Essentially devised as an emergency measure for combating economic crisis, it starts to apply sanctions and control mechanisms for limiting births in the urban areas and slowly spreads to the countryside. Because of continuing social and political resistance, birth planning progresses cautiously. Again, well-developed coastal areas take the lead. Retrospective surveys demonstrate that the educational factor now contributes substantially to the fertility decline in the cities. A huge rural-urban fertility gap and beginning regional differentiation ensues.

Nevertheless, the influence of urbanization on national population dynamics remains limited. This is due to newly instituted migration checks, which cause urbanization rates to stagnate or even fall. While fertility plunges in 1966/67, the turmoil of the Cultural Revolution causes it to rise for the rest of the decade. Between 1967 and 1970, economic decline strikes once again, and the second birth-control campaign mostly ceases. Because of these disruptions and lagging implementation in the villages, its overall influence on fertility remains muted. Massive campaigns are mostly limited to major cities, above all Shanghai. While the marriage age continues to rise, it does not show a linear relationship to fertility trends. However small the results of the second birth-planning campaign may have been, it introduces fundamental changes in thinking: the idea that the number of children per couple should be limited by the state, and the complete liberalization and cost-free provision of abortions and sterilizations.

Despite earlier groundwork, the major breakthrough for Chinese birth control comes only in the 1970s. In these years of the continuing Cultural Revolution, the economy grows only haphazardly, urbanization rates continue to stagnate, and the share of agricultural employment comes down very slowly. However, while by conventional reasoning this should point to continuously high levels of childbearing, the extent of fertility decline is dramatic. Within a decade, all birth indicators are nearly halved. Primarily affected are higher-order births beyond the second child. After the restoration of state power and the end of the anarchic phase of the Cultural Revolution, the Party forces increasingly tighter forms of birth control on all couples. With some noted delays and variations, birth control arrives in the countryside for good. Over the entire decade it may be observed how it extends from the cities to the coastal regions and then to the hinterland. Only the national minorities continue to be largely exempt. In the process, the rural–urban fertility gap decreases, while differentiation by region or nationality increases.

In view of the earlier rejection of birth control, the unfavourable economic environment and the limited financial or organizational resources for birth planning in the 1970s, the unprecedented speed of fertility decline over this decade is truly astonishing. Social factors such as the pronounced rise of educational standards for young women, the rise of female labour participation and the massive extension of a basic medical network into the countryside are certainly supportive. Still, the decisive role seems to have been played by politics. The exact mechanisms of birth-control enforcement at that time remain insufficiently documented, however. In part, this has to do with the political conventions of current times which are eager to stress distance from the Cultural Revolution. It is also connected to the tight information policies, the non-existence of a centralized birth-planning bureaucracy and the lack of comprehensive records for the former period.

There are voices who attribute part of the story to the greater willingness of Chinese peasants to cooperate in a two-child policy that offers a greater chance to produce male offspring. The newly introduced principle of providing contraceptives free of charge also plays a part, but the crucial mechanism for effecting the drastic fertility decline still seems to have been the penetration of state power into almost every aspect of life. Even if bureaucratic authority itself was shaken by the repeated mass campaigns and discreet ways for circumventing policies existed, cadres still wielded almost limitless power for denying means of subsistence to anyone disobeying their commands. The magic of Mao Zedong's final stamp of approval for a limitation of birth numbers and the end of polemics on birth control seem to have done the rest. A look at the direct determinants of fertility shows that compulsory contraception and the swift rise of the marriage age due to administrative measures have contributed about equally to the sharp fall in birth numbers, with abortions following in third place.

Nevertheless, the remarkable fertility decline reached by the two-child policy was still deemed insufficient by Mao's successors, who faced the burden of another economic crisis and two decades of retarded growth. At the end of the 1970s, it is again thus a sense of economic predicament that leads to a radicalization of population policy. Birth control is epitomized in the one-child campaign, which clearly sees different phases of implementation. A period of stringent policies between 1980 and 1983 is followed by increasing exemptions and moves for a gradual return to a two-child rule between 1984 and 1989, before a renewed tightening starts in the 1990s.

Pinning down the contribution of politics and various socioeconomic factors to the fertility dynamics of the reform period is hard. In the early 1980s, the indiscriminate application of the one-child rule to all parts of the population lessens the weight of socioeconomic differentials. But even after the Party takes social and economic discrepancies into account, the importance of such factors for fertility dynamics remains limited. The pace of urbanization accelerates, and all per capita indicators referring to private consumption or social product greatly increase, albeit with noticeable fluctuations. However, while moderately strong associations with birth figures do exist, these explain less than half of the fertility trend. Personal income, in particular, is an enigmatic factor, since instances of wealth leading to both rising and falling fertility may be cited. Moreover, establishing a clearly defined income threshold beyond which fertility decline sets in proves to be impossible. The record for education is also anything but unequivocal. Although all surveys regularly demonstrate its function in lowering fertility, the importance of this factor none the less seems to have diminished with the extension of birth control among the under-educated peasantry. Since the later half of the 1980s, most relevant surveys have education ranking only fifth or sixth place as a determining factor for the number of children per woman. Finally, nationality status continues to play a role – but, due to the introduction of birth planning among the minorities, not to the extent of the 1970s.

Everything therefore points to the continuing dominance of the political factor in the 1980s. The various, albeit unsatisfactory, attempts to measure its influence in comparison to the socioeconomic sphere point in the same direction.[2] But under closer scrutiny, the impact of governmental birth control has not been unlimited either. While the study of refined statistical indicators leaves no doubt that the one-child campaign did lower fertility still further, its performance was neither without failure nor very impressive. This is most clearly demonstrated by the slump of the average marriage age over the entire decade, by the slight resurgence of fertility in 1981 to 1982 and 1986 to 1987, and by the fact that the fertility rate at the time of the 1990 census had not dropped much beneath the level of the preceding count in 1982. Throughout the decade, the percentage of second and higher-order births remained much larger than anticipated. Furthermore, the peak period of childbearing reverted to earlier years of life. These tendencies have been exacerbated by the large cohorts of young people born between 1962 and 1970. Although their advancement into the marriageable and childbearing age groups has not influenced fertility *per se*, it has driven up the birth totals by the sheer mass of young women involved.

City and countryside have contributed to this situation in rather different ways. In the cities, the clout of the state and spontaneous social developments since the 1970s have combined to lower fertility levels and to make birth planning a success. Even though low urban fertility disguises the continued existence of two-child preferences, the long-term economic and social forces at work make a pronounced resurgence of urban fertility levels unlikely. The situation is different in the rural areas, however, where fertility levels lag behind urban standards by about twenty years. The majority of peasants do not accept the one-child norm, and numbers for second and higher-order births have continued to be much higher than intended. Most affected are the hinterland regions with their retarded development and their higher degree of traditionalism.

As a result, the actual birth figures of the 1980s have greatly exceeded the original plans. In contrast to the earlier periods with their paucity of demographic material, the improved data for the 1980s permit a precise evaluation of the factors involved. Chinese calculations for the slight increase of the birth rate in 1987 as compared to 1981 apportion +8 per cent to the unfavourable changes in age structure, +12 per cent to the rise in marriage age, −14 per cent to the drop in marital fertility and −5 per cent to interaction between these factors. The underlying method, however, cannot distinguish between spontaneous and politically induced changes, and the results are also highly dependent on data input and the years chosen for comparison. The year 1987 showed a peak in fertility resurgence. Two years later, fertility was receding again, but the impact of the extraordinarily large cohorts born between 1963 and 1966 could be felt even more. Models comparing 1981 with 1989 thus assign markedly different weights to age structure and marital fertility (+39 per cent and −51 per cent, respectively).[3]

In this way, many intervening factors have combined to thwart the original ambitious objectives of the one-child campaign. The most important direct determinants of childbearing confirm the picture of major difficulties in policy implementation. Due to the sudden slump and belated re-increase of the average marriage age, this factor did not promote further fertility decline. As the most important direct predictor of fertility trends over the decade, contraceptive prevalence could not maintain its fast rise during the 1970s after a relatively high plateau had already been reached at the end of that decade. Contraception was becoming prevalent among younger age groups, though, and it came to rely more on long-term methods. Changes in birth spacing were again a negative factor in further fertility decline; intervals shrank, partly out of fear of still tighter policies in the offing. The great and abrupt oscillations of the abortion rate, plus its soaring average of more than double the mean value for the 1970s, also testify to the problems of birth control in the 1980s and its crash-programme character. Ultimately, all these difficulties were grounded in fundamental changes in the political and economic setting, over-zealous targets, a host of implementation problems and massive popular resistance.

The fertility and birth-planning figures of the 1990s are not sufficiently reliable to reach firm conclusions for the following decade. Some recent trends of thinking have been introduced in the historical outline of birth control; together with a discussion of the political factors, they will be taken up again in chapter 16. The major problem for an assessment are strong hints for continuing, serious data manipulation that would cancel out many of the more extravagant claims. Due to the immense political pressures applied and socioeconomic developments conducive to birth control, a further fertility decline is likely, nevertheless. With respect to the direct determinants of childbearing, the renewed emphasis on late marriage, late birth and prolonged birth intervals, as well as the further increase of contraception, would be the major mechanisms involved.

How is the balance for births averted through birth-control efforts, and what have been the results for society and the economy? Numerous official statements and propaganda articles from China have pursued these seemingly simple questions, which yet turn out to be even more intricate than birth planning and demographic development *per se*. Although the few more elaborate studies on the topic demonstrate a rapid assimilation of advanced research techniques from abroad, they regularly run into a number of problems, which lead back to the inability of economics to provide clear-cut answers for the extremely complex and controversial interrelationships between demographic and economic development.

Most calculations of demographic impact rest on an assessment of potential fertility in the absence of governmental birth control.[4] For this purpose, past trends that incorporate spontaneous fertility reduction furthered by socio-economic development are projected into the period after the beginning of state-run birth control. The difference between projected trend values and actual figures is then taken to signify programme effect. This procedure requires to fix a precise year as the beginning of birth control and to rule out highly atypical years before that date. Immediately, the familiar difficulties for the Chinese case arise. The chequered history of birth control makes it hard to fix a precise start. Moreover, the fertility data for the early 1950s show an upward trend; using these figures for a projection of potential fertility would imply that no spontaneous fertility reduction but rather a continuous increase would have taken place in China – a quite unrealistic assumption. After 1958, the intrusion of political campaigns makes the figures highly erratic, so that no clear trend may be derived.

In view of these problems, Chinese demographers have discarded the first and second birth-planning campaigns as largely ineffective, and have settled for 1971 as the start of a coherent, long-term programme. They have also substituted a Chinese trend line for potential fertility with interpolation and model calculations from other developing countries in the 1960s. All these procedures are inherently unsatisfactory and mask the non-existence of sufficient information for the earlier period. Nevertheless, the few methodological alternatives are problematic, too. The present Chinese calculations result in a total of up to 340 million births averted by birth planning over the past three decades, with about 80 million for the period 1971 to 1979, 130 million for the period 1980 to 1989 and another 130 million for the period 1990 to 1999. These figures depend on later verification of the dubious birth numbers for the 1990s, but under this proviso, and as a rough approximation, they are acceptable. They imply that, in the absence of state-run birth control, China would have had a population of nearly 1.60 billion instead of the reported 1.27 billion people at the end of the twentieth century.

Another telling balance may be drawn up once the officially reported number of births under the one-child policy is compared with the hypothetical number, had the total fertility rate stayed at its 1979 level of 2.77 children per woman, the last available figure from the period of the two-child policy. An own calculation for the number of births averted by the tightening of birth control would result in nearly 25 million between 1980 and 1989 and more than 90 million from 1990 to 1999. The implied total population number for 1999 would have been 1.41 billion. Because of uncertainties posed by the repeated adjustments for birth numbers in the 1980s and by the questionable data of the 1990s, this again is a rough estimate only. Further, the difference in the 1980s probably would have been somehow greater, since it may be assumed that, without relevant counter-measures, the breakdown of collectivized agriculture during the 1980s would have driven up fertility from its level in 1979. But, no matter what the exact balance would have been, the figures once again reflect the implementation problems of birth control in the 1980s and the failure of the original plans.

The problems of demographic evaluation, however, are dwarfed by the difficulties in considering social and economic impact. The Chinese sources cited above claim that without birth control, social and economic development would have come to a halt. In particular, they credit the campaigns since 1971 with the following achievements: more than 100 million rural surplus labour averted until 1998; savings of 6.4 trillion yuan in private and 1.0 trillion yuan in social childrearing costs until 1998, with the grand total approaching Chinese gross domestic product in 1997; more than 1 trillion yuan of added national income and more than 660 billion yuan of added private consumption until 1990 (no figures are presented for the following years); raised per capita grain production instead of stagnation (293 kg in 1971, 402 kg in 1997); restrained deterioration of the man–land ratio (0.10 hectares per capita in 1978, 0.08 instead of 0.06 hectares in 1997) and of per capita freshwater resources (2275 instead of 1836 cubic metres in 1997). Further unquantified benefits are claimed for areas like household income, state investment, urban unemployment, educational attainment, health standards, life expectancy, use of energy or natural resources and environmental protection. Other studies still add transportation capacity, housing and private savings to the list. For the period 1978 to 1997, it is claimed that fertility decline contributed 26 to 34 per cent of the growth of GDP per capita, 15 to 22 per cent of the stock of fixed assets, 13 to 24 per cent of the growth of labour productivity and 25 to 40 per cent of the growth in standards of living.[5]

The difficulty with these figures is that they largely reduce the complexities of social and economic development to dependency on population growth only. This does injustice to factors such as distribution and consumption patterns, political and economic systems, technological advances, educational levels, foreign trade and so on. Moreover, the argument presupposes that, without exception, all additional births would have resulted in idle dependants making no contribution to the economy. In light of many local studies that document cases of positive value of additional manpower for household income, or that try to balance the expenses with the contributions of children, this seems questionable. No consideration is given to the social contract between generations by which parents exchange present childrearing costs for later support in old age. Furthermore, the fundamental asynchronism of birth-control measures taken now and their economic effects accruing tomorrow leads to the problem of how to discount for future changes of price and scarcity relations, how to assess the future composition of the commodity basket, and how to predict long-term economic developments with sufficient precision. Typically, the latter are measured by the month, whereas demographic change operates by decades.

In the final analysis, these considerations and many similar arguments lead back to the problems of calculating an optimum population or a maximum carrying capacity of the national territory that have been alluded to elsewhere in this study. They make it untenable to follow the practice of some Chinese studies, which derive figures for economic impact through simply dividing economic performance by either hypothetical or actual birth numbers. Other, more careful Chinese sources refrain from making such claims and limit themselves to a long inventory of economic, social and environmental problem areas with obvious links to population issues. However, nowhere do they succeed in clearly separating the demographic causes of problems from the host of other factors involved.[6]

In view of such conceptual difficulties, the attempts at drawing up a balance of birth-planning benefits versus birth-planning costs have remained tentative, too. Western analyses that have taken up the Chinese claims are forced to introduce numerous caveats, and precise estimates run into similar problems as outlined above. Nevertheless, they agree that, even if human and political costs are completely disregarded and only easy-to-measure birth-planning expenditures enter the calculations, the positive ratio of benefits over costs of birth planning has declined.[7] The exertions needed to lower China's fertility rate to replacement level that are documented in this study support this view.

While the 'big calculations' of birth control thus falter for lack of a sound theoretical and methodological basis, it seems only fair to state that there are good reasons to maintain the anti-natalist argument, if it is put in relative, historical terms and refrains from staking out precisely quantified claims. Given the low level of Chinese development in the 1960s and 1970s, it seems inconceivable that without birth planning the progress registered in the 1980s and 1990s would have been as large as it has been in the past. This applies both to social product and individual standards of living. The discussion of these problems earlier in this study and the projections introduced in Chapter 15 indicate that many severe constraints are here to stay for the foreseeable future, even if economic policies and technological advances can alleviate them. With a high degree of certainty, some of them, such as surplus labour, will still further aggravate before an improvement can be contemplated. Under the prevailing circumstances, the case for birth control, therefore, is strong. Whether it has to come in the present form of the one-child policy is another matter.

15 Looking forward: demographic projections and their implications

Defying the all too tangible pressures of the state, Chinese population developments have deviated considerably from the course anticipated and charted by politicians in the past. Starting with the surprisingly high census results of 1953, continuing with the unmet objectives of the second and third birth-planning campaigns in the two following decades, and culminating in the abandonment of the original targets of the one-child policy in the late 1980s, a continuous upward revision of population figures has taken place. In the latter case, this has entailed discarding detailed demographic projections for desirable population numbers. Each time, the revision has been in the range of 70 to 100 million or more, equal to underestimates of 11 to 12 per cent for 1953 and 1980 and, depending on whether the initial and extremely ambitious target of 1.13 billion or the more liberal 1.20 billion limit is chosen, some 5 to 12 per cent per cent for the year 2000.

These errors are substantial and well above the normal order of inaccuracies in projections over comparable time lengths for other countries with very large population sizes. Since 1991 this story of constant underestimation has been replaced by an equally unexpected overperformance of birth planning. It seems to have led to an unanticipated rapid decline of fertility, curbed an expected peak period of births and compensated past errors to some degree. However, in view of the deficiencies of the Chinese statistical system and continuing resistance to present population policies, recent trends still remain elusive and await further clarification.

Such experiences make it advisable to guard against taking politically defined target numbers at face value and expecting that actual population developments will be in close accord with them. There is no doubt that projections of population numbers based on desirable outcomes or on different fertility policies will continue to be undertaken in the future. This is because their major value consists in alerting politicians to the potential consequences of different courses of action. They also provide planners with reference points for checking plan adherence and adjusting policies in time. Nevertheless, the recognition that population development cannot be manipulated at will has gained ground in China, too. It has led the politicians and social scientists of the country to take their bearings increasingly from actual population trends under conditions of birth planning rather than from grand master plans.

In the late 1980s, this new realism, plus the shrinking distance to the target date, narrowed the range between different projections for 2000 to a minimum of 1.25 billion and a maximum of 1.31 billion. This variation continued to show up in the medium scenarios of Chinese projections from the mid-1990s, and demonstrated that some uncertainty about population developments at the end of the century remained. The discrepancies for the following decades increase with projection length to a band between 1.37 and 1.62 billion in the projections for 2050. They assume much greater proportions if low and high variants of the projections are also considered.[1]

In the long run, growing divergences result less from baseline errors than from differences in model assumptions that are seemingly negligible in the short term but entail serious consequences with the passage of time. Usually, different suppositions as to birth-control policies, marriage trends, spontaneous fertility behavior, medical advances and mortality levels, as well as the manifold social, economic, technological and cultural factors affecting them, loom behind the mathematical variations. As outlined in the preceding chapter, their interrelationships are hard to generalize and do not permit treating population as an endogenous element within an integrated model of socioeconomic change. Uncertainties in demographic projections become disproportionally large once scenarios transcend a horizon of twenty to thirty years and incorporate hypotheses about the fertility behaviour of still unborn generations. Recent projection methods employed in China have become ever more refined and often include stratification by regions, rural and urban areas or educational levels. In a number of cases, they also involve intensive discussions about the influence on population growth exerted by different ages for first childbearing or different mortality levels.[2] But while these methods are useful for demonstrating the influence of such factors on demographic change in the future, it remains doubtful whether they will yield more reliable forecasts than standard methods of cohort-component analysis for the whole population.

All projections presuppose an essentially stable environment. A final caveat, therefore, concerns the possibility of demographic quakes triggered by future epidemics, natural catastrophes, wars or political upheavals. While such a proviso often is added as a routine footnote, the dramatic fertility drop in Eastern Europe after the sudden change in the political system and the subsequent breakdown of social order shows that it is anything but superfluous. The look to the future thus invariably involves an attempt to penetrate haze. Nevertheless, projections do succeed in tracing rough contours and establishing a sense of direction. Rather than relegating future prospects to pure guesswork, they show the constraints on development. Within this framework there remains leeway to pursue different paths. The choices are not unlimited, though. Drawing on the past record of China and the experiences of Taiwan or other East Asian regions, the following variables seem to be of particular importance for Chinese population trends in the next fifty years.

The average marriage age of women is likely to rise spontaneously on a scale of slightly more than 0.1 years per annum. Late-marriage policies may accelerate this process to an increase of 0.15 years per annum. However, they may also lead to backsliding if enforcement slackens. No definite ceiling for female marriage age can be set. A late-marriage standard of 25 years has been urged in the past but unattained. An upper limit seems to be the average of 27 years presently reached in Taiwan, Hongkong and Japan. However, since these are areas with extremely high urbanization rates and income levels, much depends on whether similar conditions can be achieved in China within the projection period. Furthermore, the fact that the three areas alluded to combine the same level of female marriage age with different per capita levels of gross domestic product amply demonstrates that the link between marriage age and standards of living is anything but linear. With a per capita GDP less than Taiwan and 40 per cent of the USA, South Korea at present features an average female marriage age of more than 29 years, higher than in the USA or most Western European countries.

Social and cultural change may increase the incidence of non-marriage, prolong the interval between marriage and first birth or totally disconnect wedlock and childbearing. In present Chinese society, marriage is still upheld as a universal norm, with childbearing respected as an inalienable aspect of it. Birth-control policies have played an ambiguous role in this regard. They seem to have first strengthened the link by increasing anxieties about future childbearing opportunities and shortening the interval between marriage and first birth. In contrast, a trend towards granting earlier marriage under condition of delayed childbearing has become evident over the past decade. It remains to be seen how this interplay of birth policies and social responses will work out in the future. Marriage ideals, lifestyle preferences and role expectations for women are always involved. Politics would also require the interbirth intervals for a permitted second or higher-order child to increase, but private considerations may shorten them in order to increase individual freedom once family obligations have been met. The percentage of Chinese singles will grow conspicuously, though it will remain lower than in Western countries. The same will apply to childless couples, divorces, premarital sex or illegitimate births. They are on the rise everywhere in East Asia, but nowhere does the dissolution of traditional family patterns reach Western proportions.

There seems to be little room left for raising levels of contraceptive use. Even if they are discounted for over-reporting, the percentages for married women of reproductive age using modern methods of contraception remain among the highest in the world, and have been pushed up to their present level of more than 80 per cent by the one-child campaign. Education and intimidation in favour of contraceptive use have been all-pervading, and most women not practising contraception await pregnancies or have other reasons to be unconcerned. The only area left for improved education seems to be unwarranted trust in the contraceptive function of breast-feeding. Within the contraceptive mix, some scope exists for extending sterilization and IUD use still further, but popular opposition and lack of funding argue against such a course of action. Economic reforms have raised birth-control expenses and may necessitate a backtracking from cost-free contraception and abortion. Under such circumstances, it is also conceivable that contraceptive prevalence may fall instead of rise still further. Scientific progress is a major unknown in the picture. It may contribute improved or altogether new methods of contraception in the future, but key demands such as low price, convenient use, reliability, reversibility and freedom from medical complications are often hard to reconcile.

It is not altogether clear how the abortion issue will develop in the future. In past years, it has been linked to both the widespread son preference and the failure to establish sufficiently reliable contraception. For the leadership, there remains the dilemma to choose between sex-specific abortions of female foetuses with a high imbalance of the sex ratio at birth or acceptance of higher fertility due to an unmet demand for sons. Until now, the state has tried to strike a balance: it has condoned second-child permits for parents with only one daughter, denied further birth permits for parents of two daughters, prohibited prenatal sex screening and threatened stiff penalties against contraventions. If this course should prove to be unsuccessful and serve to perpetuate unauthorized childbearing, legalizing sex-specific abortion may be considered. While raising the sex ratio at birth and creating problems for the marriage market, it would lower fertility.

All these issues involve clashes between Western ideals of equality or personal self-fulfilment and Chinese values based on family obligations and gender inequality. The extent to which foreign models and worldwide communication will influence the latter is hard to predict. Rural society in China seems still to be firmly pitched against the inroads from outside. Judging by the surveys on their family-size preferences, Chinese city-dwellers have covered the furthest distance in bridging the gap so far. Precedents are set by urbanites in Taiwan, Hongkong or Singapore, who are increasingly emulating a Western lifestyle. The links of many urban Chinese on the mainland to the past and their rural origins are much stronger, however. It is therefore an open question whether the present family-size preferences of urban Chinese will remain stable, develop further towards a one-child ideal or revert to higher child numbers once policies are relaxed. Experiences with attitudinal surveys counsel for caution. Often, preferences professed before have not matched behaviour afterwards. Although a secular trend towards small families is likely, no clear judgement on the pace and scope of changes is possible. Especially in the rural areas, catching up on postponed births remains a distinct possibility.

Apart from fertility measured at the individual level, birth numbers will also be determined by the total number of women of reproductive age. Figures in Table 34 show that the present age–sex structure of the population still remains problematic. Although the percentages for the high-fertility age groups 20 to 34 will fall after the year 2000, the total number of women of reproductive age will continue to rise until around 2012. They will then significantly surpass the comparable cohort sizes for 1980. In 2016, women aged 20 to 34 will hail from the more than 20 million strong cohorts born between 1982 and 1996. It is a fair guess that the absolute numbers of children borne by them will stay high too, even if fertility per woman declines. Such circumstances make it likely that another peak period of births will arise after 2010, when the particularly large cohorts of women born between 1986 and 1992 enter the high-fertility age groups. Beyond 2020 the number of women of reproductive age and the number of births are less certain, since they also depend on the size of cohorts not yet born.

Mortality is another factor influencing future population growth. With a life-expectancy of 68.4 years in 1990, China has reduced mortality to a much lower level than is normal for a country at her level of economic development. However, due to higher than anticipated infant mortality, the increase in life-expectancy has slowed down since the 1980s and may even have registered temporary stagnation or reversal. Future developments will also depend on such hard to predict factors as advances in medical treatment or genetic engineering, progress in the treatment of geriatric diseases, as well as the scope of old-age support and insurance for bearing soaring healthcare expenses. Here, profound social and systemic changes are underway in the country. Finally, all mortality projections depend on a further successful containment of AIDS and other epidemics. Until now, Chinese health standards have been one of the assets of the country. But the opening up and the new freedom in Chinese society can be a double-edged sword and may lead to the proliferation of some diseases. Health risks arising from rapid environmental degradation pose another threat.

Still harder to predict are other socioeconomic background variables. Urbanization is a major factor in the picture. Associated with it are the rise of female education and occupation, growing consumption and increasing opportunity costs for raising children, as well as manifold cultural changes, which tend to postpone marriage and reduce fertility. Among them are transformations of family structure, the extension of a system of social security, rising mobility, greater economic risks for the individual and changes in lifestyle. Last but not least, the issue of different birth policies for urban and rural areas is involved. Recent projections from China have seen urbanization rates climb from their present level of more than 30 per cent to anywhere between 40 and 52 per cent in 2020, and 55 and 75 per cent in 2050. These extremely wide margins result from a number of crucial unknowns: future economic trends with their effects for the labour market, income development and employment creation in the rural areas, state policies with regard to rural–urban migrants and their chances of enforcement. Because the pace of urbanization over the past two decades has been rather uneven, it is hard to extrapolate long-term growth from recent time series.

The educational scene contributes another important element to future fertility trends. Here, trends of the 1990s are favourable, as the extension of nine years of compulsory schooling seems to have made rapid progress in the villages, too. Net enrolment rates for both sexes are near to 100 per cent at the elementary school level. At the end of the 1990s, female youth illiteracy was supposed to be down to 5 per cent. Although the enrolment of girls still trails that of boys at high school level, even here the share of girls out of school seems to have shrunk from around 55 per cent during the mid-1980s to only 35 per cent in the late 1990s. This makes it conceivable that ambitious targets for reaching universal school attendance at the junior high school level by 2010, with transition rates of more than 50 per cent from the junior to the senior high school level, may be realized.

Chart 19 presents medium variants of prominent Chinese projections from the past two decades. It also introduces five new projections based on the findings of this study. The chart shows how already in 1983 the extremely ambitious targets from the beginning of the one-child policy had been superseded by a more sober estimate from the Academy of Social Sciences. But even that estimate assumes that fertility will fall to 1.8 children per woman by 1985, decline further to a trough of 1.5 between 2000 and 2010, and then slowly reincrease to 1.9 by 2050. Although the latter trajectory already transcends the 1.2 billion limit, there still exists the belief and the wish that the population total will slowly recede after reaching a plateau of 1.23 billion in 2006. The two projections from 1986 hail from some of the most influential demographers of the country and from the State Council's Development Research Centre, respectively. They testify to the major change in outlook that took place during the mid-1980s. The recognition that fertility falls more slowly than expected gains ground. Nevertheless, reducing it to below replacement level during the critical period of the 1990s is insisted on. After the turn of the century an increase to 2.1 is permitted. This implies a later return to a modified two-child policy. The last projection from 1988 betrays the alarm over fertility rates that still show no sign of abating. Prolonging the then level of 2.2 children per woman into the indefinite future, it reaches the number of 1.62 billion people in 2050.

The new projections start from the age–sex structure and the fertility level as revealed by the fourth census in 1990. Their major shortcoming is that as yet no reliable time series for fertility rates in the 1990s, no revised schedules for age-specific fertility and mortality rates, and no new baseline for the age–sex structure in 2000 can be established. This weakness is partly remedied by combining two hypothetical fertility trends of the 1990s with the preliminary population total of the fifth census on 1 November 2000. For purposes of better comparability with the mid-year results of earlier population counts, the latter is adjusted to a total of 1.263 billion for 1 July 2000.

The projections apply age- and sex-specific fertility and mortality rates to the original age–sex distribution of the population, year on year, in order to derive new age and sex groups and to calculate future population sizes. Besides the age–sex pattern of 1990, the parameters outlined in the note to Chart 19 are used. Taking Shanghai mortality levels of 1990 as a ceiling for national mortality in 2050 is on the conservative side. It implies advances in life expectancy of more than 0.1 years per annum and a future average of nearly 75 years nationwide. The average annual gain in life-expectancy is a little higher than between 1981 and 1989 but lower than many Chinese projections, which calculate a life-expectancy of 78 to 80 years or even older by 2050. For purposes of comparison, the high curve of the chart ('delayed two-child policy, low mortality') therefore replicates the delayed two-child policy scenario with a steeply raised life-expectancy of 81 years in 2050. As shown, this increases the total population for that year by more than 100 million. Raised life-expectancy would mostly affect

Chart 19a Past Chinese projections of total population 1990–2050 (million)

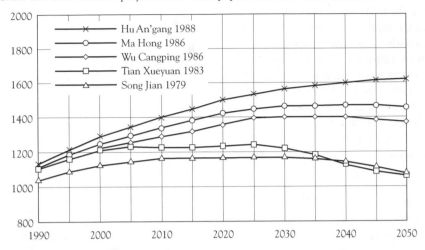

Chart 19b New projections of total population 1990–2050 (million)

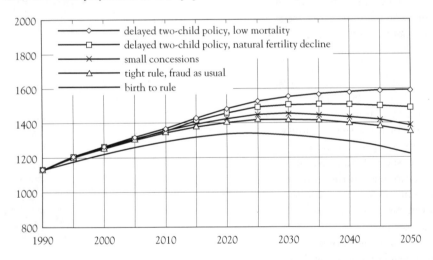

Sources for past Chinese projections according to their year of calculation:
Song 1979: Song Jian and Li Guangyuan 1980, 60–66; Song Jian et al. 1982, 180; Tian 1983: Tian Xueyuan 1984; Wu 1986: Wu Cangping 1988, 26; Ma 1986: Ma Hong 1989, 98; Hu 1988: Hu An'gang 1989a, 58. The new projections are based on the age- and sex-structure of the 1990 census. The following parameters were used for the first four models: age- and sex-specific mortality levels as of 1990 with a decline to Shanghai mortality levels within 60 years; percentage contribution of one-year age-groups to the total fertility rate as of 1989; sex ratio at birth equal to 1150. The following assumptions applied to the total fertility rate: birth to rule: sharp decline to reported values in chart 7, columns 5–6, rise to 1.80 in 2007 and thereafter; tight rule, fraud as usual: decline to 1.9 in 1993 and thereafter, 1.6 in 1999, 1.85 in 2000 and thereafter until 2050; small concessions: decline to 1.85 in 1995 and thereafter, 1.95 during 2010–15, 2.0 during 2015–25, decline to 1.85 in 2030 and thereafter; delayed two-child policy, natural fertility decline: slow decline to 1.9 in 1996 and thereafter, 2.3 during 2010–2015, slow decline to 1.85 in 2036 and thereafter; delayed two-child policy, low mortality: same scenario as above, with mortality decline twice as fast as in the other models

very young children and persons over 64 years of age. The share of the elderly among the total population would climb from 18 to 21 per cent. Also debatable is the assumption of a constant sex ratio at birth of 1150 infant boys per 1000 infant girls. It is based on Chinese surveys from the early 1990s and present levels in Taiwan. Lowering this ratio to 1100 would raise the 2050 population total by approximately 1 per cent.

The projections use the total fertility rate as the major variable. Its internal composition is modelled according to conditions in 1989 and treated as a fixed parameter. This will need to be revised once new data from the 2000 census become available. The chart includes a curve ('birth to rule') that would result if the presently valid birth-planning regulations were fully respected, and the unadjusted, officially reported fertility rates from 1992 to 1999 are taken at face value. After the turn of the century a slight resurgence of fertility rates, due to privileges for parents born as single children, is assumed. Because the assumption of full compliance is highly unlikely, this curve is likewise only added for reference, with no age structure given.

The more fully documented models start with a low projection ('tight rule, fraud as usual') that accepts high official adjustments for the total fertility rate which imply under-reporting of approximately 30 per cent. Nevertheless, fertility would still be 15 per cent less than the 1990 figure and clearly below the replacement level of 2.1. The projection further assumes a sudden plunge shortly before the new census in order to meet required population targets. After the census, the fertility rates regain a level of 1.85, where they remain. This projection reaches a peak population of 1.43 billion in 2029, with a decline to 1.35 billion by 2050. It implies a dismissal of scenarios that allow for a fertility resurgence. The low projection requires either the present population policy to continue or a massive voluntary change of marriage and childbearing patterns to set in. A speedy process of urbanization and modernization would help to promote such conditions. At the same time, the projection also implies a disbelief in even further fertility decline. Although culturally similar areas such as Taiwan and South Korea have nowadays reached very low levels of 1.5 children per woman, they boast far higher urbanization rates and economic standards than China.

The following projection ('small concessions') presupposes a stable low fertility level of 1.85 between 1994 and 2010. This leads to the same population total for 2000 as in the preceding scenario. The projection envisages a small fertility increase between 2010 and 2025 and projects a renewed decline to 1.8 within the following two decades. Such a scenario requires that birth policies are slightly relaxed after 2010. However, compensatory childbearing needs to remain controlled over the following decade. After 2025, a gradual, spontaneous fertility decline is assumed to set in. This projection resembles some Chinese assumptions about future trends. It reaches a peak population of 1.51 billion by 2030 and a figure of 1.39 billion for 2050, which is a little lower than in recent Chinese projections.

The high projection ('delayed two-child policy, natural fertility decline') finally reckons with a stable low fertility level of 1.9 between 1996 and 2010.

The population total for 2000 slightly exceeds the result of the last census. After 2010, birth numbers suddenly surge under a return to the two-child policy. Both this upward trend and the subsequent gradual decline are on a markedly higher level than in the intermediate scenario. However, although the assumed fertility rate of 2.3 for five years after the policy reversal would imply a breach of ceilings, this level would nevertheless be lower than before the introduction of the one-child policy. It would still require either some sort of relaxed birth-control policy by the state or later marriage and voluntary fertility reduction by the population. Another underlying hypothesis is that two decades of intensive birth-planning propaganda have left their mark and that large-scale steriliza-tions have reduced the scope of a potential comeback. In this scenario, it is only after 2025 that fertility gradually falls below replacement level. This would raise the population to a plateau of approximately 1.50 billion between 2024 and 2045. Although most recent Chinese projections simulate lower fertility levels, their assumptions of higher life-expectancy produce a higher population total for 2050 than calculated here.

Table 34 disaggregates the three intermediate projections of the chart for important subgroups of the population. For brevity's sake, they will be designated as the low, medium and high projections. The figures signal a long-term decline in the number of youth and their share in the total population. By 2050 their percentage in China may be as low as in present Western Europe. Although no projection sees an increase in the percentages for the young age groups, the two higher ones see a certain resurgence of absolute numbers between 2011 and 2025. The annual number of births could move up to more than 23 million over the first five years of that period. Even in the low projection, birth numbers will stay at a high level of 17 to 18 million in the mid-term until they diminish after 2020. There will be continuing fluctuations of children in elementary school age 7 to 12. This will be paralleled by similar fluctuations at the junior and senior high school levels.

All projections continue to show a steady growth of people at working age 15 to 64 over the next two decades. Depending on the different assumptions of the three projections, this segment of the population will continue to increase until around 2027. Its relative share in the total population will reach a zenith about a decade earlier. After 2027, the low projection has the working-age population recede to almost its original level in 2000; in the two other projections it remains at a markedly higher level than at the outset. The increase in the active population until 2027 may be dramatic. Between 1990 and the future peak year, it may increase by about 250 million, equal to an average annual net increment of up to 6.8 million. This trend can no longer be influenced by birth-control policies, and can be alleviated only by indirect interventions such as an extension of years in school, a reduction of female employment, a delayed entry into the workforce and still earlier retirement.

Some of these measures have already been implemented in the cities, where legal limitations of the working age and various social policies shorten the period of active life. They are largely irrelevant for the rural areas, however, where labour legislation does not apply, school attendance is markedly shorter

Table 34 Projections of age structure 2000–50

		2000	2010	2020	2030	2040	2050
Tight rule, fraud as usual:							
total population	(million)	1262	1347	1411	1430	1407	1354
infants 0–1	(million)	17	19	18	15	15	14
	%	1	1	1	1	1	1
youth 0–14	(million)	319	276	267	247	226	217
	%	25	20	19	17	16	16
working age 15–64	(million)	856	965	991	975	906	864
	%	68	72	70	68	64	64
old age 65+	(million)	87	106	153	207	275	272
	%	7	8	11	14	20	20
dependency ratio	%	47	40	42	47	55	57
women 15–49	(million)	343	362	336	315	293	270
	%	27	27	24	22	21	20
women 20–34	(million)	165	147	147	127	123	114
	%	13	11	10	9	9	8
Small concessions:							
total population	(million)	1262	1347	1423	1451	1432	1387
infants 0–1	(million)	20	19	19	16	16	15
	%	2	1	1	1	1	1
youth 0–14	(million)	319	277	278	264	234	230
	%	25	18	20	18	16	17
working age 15–64	(million)	857	964	991	980	924	886
	%	68	72	70	68	65	64
old age 65+	(million)	87	106	153	207	275	272
	%	7	8	11	14	19	20
dependency ratio	%	47	40	43	48	55	57
women 15–49	(million)	343	362	336	317	301	280
	%	27	27	24	22	21	20
women 20–34	(million)	165	147	147	127	128	122
	%	13	11	10	9	9	9
Delayed two-child policy, natural decline:							
total population	(million)	1268	1357	1463	1507	1506	1479
infants 0–1	(million)	20	19	22	17	18	16
	%	2	1	2	1	1	1
youth 0–14	(million)	324	285	311	293	258	257
	%	26	21	21	19	17	17
working age 15–64	(million)	857	966	994	1007	972	949
	%	68	71	68	67	65	64
old age 65+	(million)	87	106	153	207	275	272
	%	7	8	10	14	18	18
dependency ratio	%	48	40	47	50	55	56
women 15–49	(million)	343	363	340	330	324	307
	%	27	27	23	22	22	21
women 20–34	(million)	165	147	149	130	143	135
	%	13	11	10	9	9	9

Note: The dependency ratio gives the number of dependents in age groups 0–14 and 65+ per 100 persons of working age 15–64. For parameters and model assumptions see text and the new projections in Chart 19.

than in urban areas, and social support for old age is hardly known. The elderly continue in work, and only the household role of peasant women may lower the overall total of the rural labour force. In the cities, there are likewise sizeable numbers of old people who continue to hold informal jobs to supplement meagre pensions. Moreover, few private households can afford to have the wife stay out of work – even if that were an attractive option for younger women. About 84 per cent of the age group 15 to 64 has been in work during the 1990s. By the standards of industrialized countries and in comparison to Chinese figures from earlier decades, this is an extremely high participation rate. If it is applied to the projections of the future labour force, the latter could grow from 720 million in 2000 to 853 million in 2027. These numbers signal continuing heavy burdens for job creation. Relief is only in sight beyond the later half of the 2020s, when the cohorts in active life diminish.

After 2020, employment problems will be increasingly overshadowed by problems of population ageing. While all three projections show the same absolute cohort sizes of the elderly, their weight within total population varies. The Chinese workforce will be declining, too, with nearly 30 per cent of the employed in the final decade of their active life. The ranks of the very old above 80 years of age will likewise grow rapidly. However, due to the failure of the one-child policy to deliver its most ambitious promises, the percentages will not reach the extreme heights that would have been otherwise possible. Some earlier forecasts had people in old age attain a share of more than 35 per cent in 2050. The new projections show their percentage to approach 20 per cent by 2050 – still lower than the level of 30 per cent expected for Japan and Western Europe at the middle of the century.

The ageing of the Chinese population has already begun. It will accelerate between 2010 and 2040 and then progress at a slower pace. Until 2010 the dependency ratio will remain advantageous and decline even further to 40 per cent, so that welfare burdens for the young and old can be widely distributed. But Table 34 shows how there will later be a fundamental change in the situation. The incessant rise of this indicator signals that the reduction in the number of children and youth cannot make up for the additional number of people in old age who will have to be supported by the active population.

Regional trends will show marked variations. While many coastal areas in the East and the highly urbanized provinces of the Northeast will see rapidly falling rates of growth, with negative growth after 2020, the Western half of the country and the populous provinces of Central China will continue to show high natural growth rates in future decades. The population in these parts of the country will be much younger than in ageing regions of the East. This will be most pronounced in the Northwest. The lowest proportions of youth, the fastest decline of the labour force and the highest percentages of elderly people will be found in those urbanized regions of China where the most spectacular successes of birth planning have been recorded. In Shanghai, the natural growth rate of the resident population already started to become negative in 1994. In this, the largest metropolis of China, the elderly are expected to make up one-third of the population by 2050. Here, as in other urban areas, the future population structure will depend on the extent to which such trends are alleviated by young in-migrants.

In the foreseeable future, China thus has to prepare for shouldering two burdens at the same time: continuing high birth figures and a growing number of elderly people. In spite of strict birth planning and fertility below replacement level, China's population will continue to expand substantially. The age structure will produce an average annual growth rate of 0.7 to 0.6 per cent over the next ten years. Applied to the huge base numbers, the population momentum will generate annual additions of 8 to 10 million to the population total. These pressures will ease after 2020, when natural growth will fall below 0.5 per cent per year. According to the different scenarios, negative growth will set in only between 2030 and 2035. However, by that time an increasingly urgent new problem will have emerged.

16 Weighing the options: past experience and new ideas

The smooth figures of population projections for China disguise the huge implementation problems of Chinese birth control documented in this study. International family-planning circles tend to celebrate the fall of Chinese fertility levels that in recent years has contributed to a major downward revision of world population forecasts by the United Nations. This outlook differs from the views of many Chinese politicians, who worry about the stability of low fertility. Instead of falling after the turn of the century, the population will outgrow the originally defined ceiling of 1.2 billion, so that by 2050 more than double the size of the often proclaimed optimum figure of 700 million will be reached. More than 300 million births averted by birth control will then be matched by more than 300 million people in excess of the original plan. Seen from this perspective, Chinese birth control may be equally termed a huge success and a gigantic failure. This would apply not only to the twists and turns in the first three decades of the People's Republic but also to the original, ambitious targets of the one-child policy. While they underestimated the internal dynamics of population growth and the social resistance to radical birth rationing, they overestimated state power.

Even after the establishment of a vast birth-planning apparatus, many classic problems of the Chinese polity have persisted: strong pronouncements are followed by lagging action; a widely ramified bureaucracy escapes central control; the rural areas are hard to govern from the capital. Overall, it has taken nearly three decades to establish the present framework of a harsh birth-rationing regime, coupled with limited concessions towards family demands. The centre has constantly struggled with the difficulty of balancing the need to accommodate vastly different conditions at local level with the wish to preserve the thrust of a tight programme mandated from above. This is why it has insisted on the continued application of a dual rule by Party and government organs. Few arenas of economic and social policy still display the large degree of operational Party control that characterizes birth planning to this very day. This strong involvement of the Party has succeeded in whipping up periodic campaigns and in pushing through stern birth-planning norms, but the drive for their enforcement has often been followed by attrition whittling down many leadership decrees after a lapse of time.

The host of implementation problems surfacing in the 1980s reveals these basic contradictions. Specifically,

- the long list of birth-control sanctions led to excesses and abuses, while at the same time it became eroded from within;
- the much shorter list of material incentives depreciated and preferential treatment for single children lagged in enforcement;
- the crucial extension of social security did not materialize.

At the organizational level, many problems endure until this very day. For example,

- it has proven difficult to unify the increasingly intricate birth-planning norms at regional and local level, with ensuing problems of transparency and application;
- the coordination of various bureaucracies continues to be hard to tackle, and the extension of the birth-planning apparatus to the grass-roots level has been delayed for years;
- birth-planning funds have been hard to secure;
- recruitment, remuneration and training of specialized personnel have continued to be unsatisfactory;
- the ensuing problems of motivation have been deepened by sharp contradictions between the populace and grass-roots cadres, who are torn between their official duties and their obligations to local groups.

As a result of these constraints, birth planning has suffered the fate of all centralized planning systems, which struggle with the problem of lacking or distorted information from below. Among all Chinese statistical data, birth-planning figures are the most unreliable. While additional surveys and multiple systems of record-taking have introduced some checks, they have been unable to prevent the situation from deteriorating.

Such problems have been further exacerbated by fundamental changes resulting from Chinese reform policies. The following issues have figured most prominently:

- agricultural decollectivization and the return to family-based farm management, with the economic emancipation of peasants, the draining of collective welfare funds, manpower demand for petty peasant activities, and a prevalent neo-traditionalism following from it;
- the growth of the private sector, the slow revival of a labour market, increasing social mobility and new personal freedom;
- a new marriage law with a consequent drop of the marriage age;
- the increasing regional differentiation throughout the country, the waning of the central government budget, the growth of extra-budgetary revenues at provincial level, and ensuing control deficits of central government;
- ideological disintegration, mounting corruption and the erosion of Party leadership.

In consequence of such development:

- the number of official second-child permits continually increased in the 1980s, and the number of additional, unauthorized births has remained very high;
- the 1.2 billion population target for 2000 has been breached and greatly exceeded;
- demographic planning has become ever more complicated;
- population policy has turned into a highly ambivalent affair, since, while the one-child norm continues to be officially proclaimed, it often disguises a factual two-child situation.

A look behind the scenes of Chinese birth planning in the 1980s thus reveals the existence of many compromises and contradictions. Improvised rules and passive resistance were prevalent in the villages. Only the Chinese cities accomplished an effective network of birth control, but, even here, growing problems arose due to the gradual dissolution of socialist work units with the close supervision guaranteed by their government and joint-family functions.

The reaction of the leadership has been a general tightening of birth control in the 1990s. It has included the following measures:

- the increased specification of birth-planning regulations, the creation of a body of contextual population law, and the buildup of a rule-enforcement system independent of work unit-administered self-justice;
- additional restrictions for childbearing and sharply increased penalty sums for non-compliance with birth-planning rules, plus regular cadre evaluations and liabilities for birth-control enforcement;
- increased funding, an extension of the birth-planning apparatus and the medical network and more economic benefits for peasants with only one child;
- increased substitution of short-term contraception with IUD insertion and sterilization;
- renewed propaganda activities and the reintroduction of some techniques of mass mobilization.

The paradigm underlying these measures was forcefully reformulated at the start of the renewed tightening. It is contained in a book published during the turmoil of 1989 by Hu An'gang, a young Chinese economist who has since risen to become a policy adviser to Premier Zhu Rongji. While clearly following a line of reasoning discussed earlier in this study, Hu's book also digested the difficult experiences of the past and adopted a more realistic stand. It perceived China as a poor developing country, having to cope with a continuous, huge excess population in the course of her modernization. A low standard of living would therefore prevail for the foreseeable future, and the country would not be able to join the ranks of middle-income countries within the next decades. Millions of poorly educated peasants with low incomes would swell the ranks of marginalized labourers, and a low-wage policy would have to counter the reality of massive, long-term, structural unemployment and underemployment.[1]

Such fears were intensified by worries about long-term trends in grain production and food consumption. Hu An'gang viewed the provision of adequate food supplies as 'the most pressing problem' of Chinese politics and a permanent 'sword of Damocles' hanging over the country during the first half of the twenty-first century. He forecast a sluggish increase in grain production, a dramatically shrinking man–land ratio and a widening gulf between supply and demand. Clear limits of self-sufficiency would soon be reached, and these could be stretched only by a combination of massive agricultural investment, sharp price rises, food imports, changes in land use, continued rationing and a lowering of consumption standards. The constraints would be all the tighter, as both the dangers of population ageing and the fertility trends of the 1980s would make the original targets of the one-child policy unfeasible.

This then is the Chinese nightmare vision. Ultimately, it promotes a philosophy that perceives the country's huge population as the one decisive obstacle for the ascent of the nation and declares a demographic revolution from above as the most important prerequisite for future progress. Having internalized a low expectation of future economic performance, it reaches the following conclusion:

> We have to tell the people frankly and honestly that under no circumstances can we compete with the resource consumption of the USA and other developed countries. Not even with the Chinese compatriots living in Hongkong, Taiwan and Macao. . . . We should not make unrealistic promises to the people in regard to the future and thereby produce barriers of expectation that are hard to overcome in the following generation.[2]

In the final consequence, this line of reasoning promotes an enlightened demographic despotism and establishes a new basis for legitimizing communist rule in China. Rather than the herald of future freedom from want, the Party is presented as a strong authority enforcing individual sacrifices, providing collective ersatz solutions, steering the course against the threat of chaos and imposing the continuation of strict birth control. The explicit message is the need to halt further liberalization and to force the fertility rate down to 2.0 – clearly below the 1987 level of 2.6 but also clearly above the former target of 1.5 to 1.7.[3]

The arguments of this study have been echoed by a chorus of other voices from academic circles and the birth-planning bureaucracy. Here they will be labelled the pessimist camp. In their eyes, the economic burdens of overpopulation continue to be more menacing than the future dangers of over-ageing. According to them, the low fertility level of the 1990s is deceptive and highly unstable, as it largely relies on constant political pressure. Moreover, it does not prevent actual birth numbers from being excessively high. The pessimists hold that past policy changes produced only negative results;

proclamation of a two-child policy would trigger an immediate resurgence of fertility and quickly lead to a three-child reality. Moreover, it would also arouse the wrath of those who have had to obey the strict rules of the past.

These opinions have led the pessimists to believe that only a continued one-child policy with few exemptions can lead China out of her predicament and help her to approach population numbers requisite for the desired levels of well-being. They therefore counsel to keep fertility clearly below replacement level – at least for the next few decades, better still for a whole century. Many members of the camp feel provoked by the two-child exemptions for one-daughter households, which potentially involve half of all young peasant couples. Even more irritating to them are routine permits for a second child after late marriage and prolonged spacing, and the Yicheng experiment embodying these principles is whole-heartedly condemned. Cities with ageing populations are advised to lower barriers against in-migration from the villages instead of clamouring for a liberalization of birth policies. Some proposals also seize on the eugenic argument and the policies of Singapore's elder statesman Lee Kuan Yew. While advocating preferential second-child permits for intellectuals, they explicitly want to exclude illiterates and disabled persons from the number of eligible persons.[4]

More moderate voices also counsel against a policy change. They stress that constancy and gradualism produce better results than abrupt breaks, and they point to the fact that most birth-planning regulations contain a clause that explicitly permits second births for parents who are themselves single children. The number of such couples would constantly grow; by 2005 they would automatically bring about a transformation of the one-child policy for urban areas. This appealing argument generates uneasiness. A case in point is Beijing, where the city administration confirms the relevant clause while it hands out bonuses to couples not invoking it. And the logic of the rule is contested. Critics claim that the majority of better-educated single children would themselves only produce single children anyway.[5]

In essence, the arguments of the pessimists rest on continued scepticism about the prospects in policy arenas with strong demographic content. This is why a brief look at recent trends in some crucial areas is indispensable.

With an average increase of 1.5 per cent between 1990 and 1999, grain production has outpaced population growth. However, growth was less than half that of the preceding decade. In 2000 it saw the biggest slump since 1960 – against the background of ample grain reserves however. These trends caused per capita production to climb steeply in the 1980s and edge up only slightly in the 1990s, before it fell back to the level of the mid-1980s in 2000.

There are manifold political, economic and ecological reasons for these developments, which have been intensely discussed. American environmentalist Lester Brown's 1994 prediction of major Chinese food shortages and a coming crisis for the global grain market renewed the debate in China and abroad. While specialists differ as to the precise extent of future growth, most tone down Brown's arguments and conclude that the country will be able to feed its growing population. Trust exists in the potentials of agro-technical improvement, and consolation is offered by a new land census that has revealed the existence of nearly 40 per cent more cultivated area than hitherto reported. Although much of this seems to be marginal land, it has lowered the calculations for unit yield and raised the man–land ratio. By implication, it has also opened up more room for future advances. Achievements in slowing down land losses or in offsetting them by agricultural intensification have further contributed to a more optimistic picture.

The breach of population targets for 2000 has thus not produced the dreaded food crisis, and the diet has substantially improved. However, the demographic factor has certainly diminished per capita gains and contributed to the high level of Chinese grain prices. Complicated political choices and huge challenges still lie ahead for Chinese agriculture, and the problems are far from being solved. Besides future fertility, agricultural investments and rural policies, trends in the food balance, urban–rural distribution and import volume will be the major variables. It is most likely that population growth in the next two decades will cause per capita production and consumption to either stagnate or rise only gradually beyond the moderate standard of today.[6]

While food projections justify some guarded optimism, recent employment trends afford reason for anxiety. Although China has made Herculean efforts for the re-allocation of rural surplus labour, the record for the 1990s has been disappointing, and the outlook for the next two decades is bleak. During 1990 to 1999, the increase in overall employment has trailed that of population in working age and has remained far below growth in the 1980s.

The reality behind these statistics has been a decline in agricultural work and three retrenchments for township and village enterprises, which applied the breaks to their former upsurge. Today, such enterprises, plus private companies and the self-employed in the non-agricultural sector of the villages, employ one-third of the total rural labour force – a remarkable change from the less than 10 per cent of the pre-reform period but still insufficient to solve the problem of surplus labour. Although the true extent of rural employment and underemployment is notoriously hard to calculate, most current estimates still reckon with a minimum 120 million and a maximum 200 million surplus labour, equal to between 25 and 40 per cent of the entire rural labour force at the end of the twentieth century. Many of them joined the 50 million to 80 million migrant workers in the mid-1990s. In the long run, agricultural employment, which has declined from 70 per cent of total employment at the outset of economic reforms to about 50 per cent, will have to shrink further to some 10 per cent.

Urban employment has fared little better. Even though an average growth rate of 2.6 per cent between 1990 and 1999 looks impressive, it is also below the record for the 1980s and former expectations. A sharp drop in formal employment during the late 1990s has lowered the figures, and only a massive shift towards jobs in the informal private sector has prevented worse. High investment has not been able to turn the tide: it has favoured capital-intensive industrialization more than would be desirable for China. The problems have been exacerbated by surfacing unemployment. First news of non-renewed work contracts shocked the country in 1988. Since 1996, streamlining of overstaffed bureaucracies and state-owned enterprises has resulted in at least 7 million laid-off workers formally still on the payroll but in reality on the dole. If these people, plus millions of workers discharged by town and township enterprises, were added to the artificially low number of about 6 million urban unemployed who are officially registered, a number twice to three times as large would ensue. After all the book-keeping has been done, the grand total for all types of rural and urban unemployment and underemployment in China could soar to one-third of the working-age population, equal to between 250 million and 300 million people. Social policies such as retraining, prolongation of schooling or early retirement may reduce some of the pressure, but the heat will be on until the cohorts in working age decline after 2020. While creating an abundant pool of cheap labour as a principal asset of the country's investment environment, this setting also lowers productivity, retards technological and economic change and produces huge potential for social and political unrest.[7]

The extent of labour redundancy and the approaching problems of over-ageing have heightened the need for a new system of social security. The absolute size of the old population over the next fifty years is already a largely foregone conclusion, and the number of dependants in relation to persons in working age will increase under any scenario. Even if birth-planning rules were relaxed, the responsibilities for wage earners in their prime would sharply increase. It is most likely that increasing urbanization and many other social changes underway will weaken traditional arrangements of co-residence in multi-generational households. A greater number of surviving parents with raised life-expectancy will prolong periods of old-age support and add to steeply rising health expenses. In addition, economic reforms with changes in property relations, employment policy and state-run pension schemes will transform the erstwhile fabric of old-age care.

The past two decades saw the ratio between pension payments and total wage expenditures climbing from 6.5 per cent in 1980 to more than 22 per cent in 1998. The ratio of retirees to active workers and employees likewise increased from under 8 per cent in 1980 to more than 31 per cent in 1999. Projections for 2050 forecast nearly 50 per cent. Such figures mirror the squeeze between declining employment plus lagging contributions in the formal sector and an increasing number of pensioners. It has prompted fundamental changes in the system of old-age security. A new system announced in 1997 envisages increasing contributions with decreasing benefits; it will force down the level of pensions from an average 88 per cent of the pre-retirement wage to roughly 50 per cent of the past wage average in real terms. Under this system, a basic standard of living for workers earning low wages can hardly be guaranteed, and the majority of the rural population will continue not to be covered. Even so, serious deficits in pension funds are anticipated for the future and have already materialized ahead of schedule in 1998. While delayed retirement and various new policies for social security may alleviate some pressures, the role of pensions in old-age support will therefore stay limited. Family care for the elderly will have to remain an indispensable part of the picture.[8]

China's phenomenal economic growth during the reform period brightens this bleak outlook. It has overcome all intermittent slumps and has left behind the expectations of both domestic planners and foreign observers. The average annual increase of gross domestic product (GDP) of 9.7 per cent between 1980 and 2000 has thus been much higher than the approximate 7 per cent projected before. Even a downward revision of the official figures would still result in an impressive achievement. This has created the paradox that, while population targets have been seriously breached, most economic targets have been surpassed. The often derided goal of quadrupling per capita value of social product until the end of the century was realized three years ahead of schedule. In the year 2000, GDP per capita stood at about 2250 yuan; it had far outstripped the 460 yuan of 1980 and was nearly 60 per cent higher than in the gloomy forecasts of the late 1980s.[9] With the exception of grain production and rural income, all other indicators of personal consumption were much higher than anticipated before. Even the notorious bottle-neck sector of urban housing performed unexpectedly well.

Various economic factors make it likely that the fast growth of recent years will slow down in the future. However, should the country succeed in attaining real growth rates of 4 to 7 per cent over the next five decades, it could reach present standards of the upper-middle-income group of countries. Depending on future population size, gross national product per capita in the mid-twenty-first century would range between the levels of Argentina and Portugal during the mid-1990s.[10]

By necessity, such model calculations conceal many uncertainties and glaring discrepancies within a huge country. Nevertheless, they have had their repercussions. As the terminal point for officially announced policies up to the turn of the century drew near, the opponents of the one-child policy felt emboldened to become active again. Their views have been published in many specialist journals and document the limits within which dissent has become tolerated in Chinese political discourse. The dissenters from the optimist camp take issue with neo-Malthusianism: according to them, it is not overpopulation breeding poverty but rather poverty breeding overpopulation. Economic revolution should therefore precede demographic change.

An invisible force behind their views has been international revisionism in population theory that has been fuelled by rapid economic growth and steeply falling fertility in other Asian countries without compulsory birth control. In a radical version, demographic revisionism posits that population increase may stimulate economic growth. More moderately, it believes in the power of market forces to regulate population increase. The inroads of market economics in Chinese thinking on demographic issues may be gauged from a proposal submitted by Tian Xueyuan, the former head of the Academy's Institute of Population Studies, who started as one of the leading proponents of the one-child policy before modifying his stand later on. In August 1993 he wrote:

> In birth planning we should strive for a gradual change from administrative regulation to behavior guided by interest . . . . Those who have fewer

children pay less, and their children get more, while those with a higher number of births pay more and do not get any benefits for their children.[11]

The fact that this view was published by the Party newspaper documents that it has been discussed within the leadership. It can amount to a population tax, which has been debated in China's demographic circles for years; alternatively, it can also imply drastically raised penalty sums for deterrence. But fines are not identical to taxes, since the latter refrain from criminalizing excess births as long as the persons concerned voluntarily accept higher payments. The taxation of births, however, raises the sensitive question whether a higher number of births until the advent of the longed-for son should be the reserve of the rich, or whether there should be equity in the vital sphere of childbearing. Such considerations apart, the pragmatic issue remains whether a population tax might be raised effectively and whether it would suffice to limit demographic growth.

This is not the main concern of the optimists, who hold that income growth and broadly rising educational attainment are promoting a sufficiently large, voluntary reduction of family size. Such gradual change would produce more balanced population structures than the sharp ruptures caused by political intervention. Because fertility in cities and towns tends to be low anyway, some specialists also recommend a faster pace of urbanization with more in-migration from the countryside. In view of the country's record over the past twenty years, the optimists discern no clear-cut, negative correlation between demographic and economic growth and are willing to accept higher population totals than their opponents. While the one-child policy for them has only uncertain economic benefits, they blame it for accelerating population ageing and causing grave problems of old-age support. Peasants would not comply with policy for need of manpower and lack of pensions. The cities would likewise suffer from labour shortages and particularly acute over-ageing, with biased population and family structures. Other arguments focus on negative side-effects of strict birth planning such as the biased sex ratio at birth, abuses in policy implementation and strained relations between cadres and the population at large. In contrast to their adversaries, the optimists claim that earlier periods of relaxation did not trigger any major problems. Quite the opposite: difficulties are said to have been caused by excessively tight policies.

Reviving earlier proposals from the mid-1980s, the optimists propose to allow a second child, if late birth beyond age 24 and an interval of more than five years after the first birth are respected. The necessity of insisting on late marriage is under dispute, and some proponents of a relaxation accommodate the widespread wish for earlier marriage. However, late birth and extended spacing are always insisted on. In order to give more clout to these often disregarded provisos, a linkage to housing allocation is suggested. The optimists have many followers in the highly urbanized coastal areas, where problems of ageing are particularly acute. While they argue in favour of a general second-child permit for the whole population, their special attention is focused on Shanghai and other cities which are said to be in urgent need of relaxation.

Their minimal demand has therefore been to abolish the one-child rule in all low-fertility regions by 2000.[12]

With a host of internal presentations and articles published between 1993 and 1997, the optimist camp launched yet another initiative for the introduction of a modified two-child policy. The arguments left their imprint. During the mid-1990s, Chinese politicians began to express confidence in the potentials of economic growth and the success of birth planning. Instead of warning against population increase devouring all economic progress, they now confined themselves to citing the beneficial effect of birth planning for more economic growth. The former minister of the Birth-Planning Commission, who herself had expressed sympathy for a policy change before, underlined her firm intention to 'gradually change the previous approach, which relied on administrative methods, remedial measures [i.e. abortions], and shock campaigns'. As the sense of predicament started to fade, a debate on the problems of depressed fertility commenced in scholarly articles. When in early 1996 a leading demographic journal featured a symposium under the headline question 'Is Overpopulation the Main Obstacle For China's Modernization?' and allowed some contributors to answer in the negative, everything seemed ready for a break with the fundamental paradigm. One year later, the same journal published projections for a modified two-child policy that once again recommended the raising of fertility levels after the turn of the century. The belief in an imminent change of policy became so widespread that in a Chinese public opinion survey of late 1997 more than 70 per cent of the respondents thought that second children would be universally allowed by 2000.[13]

Instead of meeting these expectations, the small circle of China's highest leaders turned down the demands for an end to the one-child policy for the fourth time since 1981. A decision of the Politburo's Standing Committee from February 1998 endorsed a long-term population plan submitted by the Birth-Planning Commission for the period until 2050. This plan set population targets of under 1.33 billion by 2005, under 1.40 billion by 2010, and under 1.60 billion by 2050. Continued birth planning was declared to be essential for the next five decades, and an imminent policy change was explicitly renounced. There is some room, though, for a measured transformation, as the targets are on the generous side. This is also signalled by the fact that six months after the February 1998 decision, the Birth-Planning Commission started a research project on future population policy and dispatched a new investigation group to the two-child trial area of Yicheng county. Weighing the pros and cons of different policies, it came down in favour of a slow change to general second-child permits for parents who were both single children. The four discarded alternatives were an unlimited continuation of present policies, general second-child permits for parents among whom only one spouse was a single child, a general second-child permit for all peasants, or a return to a two-child policy for the whole population.[14]

The February 1998 decision has silenced the voices in favour of a two-child policy for the time being. The publication of a new Central Committee decision on 'Strengthening Population and Birth-Control Work and Stabilizing the Low

Fertility Level' in March 2000 made their defeat all the greater. This decision warns against 'blind optimism' and a potential resurgence of fertility; it speaks of 'aggravating problems' of employment and population ageing as well as 'acute contradictions' between population numbers, economic, social and environmental problems; finally, it announces the gradual introduction of pension schemes for single-child or two-daughter households 'according to circumstances'. In a thinly veiled reply to the provocative question of 1996, it also contains the sentence 'Overpopulation is still China's biggest problem'. This has been taken up by a new government White Book of December 2000 which again defines population as 'the key factor and number one problem constraining China's economic and social development'.[15]

One can only speculate on the reasons for the reaffirmation of the one-child policy, which is all the more unexpected since the results of the new population census of November 2000 were not yet known. It is probably not far-fetched to assume that, just as on previous similar occasions, the reluctance to effect a major policy reversal under conditions of uncertainty played a major role. China's leaders are no demographers. Faced with contradictory advice from the specialists, a heap of unreliable figures, unknown consequences of an about-turn and some aggravating population issues before their very eyes, they have tended to focus on the immediate problem and to opt for established procedure. It is likely that the acute unemployment problems of the late 1990s, the sombre projections for a huge increase of job-seekers over the next two decades and the outlook of another 300 million people until the mid-twenty-first century have been important factors in their resolve. Thus the old fear that, under the concrete conditions of present China, a two-child policy could easily lead to a three-child reality held sway.

The political background will have influenced the decision, too. All basic guidelines of the one-child policy have been decided by a group of veterans, who in 1978, after the end of the Cultural Revolution, resumed governing the country. Hard-line birth planning is inseparable from the names of Deng Xiaoping, Chen Yun, Li Xiannan, Bo Yibo, Hu Qiaomu and Wang Zhen. These influential politicians shared basic convictions that prompted the one-child campaign in 1979. A decade later, a firm stand on population policy seems to have ranked among the important qualifications of their hand-picked successor Jiang Zemin, who replaced former concession-makers Hu Yaobang and Zhao Ziyang. Ever since 1994, Jiang Zemin has turned down the idea of steering population development by the application of market economics. Instead, he has insisted on the strict implementation of birth-planning rules. During recent years, he has been repeatedly quoted with the rebuke to 'strengthen birth planning instead of putting a break on it'. In a meeting with Hongkong representatives in March 1999, he described population pressures as 'a matter of life and death'.[16]

Despite its well-known problems and widespread unpopularity, the one-child rule thus stays in force. Although in practice it has been largely modified to a one-and-a-half-child policy, the regulations and enforcement procedures governing it continue to tighten since the end of the 1980s. A case in point is Guangdong province, which in September 1998 at long last yielded to years of pressure by abolishing its general second-child permit for peasants. Another example is furnished by the introduction of levies for second-child exemptions in a number of provinces. These have 'solved' the conflict between market and command approaches in a manner typical of present-day China: they have added new taxation without giving up old sanctions. A few carefully measured concessions have balanced these developments. Examples are the slow advances for contraceptive choice, the growing recognition of a private sphere and the newly acquired right to sue the birth-planning bureaucracy for breach of law.

But the debates among China's demographers and the manoeuvres of her political leaders are only one side of the picture. There can be no doubt that since 1990 the birth-planning regulations, sanctions and controls have hardened. Implementing them, however, becomes equally harder, as the powers of intervention in social life slip away from the state. All new administrative inventions have not been able to reverse this fundamental change in the nature of things. The conflict remains between a state driving home the rationale of birth planning with ever tougher enforcement and a society reacting with ever more deft evasion. Against this background, views on the present state of Chinese birth planning have become extremely divergent. On the one hand, they include rural cadres who count on the determination of the state and who contribute comment on the birth-planning behaviour of Chinese peasants as such:

> They will all eventually comply with this new policy . . . . The first time was the most difficult, just like when you put a yoke on an ox's back for the first time. It will resist and struggle. But once the yoke is accepted by the ox, you can tighten it repeatedly, even to the point of choking it to death. Peasants are like oxen. Once they accept something as inevitable, you can continue to tighten the screw.[17]

Since the population count of 1990, this tightening of financial, legal and administrative screws may be observed everywhere. It may explain the most astonishing figures for Chinese fertility in the 1990s. China claims to have accomplished what could not be attained during the entire decade of the 1980s – the achievement and over-achievement of population plans, fertility spectacularly below replacement level, and a steeply falling number of births during a period when large cohorts of young women entered marriageable age.

Is this assumption realistic? Already in 1992, the Birth-Planning Commission and the State Statistical Bureau adjusted the results of the last national fertility survey, so that the total fertility rate was raised from 1.4 to 1.9 children per woman. The same step was taken with regard to the micro-census of 1995, which gave approximately the same results. In plain language, this means that the under-registration of births is estimated at 20 to 30 per cent, rising to 50 per cent for third- and higher-order births. But even a total fertility rate of 1.9 is low. The large increase of sterilizations, including surgery after the first child, the stronger enforcement of late marriage and late birth, the wide extension of grass-roots organization and the drastic increases of penalty sums, the weaving of an ever-tighter net of legal stipulations, administrative liabilities and mutual controls during recent years might explain it.

Social and economic trends triggered by Chinese reform policies may also have contributed to such a trend. The spectacular drop of fertility rates in a number of Asian countries over recent years gives reason to suspect that similar developments will happen in China. But neither is there a magic formula for predicting the timing and scope of such a trend, nor is it possible to accurately gauge how a long-term, secular fertility decline balances with the forces promoting temporary resurgences. In fact, the tight controls applied by Chinese birth planning are hindering all attempts to arrive at exactly such a measurement. There remains the distinct possibility that a vicious circle of pre-emptive posturing, birth-control fines spiralling in reaction to large numbers of above-quota births and data falsification rising in response to increasing penalties, is operating. Chinese fertility trends during the 1990s remain an opaque issue. For many years, the fertility rate may have amounted to anything between 1.4 and 2.1 children per woman – an extremely high margin, indicating how transparency is lost if hard-line population policies combine with a continuing deregulation of economic and social life.

The picture of the Chinese oxen trotting under the yoke of birth planning could therefore acquire quite different shades. Because Chinese political culture nurtures coercion from above coupled with evasion from below, a famous series of paintings from the Song dynasty may also contain the appropriate imagery. The picture scrolls show a wild ox being caught, disciplined and harnessed, before it suddenly dissolves, vanishes from sight and leaves the oxherd alone with the solitary moon.

The oxherding pictures express ideas of Zen-Buddhism and not of population development. But if in 1990 we still read reports on a coming population crisis, only to witness the miracle of a stable low-fertility level materializing within the short span of a year, there may be hidden links between Zen-Buddhism and demography. The oxherds will have a tough time making the oxen visible again. Their next chance to do just that will be the census of November 2000. Nobody knows what it will reveal: the old scenery, new horizons, or, once again, the moon in the mist. The answer will be decisive for the prospect of Chinese population policy to move beyond the present torments of forced birth control. It will indicate how far the country has progressed to a new era in which the limitation of population and family size will be an accomplished fact – and both long-term aspirations of Chinese political effort and deep-rooted anxieties of Chinese society may be fulfilled.

Epilogue: The population census of November 2000

Scheduled for a highly unusual time of the year, China's fifth national population census was held on 1 November 2000. The census ran into major problems of non-cooperation among couples with unauthorized births, migrants and other persons with vested interests in evading correct registration, whose numbers had constantly grown in recent years. Amidst a flurry of relevant reports, the period of enumeration had to be prolonged for five days. Even so, a first quality check in a random sample of 602 census blocks revealed an undercount of 1.81 per cent. Calculated for the whole population, the percentage is equal to roughly 23 million people. This number is already included in the preliminary census results, which have been published sparsely and with considerable delay. The publication of preliminary data is still incomplete and does not conform to previous practice. In particular, information on the precise age and sex structure or the birth and death rate during the twelve preceding months is lacking. It may be speculated that raw figures show the latter ones to be implausibly low. The information available to date is collected and compared to previous counts in Table 35.

The reported population number for November 2000 implies an annual increase of 10.89 per thousand and a total fertility rate of an average 1.9 children per woman between July 1990 and July 2000. These are average figures that could conceal different circumstances in various years. The calculation of a precise time series for the 1990s requires more detailed data. Initial examination of component groups within the total population shows a number of irregularities. The percentages for the three broad age groups thus conform exactly with the annual sample survey of 1999 but not with model calculations for fertility trends. While the figure for youth aged 0 to 14 still seems too low, the subtotal for the adult population aged 15 to 64 seems too high. It remains unexplained how broad age groups can be calculated, if precise data for the age structure are lacking. The urbanization rate has risen to 36.1 per cent because of a major definitional change in counting migrants without permanent household registration. They are now included in the urban census population after a stay of at least six months in cities or towns. The resulting urbanization rate is 5.2 percentage points higher than the 1999 figure from the annual sample survey on population dynamics, which used the old definition and required at least one year's stay. The illiteracy rate of the census was officially reported as 6.7 per

Table 35 Major results of the November 2000 census and the preceding counts

		7/1953	7/1964	7/1982	7/1990	11/2000
Total population	(Million)	582.60	694.58	1008.18	1133.71	1265.83
Infants 0–1	(Million)	19.26	28.59	20.81	23.22	
	%	3.3	4.1	2.1	2.0	
Youth 0–14	(Million)	207.99	281.31	337.25	313.00	289.79
	%	35.7	40.5	33.5	27.6	22.9
Working age 15–64	(Million)	348.98	388.27	621.62	757.68	887.93
	%	59.9	55.9	61.7	66.8	70.2
Old age 65+	(Million)	25.63	25.00	49.28	63.02	88.11
	%	4.4	3.6	4.9	5.6	7.0
Dependency ratio	%	66.9	78.9	62.2	49.6	42.6
Women 15–49	(Million)	135.09	152.81	248.59	306.35	
	%	23.2	22.0	24.7	27.0	
Average private household size		4.3	4.3	4.4	4.0	3.4
Minority population	(Million)	35.32	39.92	67.24	91.32	106.43
	%	6.1	5.8	6.7	8.1	8.4
Urban population	(Million)	77.26	127.10	206.31	296.15	455.94
	%	13.3	18.3	20.5	26.2	36.1
Marital status, age 15+						
Unmarried	%	n.a.	n.a.	28.6	25.1	
Married	%	n.a.	n.a.	63.7	68.2	
Widowed	%	n.a.	n.a.	7.2	6.1	
Divorced	%	n.a.	n.a.	0.6	0.6	
Illiteracy, age 15+	%	n.a.	52.5	34.5	22.2	8.7
Educational attainment, age 6+						
Elementary School	%	n.a.	34.1	39.9	42.3	
Junior High School	%	n.a.	5.6	20.0	26.5	
Senior High School	%	n.a.	1.6	7.5	9.0	
College and University	%	n.a.	0.5	0.7	1.6	
Births in preceding year	(Million)	n.a.	n.a.	20.69	24.07	
Birth rate for preceding year	‰	n.a.	n.a.	20.9	21.6	

Notes: Data include the military but exclude Hongkong, Macao, Taiwan and Overseas Chinese; age-specific data for 1953 and 1964 with adjustments for the military and unrecorded age by A. Coale. The dependency ratio gives the number of dependents in age groups 0–14 and 65+ per 100 persons of working age 15–64. The definitions for urban population of the various censuses are not strictly compatible. Figures for educational attainment include persons attending school at a specified level and do not include persons with unknown educational levels. The 1964 census gave the illiteracy rate for population age 13+ and the figures for educational attainment for population age 7+.

Sources: Coale 1984; Zhongguo 1982 nian renkou pucha ziliao; Zhongguo 1990 nian renkou pucha ziliao; Kua shiji de Zhongguo renkou (Zonghe juan) 1994; *RR*, 29 March 2001. For data on births and birth rate in preceding year see Chart 3.

cent. It has been recalculated here with reference to the population at and above age 15 only and raised to 8.7 per cent. This remains abnormally low. The last annual sample survey gave an illiteracy rate of 15.1 per cent.

In the coming years, all figures will need to be intensively cross-checked once the detailed final census results become available. The birth figures will be submitted to particularly close scrutiny since the discovery of a still greater undercount than reported so far remains possible. Future adjustments may also affect some figures from the 1990 count.

Notes

1 Levels of understanding

1 Ji Yi 1989, 59–60.
2 *RR*, 20 March 1983; Crane and Finkle 1989; UNFPA 1997.
3 ZJSN 1993, 31.
4 He Bochuan 1990, 228.
5 For a perceptive analysis of this problem see also Herrmann-Pillath 1991.

2 Moral and cultural dimensions

1 *Xinhua*, 8 July 1987.
2 *BR*, No. 31/1994, 8–12. For official statements on Chinese birth control compare also the following comprehensive and programmatic documents of the government: Zhongguo 21 shiji yicheng (China's Agenda for the 21st Century, White Book on China's Population, Environment, and Population in the 21st Century) 1994; Zhonghua renmin gongheguo renkou yu fazhan baogao (Report on Population and Development), in: ZRB, 17 August 1994; Zhongguo jihua shengyu gongzuo gangyao (A Program for Birth Planning in China) 1995; *RR*, 24 February 1995; Zhongguo jihua shengyu baipishu (White Paper on Family Planning in China), in: *RR*, 24 August 1995; ZRB, 3 January 1996 (English translation in: *PDR*, No.2/1996, 385–390); Zhongguo 21 shiji renkou yu fazhan baipishu (White Paper on Population and Development in China During the 21st Century), in: *Xinhua*, 19 December 2000.
3 Aird 1990, 1, 89. See also Aird's statement to the US Congress in Aird 1986.
4 On Chinese population history since the eighteenth century see Chen Ta 1946, Ho Ping-ti 1959, Perkins 1969, Elvin 1973, Schran 1978, Chao Kang 1986, Zhao Wenlin and Xie Shujun 1988, Jiang Tao 1993, Harrell 1995. For a revisionist discussion of causes and effects in Chinese population development see Lee and Wang Feng 1999. An antithetical argument on Chinese population issues is also contained in Johnson 1994.
5 The passages of the White Paper on population policy are available in: ZJSN 1992, 13–14.
6 Interview 1186; ZRTN 1993, 283.
7 *RR*, 10 February 1989.
8 Potter and Potter 1990, 230.
9 Mengzi, chapter Li Lou, paragraph 26, here in the translation of James Legge, Chinese Classics, Vol.II, part 2, p. 313. The two other unfilial types of behaviour alluded to are flattering assent to encourage parents in unrighteousness and failing to succour their poverty and old age by engaging in official service.

10 On the socio-psychological background of rural childbearing behaviour in current times see also Zhang Yuanping 1991, Peng Xizhe and Dai Xingyi 1996, 208–227, 256–280. For background literature on roles and norms in Chinese family life see Lang 1946, Freedman 1970, Croll 1985, Hsieh Jih-chang and Chuang Ying-chang 1985, Linck 1988, Leutner 1989. On past intervention in natural fertility see the references in chapters 6.5, 7.1.6, 13.1 and: Fei Hsiao-tung 1939, 32–35; Hsu 1971, 108–110; Wolf and Huang 1980, 230–241; Lee and Campbell 1997; Zhao Zhongwei 1997; Lee and Wang Feng 1999. A good overview of fertility decisions and family-based advancement strategies in both late imperial and modern China can also be found in Greenhalgh 1988.
11 Compare also Pan Yunkang 1988; Liu Dalin 1992; Evans 1997.

4 Motives and goals of Chinese birth control

1 Mao Zedong 1964, Vol. 4, 452–453.
2 *RR*, 25 April 1952; Shi Chengli 1988, 113.
3 Zhang Guangzhao and Yang Zhiheng 1988, 395–466. For a recent revisionist discussion of historical trends in subsistence levels see: Lee and Wang Feng 1999, 27–41.
4 Heuser 1999, 331; Zhang Xibo and Han Tinglong 1987, Vol. I, 309, 345, 372; *RR*, 25 June 1951.
5 Hershatter 1997, 174–175; *RR*, 7 August 1954; ZJSQ 1997, 889.
6 ZJSQ 1997 1997, 131–132; *RR*, 5 March 1957. Cf. also Chandrasekhar 1959 and Tien 1973, 163–231, and Ma Yinchu 1979.
7 The Liu Shaoqi-quotation is taken from his conversation at the *Beijing Daily* on 30 June 1958 as reported in a Cultural Revolution tabloid and translated in Schoenhals 1987, 88–87. Politically selected quotations of Mao Zedong and other leaders from the 1957–58 period may be found in ZJSQ 1997, 4–5, 131–139, 146–148.
8 ZJSQ 1997, 39, 134–135, 148–151. Cf. also Orleans 1979 and Tien 1980.
9 Beijing jingji xueyuan 1977; Tien 1980; Shi Chengli 1988, 158, 168; Jihua shengyu guanlixue 1992, 27–34; Blayo 1997, 155–157. On the rustication link see *RR*, 17 January 1977, 26 January 1977; Scharping 1981, 111–116, 345, 417–421.
10 Scharping 1985–86, Vol. II, 11–12, 23–24.
11 Premier Li Peng on 27 February 1989 during a conference of directors of regional birth-planning commissions (ZJSN 1990, 4–8).
12 Sun Muhan 1987, 391. On a similar statement of Wang Zhen in January 1980 see Shi Chengli 1988, 186.
13 Shi Chengli 1988, 236–237.
14 Cf. the early essays on population economics by Zhang Huaiyu 1981, Zhang Zehou and Chen Yuguang 1981.
15 Remarks by the influential vice-chairman of the Party, Chen Yun, to the Politburo on 21 March 1979 (Chen Yun wenxuan 1956–1985, 226–227).
16 Shi Chengli 1988, 78.
17 Ibid., 219.
18 Own calculations according to data in ZTN 1993.
19 Ma Hong 1989; World Bank 1985; see also Gongyuan 2000 nian de Zhongguo 1984.
20 For a synopsis of historical trends see Perkins 1969.
21 Ashton *et al.* 1984; Scharping 1985–86, part IV; Peng Xizhe 1987; Kane 1988; White 1994, 261–262.
22 Cf. projections of the Academy of Sciences in Xiao Jiabao 1989.
23 Shi Chengli 1988, 173; *RR*, 6 October 1978; ZJSQ 1997 1997, 13
24 Sun Muhan 1987, 381.
25 Shi Chengli 1988, 188–189; ZJSQ 1997, 139. For an early Chinese discussion of the food and population connex see Sun Jingzhi 1957.
26 Chen Yun wenxuan 1956–1985, 276.

27 *RR*, 24 September 1985.
28 ZJSQ 1997, 70–71.
29 Data on cultivated area in China are contested and have varied enormously due to the lack of reliable records. Low figures of 99 to 95 million hectares based on the reports of lower units were used by the official *Statistical Yearbook* until 1999. The 2000 edition of the yearbook reported the results of the 1985 land census and the 1996 agricultural census, which instead gave totals of 132,06 million hectares for 1985 and 130,04 million hectares for 1996: Zhongguo tudi ziyuan shengchan nengli ji renkou chengzailiang yanjiu 1992, 14, 105–162; ZTN 2000, 5, 373. Such numbers are also confirmed by satellite surveys. The adjusted 1979 value for cultivated area per capita total population is an own estimate based on the 1985 figures. For historical trends see Chao Kang 1986.
30 See among a host of similar references Chen Qi 1988, 27–35; Liu Hongkang 1988, 154; *RR*, 10 March 1983; *BR*, No. 38/1996; and the talk of the then Minister of the State Birth-Planning Commission, Qian Xinzhong, to Hebei birth-planning cadres of July 1982 (in Shi Chengli 1988, 238–239). For the current debate and re-evaluation of land and food problems see Chapter 16.
31 Deng Xiaoping wenxuan 1975–1982, 149–150; Chen Yun wenxuan 1956–1985, 226–227.
32 Scharping 1981.
33 Shi Chengli 1988, 186–187.
34 Tien 1973, 195–198; Ma Yinchu 1979. See also Scharping 1981.
35 Own calculations according to data in ZTN 1993.
36 Ma Hong 1989, 14–15.
37 Xiao Jiabao 1989. See also Kirkby 1985; Taylor 1988; Scharping 1997.
38 Numbers according to ZTN 2000. See also Lee Yok-shiu 1988; World Bank 1992a.
39 *Wenhui bao*, 23 February 1986; Lin Fude and Zhai Zhenwu 1996, 113–149.
40 *RR*, 16 March 1998; ZJSN 1998, 5–7, 9–12.
41 Chen Qi 1988; Xiao Jiabao 1989.
42 On ecological problems see Smil 1993; Edmonds 1994; Qu Geping and Li Jinchang 1994; Lin Fude and Zhai Zhenwu 1996, 196–310; Betke 1998.
43 See the statements of Jiang Zemin and Li Peng in *RR*, 23 March 1994. On the link between birth control and socioeconomic development see also Sun Jingxin 1993.
44 *RR*, 17 March 1957, 11 May 1957. See also Tien 1973, 191–199, 223–224; Shi Chengli 1988, 118.
45 The relevant passages of Mao speeches of 9 October 1957 and 28 January 1958 have been altered or expurgated from both the official, edited version of his *Selected Works* and the unofficial collections of Mao texts from the Cultural Revolution. They are reprinted in: ZJSQ 1997, 132.
46 The targets for natural increase and the draft plan are contained in a speech by Vice-Minister of Health Xu Yunbei before the conference on 18 September 1963. See ZJSQ 1997, 291, 471. The targets for total population are derived by own calculation.
47 In 1994 the official *Beijing Review* printed a special article by Song Jian outlining his views on China's developmental problems; see *BR*, No.34/1994.
48 Shi Chengli 1988, 210–211; *GR*, 13 Febuary 1980; Song Jian and Li Guangyuan 1980; Song Jian *et al.* 1982. See also the authors' earlier mathematical model in *Ziran zazhi* (Nature Magazine), No. 2/1979, and the abridged English version of their projections in Liu Zheng *et al.* 1981, 25–31.
49 Ibid.
50 Hu Baosheng *et al.* 1981.
51 Song Duanyu *et al.* 1981.
52 He Bochuan 1990, 196–229; Song Duanyu *et al.* 1981.
53 *Zhongguo jihua shengyu bao*, 18 December 1987; Hu An'gang 1989a, 13, 235–240.
54 Mao Zhifeng 1995, 316; Zha Ruichuan *et al.* 1996, Vol. II, 422–423.

55 Li Peng and Peng Peiyun in speeches on 18 March 1995. See ZJSN 1995, 15; ZJSQ 1997, 222–223. See also Hu An'gang 1989a, 189; *RR*, 19 January 1995; State Family Planning Commission 1997, 111.
56 Song Jian *et al.* 1985, 201, 209–210.
57 Ibid., 267.

5 Phases of the one-child policy and its forerunners

1 For earlier work on Chinese birth planning before the one-child policy see also Orleans 1960; Tien 1973, 163–296; Orleans 1979; Wolf 1986; Banister 1987, 145–182; Sun Muhan 1987, 84–103, 117–135, 142–150; Shi Chengli 1988, 115–172; Tien 1991, 81–97; Peng Xizhe 1991, 16–45; White 1994; Blayo 1997, 138–166. For a collection of contemporary estimates of China's population during 1949–53 see Aird 1961, 11.
2 The documents may be found in ZJSQ 1997, 146, 1405. For the background see Sun Muhan 1987, 330; Shi Chengli 1988, 118; White 1994, 256–257; for press reports on women's problems see *RR*, 7 March 1951, 30 August 1951, 8 March 1956; on the 1953 census and the reliability of earlier population figures see Aird 1961; Scharping 1985–1986, part II.
3 Guojia jihua shengyu weiyuanhui 1999.
4 *RR*, 18 September 1954; *GR*, 19 December 1954.
5 The full text of the Liu-speech, the proposals of the Ministry of Health and the *ad hoc* commission and the CC directive are reprinted in ZJSQ 1997, 1–3, 146–147, 1405; ZRN 1985, 4–5; for typical specimens of press reporting on Women's Day see *RR*, 8 March 1955; on the general background see Orleans 1960, 60–61.
6 The internal directives and reports of the Ministry of Health on the first birth-planning campaign are collected in: ZJSQ 1997, 1–3, 59–61, 125–128, 146–147, 269, 889–894, 1035. The text of the Ministry's 1954 and 1956 directives on abortion and sterilization are available in ZRN 1985, 4–8 (English translations in Scharping 2000a, 18–23); text of the revised directive of May 1957 in ZJSQ 1997, 893–894. See also Sun Muhan 1987, 94–96; Shi Chengli 1988, 113, 118–123, 131. On the Ministry of Health and health politics in the early 1950s see Lampton 1977, 22–24, 46–49.
7 See also the overviews in Croll *et al.* 1985, 87–89; Peng Xizhe 1991, 27–29; White 1994, 268–273.
8 For the original contributions to the debate see *RR*, 21 February 1957, 3 March 1957 to 20 March 1957, 5 July 1957; *Wenhui Bao*, 8 to 9 April 1957, 27 April 1957; Chen Da 1957; some are reprinted in Ma Yinchu 1979 and ZJSQ 1997, 530–561. For synopses and background comments see Orleans 1960, 62; Tien 1973, 185–231; Zhang Guangzhao and Yang Zhiheng 1988, 473–486. On individual participants in the debate and Chinese social science in the pre-communist period see Gransow 1992. Cf. also sections 4.1 and 4.2.
9 ZJSQ 1997 1997, 131–132; *RR*, 14 October 1957; White 1994, 271–273.
10 Documents on the national birth-planning conference of 1958 in ZJSQ 1997 1997, 125–128, 289–291; for further 1958 reports on birth-planning issues see *Liaoning ribao*, 26 March 1958; *RR*, 6 June 1958, 12 June 1958; Shi Chengli 1988, 137.
11 For excerpts from Mao speeches, relevant passages from CC documents, and the political background to birth planning in the Great Leap see ZJSQ 1997, 4, 131–132; Zhonggong dangshi ziliao 1993, 216; Shi Chengli 1988, 125–140. On the Ma Yinchu case see also Orleans 1966; Ma Yinchu 1979. For further discussion of different views in the leadership see section 4.1.
12 See texts of the Zhou speeches in ZJSQ 1997, 134–135, 148–152. On the resettlement programme see Scharping 1981. On the demographic consequences of the Great Leap see Ashton *et al.* 1984; Banister 1987, 85; Peng Xizhe 1987; Kane 1988.

13 For the text of the 1962 CC directive, the resolutions of the 1963 work conference and relevant internal reports from the Ministry of Health see ZJSQ 1997, 4–6, 128, 291–292, 894; for the text of the newly revised regulations on abortion and sterilization of October 1963 see ZJSQ 1997, 894; for a work report of the Shanghai Party committee on birth planning in the city between 1962 and 1965 see ZJSQ 1997, 6–8, 1297.

14 Official summaries of the second birth-planning campaign may be found in 1964 and 1965 work reports of the Ministry of Health and the newly founded State Birth-Planning Commission in ZJSQ 1997, 8–10, 293–296, 895–897; further contemporary documents on financial and technical aspects of birth control in ibid., 61–64, 897–899. On birth planning in the early 1960s see also Myrdal 1963, 292; Shi Chengli 1988, 142–153; Jihua shengyu guanlixue 1992, 29; Peng Xizhe 1991, 19–26, 30–45.

15 *RR*, 27 November 1968.

16 The ministerial reports and directives on birth planning from 1970 to 1972, the State Council approval of July 1971, the relevant passages from the fourth five-year plan, and summaries of the 1971 and 1972 work conferences on birth planning are available in ZJSQ 1997, 10–12, 64–65, 129–130, 296–298, 482, 1035.

17 Contemporary press reports in *RR*, 25 August 1973, 4–5 September 1973, 26 June 1974, 10 December 1975; documents on the birth-planning work conferences of 1973–77, the Shanghai model, and regulations on contraceptives from 1974 and 1975 in ZJSQ 1997, 10–11, 65–67, 482–484, 1036–1037. On third-birth permits in Liaoning see Scharping 2000a, 107. For background literature on the development of birth planning in the 1970s see also Parish and Whyte 1978, 138–154; Orleans 1979; Banister 1987, 151–170; Shi Chengli 1988, 155–171; Blayo 1997, 155–166. On the politics of marriage see Croll 1981.

18 *RR*, 2 March 1978, 6–8 March 1978. See § 57 of the constitution of 1978.

19 Jihua shengyu guanlixue 1992, 30–31; ZJSQ 1997, 12–14, 437–438.

20 Shi Chengli 1988, 180.

21 Shi Chengli 1988; Chen Yun wenxuan 1956–1985, 222, 226–227; Deng Xiaoping wenxuan 1975–1982, 149–150; ZRN 1985, 125; Tien 1991, 101; *RR*, 11 August 1979.

22 Scharping 1985–1986, part III; ZRN 1985, 1269; Shi Chengli 1988, 191–192; *RR*, 25 September 1979.

23 Tien 1991, 117; Shi Chengli 1988, 174–176; ZJSQ 1997, 12–14.

24 *RR*, 27 January 1979; Xinhua, 22 December 1979; Shi Chengli 1988, 177.

25 Mosher 1982, and 1983, 241–245.

26 Potter and Potter 1988, 225–250.

27 Shi Chengli 1988, 185–186.

28 Tien 1991, 123–129; ZJSQ 1997, 575–577.

29 Liu Zheng, Wu Cangping and Lin Fude 1980; ZJSQ 1997, 565–568.

30 *RR*, 3 February 1980, 14 February 1980; Shi Chengli 1988, 180.

31 GR, 13 February 1980; Shi Chengli 1980, 48; *Banyuetan*, 10 August 1980.

32 *Wenhui bao*, 25 May 1981.

33 ZRN 1985, 1270.

34 The Open Letter was published by all Chinese dailies on 26 September 1980. It is reprinted in ZRN 1985, 27–29, and in all other similar compendiums.

35 Examples are speeches by Party leaders Wang Heshou and Wang Renzhong to the Central Disciplinary Commission and to the Women's Federation of 4 May 1980 and 20 November 1980 (Shi Chengli 1988, 192, 205–206).

36 Shi Chengli 1988, 196.

37 Ibid., 210–211.

38 Ibid., 214; GR, 11 June 1981, 27 August 1981; *RR*, 16 June 1981.

39 ZRN 1985, 32.

40 The case was first published in the Hongkong paper *Zhengming ribao* on 27 July 1981. It is described in Aird 1986, 208–211.

41 *RR*, 8 September 1980; *GR*, 11 September 1980; Tien 1983; Zeng Yi 1991. Compare also section 11 and ZSTZ 1990.
42 Shi Chengli 1988, 214. For a differing perspective on decollectivization and birth control see Zeng Yi and Schultz 1998.
43 Ibid., 223–224; ZRN 1985, 33; *Xinhua*, 8 December 1981.
44 Sun Muhan 1987, 400.
45 ZJSQ 1997, 707–708; Interview 386.
46 Text of the directive circulated as Zhongfa 11/1982 in ZRN 1985, 45–48. See also *Renkou*, No. 1/1985, 49.
47 Sun Muhan 1987, 184–195; Shi Chengli 1988, 240–241; *RR*, 23 August 1982; ZJSQ 1997, 21–23.
48 Sun Muhan 1987, 408.
49 Ibid., 199.
50 *RR*, 5 December 1982. See paragraphs 25, 49 and 107 of the constitution of 1982.
51 Shi Chengli 1988, 251. See also Qian's article in the central Party organ *RR*, 2 January 1983.
52 *Guowuyuan gongbao*, No. 21/1982, 1063–1064.
53 Sun Muhan 1987, 200–203; Shi Chengli 1988, 257–261.
54 Shi Chengli 1988, 276.
55 ZRN 1985, 57.
56 Shi Chengli 1988, 266; Xinhua, 5 August 1983; ZJSQ 1997, 70–71.
57 Ibid., 278.
58 Tian Xueyuan 1984.
59 Sun Muhan 1987, 235.
60 Excerpts of the report are available in ZJSQ 1997, 573–575.
61 Indirect clues to the change may be gleaned from reports in *RR*, 8 March 1984. More precise references to the meetings may be found in Sun Muhan 1987, 234–235; Shi Chengli 1988, 292–293.
62 For the full text of Zhongfa 7/1984 see ZJSQ 1997, 24–27; English translation in White 1992, 27–39. For earlier synopses see also Aird 1990, 35–38, and Tien 1991, 134–138. For earlier Chinese commentaries and reports see Shi Chengli 1988, 296–297; ZJSN 1986, 70ff., 209–211, 307–314; ZJSN 1987, 30, 288; ZJSN 1988, 23–24; ZWN 1985, 123.
63 ZJSQ 1997, 702–706, 708, 711–714, 716–717.
64 Interviews 1286, 1386, 1486, 1390, 2390, 2490. See also the detailed discussion in Aird 1990, 35–38.
65 Liang Jimin and Peng Zhiliang 1984. The experiments in Mian County later became widely noted and obtained the support of the UNFPA. See *RY*, 6/1982, 27; *Jiankang bao*, 2 March 1984; *RD*, No. 1/1986, 17–20; Shi Chengli 1988, 308–309.
66 Field research.
67 Ma Bin 1990.
68 All information on this conference from field research.
69 Shi Chengli 1988, 306–307.
70 Ma Hong 1989, 6–7. See also Gongyuan 2000 nian de Zhongguo 1984, 5–6; Hu An'gang 1989b; Ma Bin 1990.
71 ZJSN 1987, 34–41; ZJSN 1989, 64–66; ZJSN 1991, 270–275, 284–291; ZJSN 1992, 494–496; Xinhua, 26 January 1988.
72 *RR*, 13 December 1985.
73 *Jingji ribao*, 5 November 1985; Ma Hong 1989, 13–16, 97–100.
74 Ma Bin 1990.
75 Bongaarts and Greenhalgh 1985; Greenhalgh and Bongaarts 1987; Interview 2186. Compare also Chen and Tyler 1982. For an indirect rebuttal of the Bongaarts/ Greenhalgh proposal see Jiang Zhenghua and Chen Songbao 1988.
76 *RD*, 1/1986, 1–3; ZJSN 1986, 45, 307–314.
77 Yu Jingyuan *et al.* 1990.
78 ZRN 1985, 57; ZTN 1993.

352 *Notes*

79 ZRTN 1988.
80 The published version of the seventh five-year plan with the absolute target number can be found in Zhonghua renmin gongheguo guomin jingji he shehui fazhan di qi ge wunian jihua, Beijing 1986, 179–180. The underlying vital rates of the plan are given in: ZJSN 1987, 28–29.
81 The numbers cited are based on own calculations. See also later analyses in ZJSN 1991, 257–261; Yu Jingyuan *et al.* 1990; Zeng Yi *et al.* 1991.
82 Interview 1286, 1386, 1486.
83 The full text of Zhongfa 13/1986 is available in ZJSQ 1997, 27–30; English translation in White 1992, 41–50. See also Guojia jihua shengyu weiyuanhui 1992, 544–545; Aird 1990, 59–87.
84 *Zhongguo keji bao*, 20 July 1986.
85 Ma Hong 1989, 98; Ma Bin 1990.
86 Shi Chengli 1988, 432.
87 Xinhua, 4 December 1986; Shi Chengli 1988, 345; White 1992, 59–60.
88 ZJSN 1987, 6–12.
89 ZJSN 1987, 124–125.
90 GR, 6 March 1988. See also Hu An'gang 1989b.
91 Qu Yibin 1988; Zeng Yi *et al.* 1991; Wei Jinsheng and Wang Shengling 1996, 80–96. For additional analyses of the resurgence of birth numbers see Zhang Xinxia 1987; Wei Jinsheng 1988; Ma Yingtong 1988; Sha Jicai 1994, 113–123.
92 ZJSN 1987, 23–24; Guojia jihua shengyu weiyuanhui 1992, 666.
93 Random survey results in CD, 1 July 1987, ZRTN 1990; first results of the microcensus in *Xinhua*, 12 November 1987. On the estimates from late 1986 see Xiao Jiabao 1989; Ma Bin 1990.
94 Interview 3190.
95 ZJSN 1988, 22–24.
96 *Xinhua*, 31 March 1987, 4 April 1987.
97 ZJSN 1988, 4–8; Hu An'gang 1989b.
98 ZRZS 1988, 3.
99 ZJSN 1988, 15.
100 Ibid., 12–16.
101 ZJSQ 1997, 75–76.
102 Ma Bin 1990; GR, 6 March 1988.
103 Interview 1292.
104 Ma Bin 1990.
105 *RR*, 14 January 1988.
106 GR, 6 March 1988.
107 Field research.
108 CD, 4 May 1988; *RR*, 4 May 1988.
109 ZJSN 1989, 3–4. The dissension is noted in Ma Bin 1990.
110 ZJSN 1989, 27–28.
111 On the experiments in Yicheng county, Shanxi province see Yang Zhuquan 1995, 132–134; Liang Zhongtang and Tan Kejian 1997. For Liang Zhongtang's views see also ZJSQ 1997, 573–575.
112 ZRZS 1988, 21; Hu An'gang 1989b; ZJSQ 1997, 711, 716–717.
113 Field research.
114 Field research.
115 See the circular of the Birth-Planning Commission on combating corruption of 10 June 1988 in Chang Chongxuan, 409–410. For the survey see ZJSN 1989, 15–21. First data from this survey were reported in ZRTN 1989, 128–141; full documentation in Liang Jimin and Chen Shengli 1993. Compare also sections 8.2 and 10, Chart 1 and Table 21.
116 On the circular see *RR*, 13 December 1988. The list of the eight main problems may be found in Zou Ping 1988b.

117 ZJSN 1990, 92–94. See also the earlier projection in Jiang Zhenghua and Chen Songbao 1988.
118 ZJSN 1990, 11, 67; Ma Bin 1990.
119 ZJSN 1990, 4–8; ZJSQ 1997, 171–173; Zeng Yi 1994, 22–23.
120 Ibid., 4–8, 18–31, 211; ZJSN 1992, 47; ZJSN 1991, 18–31; ZJSQ 1997, 733–734; ZRGFFQ 1994, 910–911.
121 Ma Bin 1990.
122 ZJSN 1990, 9–12; Ma Bin 1990; ZJSQ 1997, 171–173.
123 ZJSN 1990, 13; Ma Bin 1990.
124 Ma Bin 1990.
125 For a field report on changes in a Shaanxi area between 1988 and 1993 see Greenhalgh *et al.* 1994.
126 Ibid.; Yu Jingyuan *et al.* 1990.
127 Aird 1990, 83; Kuang Ke 1989.
128 ZJSN 1994, 31, 190, 224, 228; ZJSQ 1997, 732; *Renkou bao*, 15 May 1995. Cf. also section 7.1.4.
129 ZJSN 1992, 6–9.
130 Interview 1192.
131 ZJSN 1991, 40–42, 48; ZJSN 1992, 46–56.
132 ZJSN 1991, 18–31; ZJSN 1993, 47–50; ZJSN 1992, 36–46; Chen Jian 1993.
133 The regulations are available in their order of mention in the following sources: ZJSN 1991, 105–108; ZJSN 1991, 193–196; ZJSN 1991, 175–187; ZJSN 1991, 187–192; ZJSN 1991, 102–105; ZJSN 1992, 10–12.
134 *Guowuyuan gongbao*, 24 November 1992; ZJSQ 1997, 89–90.
135 ZJSN 1991, 18–31; ZJSN 1994, 65; ZJSQ 1997, 744–745.
136 ZJSN 1993, 6–11; ZJSN 1996, 115–116; ZJSN 1997, 121–122; ZRGFFQ 1994, 918–1003; ZJSQ 1997,51,54–56.
137 *RR*, 21 December 1993; *FEER*, 13 January 1994; Yang Zhuquan, 276–282. For the eugenics issue see also Croll 1993; Döring 1997; Dikötter 1998; and *PDR*, No.3/1995, 698–702.
138 Interviews 1386, 3190; ZJSN 1991, 71; ZJSN 1995, 112–113; ZJSN 1999, 85; Yang Zhuquan 1995, 9–10; *Ming Bao*, 22 June 1999; Cai Fang 2000, 184–185; *RR*, 8 May 2000; *Jiancha ribao*, 20 December 2000; *Xinwen wanbao*, 13 April 2001; *Xinhua*, 29 December 2001. Cf. also section 6.1 below and the texts in Scharping 2000a and 2000b.
139 Yang Zhuquan 1995, 123–127; ZJSQ 1997, 89–90, 92–93.
140 ZJSN 1991, 187–192; ZJSN 1992, 36–56.
141 ZJSN 1991, 99–100; ZJSN 1992, 1–5, 36–46, 267–268; ZJSN 1996, 7; *RR*, 8 May 2000, 13 June 1991. See section 7.3 below.
142 ZJSN 1992, 138–144; ZJSN 1993, 17–25. Cf. also sections 7.1.4 and 7.1.7 below.
143 ZJSN 1993, 53–56; ZJSQ 1997, 748–749; ZJSN 1995–97; Li Chengxun 1999, 377; Cai Fang 2000, 106.
144 ZJSN 1993, 51–53; Xu Xifa 1995, 230–240; English translation in Scharping 2000b. For further details see section 4.9.1.
145 Guojia jihua shengyu weiyuanhui 1992, 813–815; ZJSN 1993, 17–18. See also section 7.1.3 below.
146 Interview 3292; ZJSN 1992, 36–46; ZJSN 1993, 34–39.
147 Interview 1190.
148 Zhai Shengming 1994; Yang Zhuquan 1995, 132–138.
149 ZJSN 1992, 150.
150 ZJSN 1993, 17–25.
151 Jiaozhou jihua shengyu weiyuanhui 1997. For further discussion of fertility trends see Chen Jian 1993 and section 12 below.
152 ZJSQ 1997, 662–664, 735–736, 984, 1434; ZJSN 1996, 5–7.
153 ZJSN 1995, 7.

154 *Xinhua*, 24 January 1994, 19–8–1994; *RR*, 22–23 March 1994, 4 January 1996; ZJSN 1996, 4–5; ZJSN 1998, 5–7. For the quotation from Peng Peiyun see ZJSN 1995, 19.

155 ZJSN 1991, 99–100; ZJSN 1992, 188–189; ZJSQ 1997, 84. A detailed time series of the original plan targets for 1991 to 2000 may be found in Chen Shengli and Zhao Shi 1991, 313.

156 ZJSN 1992, 20–21; ZJSN 1993, 27. The revised annual plan figures for natural increase between 1993 and 1996 are given in ZJSQ 1997, 53–58.

157 ZJSN 1995, 28–32; ZJSN 1997, 33; ZJSQ 1997, 51–58, 107–111.

158 *ZRB*, 3 March 1993; *RR*, 22–23 March 1994; ZJSN 1996, 16–20. For a further discussion of current policy up to the end of 2000 see section 16 below.

6 Legal norms and practice in flux

1 A summary list of sources for approximately 130 provincial regulations and seventy other relevant documents discussed in the following sections is given in Table 2. For the evolution of regional birth-planning norms see also Greenhalgh 1990; Scharping and Heuser 1995; Scharping 2000a, 2000b.

2 *Xinhua*, 22 December 1979; Shi Chengli 1988, 177. The Anhui regulations may be found in *FBIS*, 20 April 1979.

3 Zou Ping 1993, 258–272; ZJSQ 1997, 719–723; Hebei sheng jihua shengyu xingzheng peichang shishi banfa.

4 Scharping 2000b, 9–10; ZJSN 1988, 37–40; Zou Ping 1988b, 8.

5 *CND*, 2 August 2000.

6 See also Chen Changbin and Deng Jianming 1994.

7 An example of additional lower-level regulations on penalties may be found in Aird 1990, 71–72. See also the birth-planning measures of Harbin city in Scharping and Heuser 1995, 360–369, and of Qingtian county (Zhejiang province) in Scharping 2000a, 88–100.

8 Compare also section 5.5.

9 ZJSN 1994, 37; ZJSN 1996, 114–115.

10 For traditional marriage norms and their modern transformation see Lang 1946; Levy 1949; Domenach and Hua Chang-ming 1987; Wang Yuesheng 1995. On the politics of marriage in earlier periods of the PRC see Croll 1981.

11 ZJSQ 1997, 291. Compare also sections 6.8 and 11 (below) as well as Parish and Whyte 1978, 162–169; Saith 1981, 493; Tien 1983; Song Zexing 1987, 330–331; Banister 1987, 152–165; Tien 1991, 26–34.

12 *RR*, 8 September 1980; *GR*, 11 September 1980; Interview 1186; Yang Zhuquan 1995, 123.

13 Greenhalgh 1993, 233–237.

14 Scharping and Heuser 1995, 337–343.

15 Ibid., 360–369; Guangzhou shimin shouce 1992, 175; Zeng Yi 1994, 41–52; Scharping 2000a, 88–89.

16 Shi Chengli: 1988, 177; see also Mosher 1982 and 1983.

17 Scharping 2000a, 53, 57,63,79; Huang Shu-min 1989, 179; Hebei sheng renkou diaocha dui 1996, 15–16.

18 Greenhalgh 1993, 243.

19 See *inter alia* Hebei sheng renkou diaocha dui 1996, 1, 19–20.

20 Zhonggong Beijing shiwei 1992, 508–510, 559–561; Guangzhou shimin shouce 1992, 175–180.

21 Song Jianhua 1994; Zeng Yi 1994, 42; Yang Zhuquan 1995, 147–149; Scharping 2000a, 89–93; Hebei sheng renkou diaocha dui 1996, 40–43; field research.

22 Chen Yun 1986, 59; ZJSQ 1997, 4–5, 129–130, 291–292, 296–298. For references to a two-child restriction for workers and staff in 1973 see the Liaoning documents of 16

June 1979 (translated in Scharping 2000a, 107) and 1 March 1989 (translated in Scharping 2000b, 38).
23 ZRN 1985, 29.
24 Shi Chengli 1988, 240–241.
25 The Guangdong regulations from 1980 and 1986 are translated in Scharping and Heuser 1995, 304–312.
26 See also ZJSN 1989, 62; Peng Peiyun's remarks in *Xinhua*, 29 May 1997; or Yang Zhuquan 1995, 138.
27 Information from field studies and interviews 1386, 1486; Sun Muhan 1987, 236–237; *RD*, No. 1/1986, 1–3; ZJSN 1986, 45, 307–314.
28 Interview 1186; ZJSN 1987, 343; ZJSQ 1997, 711.
29 Zou Ping 1988b.
30 Li Jiali 1995, 567–569.
31 Some of these new rules may be found in ZRGDFH 1995, Vol.2, 589; ZRGFFQ 1994, 936–939; ZRGFFQ 1996, 1113–1119; Scharping 2000a, 78, 91; Scharping 2000b, 48. Cf. also section 6.8 below.
32 See Table 2; cf. also Nygren and Hoem 1993, 21.
33 Own calculations; for different Chinese appraisements see Yang Zhuquan 1995, 37, 140; Zeng Yi 1997, 1407–1411.
34 Hsu 1971, 108–110; Kane 1987, 67; Linck 1988, 63–64; Goodkind 1991, 669–671; Bray 1997, 321–326; Hershatter 1997, 316, 463; Lee and Wang Feng 1999, 91–92. For Chinese discourse on sex and reproduction during the early twentieth century see Diekötter 1995; since 1949 Evans 1997, 33–55. For research on traditional contraceptives cf. also section 7.1.6 below.
35 On policies for contraception see also Orleans 1960, 66–67; Snow 1973, 44; Tien 1991, 153–174. For 1970–78 contraceptive rates see ZRN 1991, 529; International Statistical Institute 1991, 73–101. Own estimates for contraceptive rates in the 1950s and 1960s on the basis of census figures for women of reproductive age, fragmentary data for marriages and production of contraceptives, as well as standard values for couple years of protection.
36 For data on contraceptive operations from the Ministry of Health see ZWN 1993. Notes to the Ministry's figures specify some provinces that did not provide data for certain years, but these missing cases do not seem to explain the full range of discrepancies with the Birth-Planning Commission data.
37 Mosher 1982; Mosher 1983.
38 Aird 1990, 32.
39 *Henan ribao*, 10 May 1990; Guangdong sheng jihua shengyu tiaoli, 18 September 1998; Heilongjiang sheng jihua shengyu tiaoli, 18 December 1999.
40 ZWN 1984, 131; Wu Jieping and Xiao Bilian 1985; UNFPA 1984a; ZJSQ 1997, 907, 927, 937, 1061; Chang Chongxuan 1991, 161–167, 174; Blayo 1997, 253–255.
41 GR, 11 June 1981, 27 August 1991. See also section 10 (below) and Huang Shu-min 1989, 181.
42 Shi Chengli 1988, 214–215; Guojia jihua shengyu weiyuanhui 1992, 315–319; ZJSQ 1997, 701.
43 Ibid., 221–222.
44 On the compulsory tests see e.g. Huang Shu-min 1989, 181; Scharping 2000a, 80, 92–93; Scharping 2000b, 49. Cf. also section 7.1.4 below.
45 International Statistical Institute 1991, 259; Blayo 1997, 262–264; Chang Chongxuan 1991, 171–173. On policy guidelines from 1994 and 1996 see ZJSN 1995, 108; ZJSN 1997, 121–122.
46 See also section 7.1.6 below.
47 ZJSQ 1997, 292.
48 Mosher 1982, 356; Mosher 1983; Potter and Potter 1988, 250.
49 PDR, No. 3/1983, 560–561.
50 Sun Muhan 1987, 237.

51 Until the latest round of revisions, provincial regulations or implementation rules from Shanxi, Inner Mongolia, Heilongjiang, Shanghai, Anhui, Jiangxi, Henan, Hunan, Guangdong, Guangxi and Guizhou worked with the formulation that sterilizations after the second child 'should' be practised, Gansu used the word 'must'. Shandong, Hubei, Sichuan and Ningxia lay down the obligation to 'propagate' or 'mobilize for' sterilization after the second child. Yunnan leaves an option to resort 'mainly to long-term contraception or sterilization'.

52 Ma Bin 1990; Yu Jingyuan *et al.* 1990; ZJSN 1992, 36–46; Radio Guizhou, 9 April 1993; Scharping 2000a, 98.

53 On the revisions see also ZJSN 1995, 108; ZJSN 1997, 121–122, 293; Scharping 2000b, 106.

54 For the 'unsettled debt' between 1994 and 1999 see Cai Fang 2000, 13–14. For an admission of forced sterilizations see Zhongguo jihua shengyu zhixing xiaoguo yanjiu ketizu 1996, 35. On provincial and county regulations in Zhejiang see Scharping 2000a, 33, 47, 55, 64, 91. See also paragraphs 19, 20 and 34 of the new Law on Population and Birth Planning in *Xinhua*, 29 December 2001. This law contains ambiguous clauses. While it decrees that 'the state creates the conditions to safeguard citizens making an informed choice of safe, reliable and suitable methods for contraception and birth prevention', it also stipulates that 'couples of reproductive age shall self-consciously implement methods of contraception and birth prevention and accept service and guidance in birth-planning technique'. Furthermore, it urges 'the choice of contraceptives with long-term reliability for couples who already have a child'.

55 All contraceptive rates in this and the following paragraphs according to Chinese data and own calculations from survey and report figures in ZJSN 1986ff.; ZRTN 1988ff.; Liang Jimin and Chen Shengli 1993, Vol. 3; ZJSN 1993, 169; Jiang Zhenghua 1995; State Family Planning Commission 1997, 27–57. Cf. also the similar results of the 1985/87 in depth-fertility survey in nine provinces: State Statistical Bureau 1986, Vol.1, 101–128; State Statistical Bureau 1989, Vol.1, 185–211. A very detailed survey for contraceptive use in the rural areas of Jiangsu province is available in Qiu Shuhua *et al.* 1994. For a summary of trends in contraception and abortion in the 1970s and 1980s see also Blayo 1997, 245–273.

56 Wu Jieping and Xiao Bilian 1985.

57 Gu Shengzu and Xu Yunpeng 1985. See also sections 7.1.6 and 7.3 below.

58 See also Zhang Fengyu 1997, 125–153.

59 For total numbers of contraceptive surgery at national level see Table 7.

60 For the relevant stipulations of the Anhui birth planning regulations see section 6.6; on Fengyang County see Wang Jiye and Hull 1991, 83–84; Peng Xizhe and Dai Xingyi 1996, 228–280.

61 See the detailed cross-tables in ZRTN 1989, 138–139, where current pregnancies are eliminated from the list of reasons.

62 Yuan Yongxi 1991, 130–133.

63 ZJSQ 1997, 9, 292, 898, 1297. For abortions in the earlier period see also Tien 1987; Tien 1991, 175–196.

64 Yang Zhuquan 1995, 37.

65 See Scharping 2000b, 76.

66 Field research.

67 Field research.

68 Field research.

69 See Scharping 2000a, 117.

70 *Henan ribao*, 10 May 1990.

71 For an open acknowledgement of such cases in recent survey reports see Zhongguo jihua shengyu zhixing xiaoguo yanjiu ketizu 1996, 35.

72 Cf. also section 10 below.

73 ZJSQ 1997, 895, 920–921.

74 Rival data on contraceptive surgery and abortions hailing from the State Birth-Planning Commission may be found in ZRTN 1994.
75 Own calculations for 1982 to 1990.
76 Chang Chongxuan 1991, 63, 170; Blayo 1997, 267–268.
77 Ibid; cf. also section 13.1 below.
78 A very divergent series with notably lower provincial rates for January to September 1992 is also available from the 1992 fertility survey: Jiang Zhenghua 1995, 292. The differences to the calculation in Table 8 are either caused by the different reference period or again indicate large-scale data falsification.
79 Zou Ping 1985; Chang Chongxuan 1991, 169–170; Chen Gaoyi and Wan Xiuzhen 1991; Blayo 1997, 270–273; Interview 397.
80 RN 1985, 996; *FEER*, 19 July 1990.
81 White 1985, 330.
82 Guangzhou shimin shouce 1992, 176–177.
83 Birth-planning report data for 1982 may be found in ZJSN 1983.
84 Arnold and Liu Zhaoxiang 1986, 227–229; Liang Jimin and Chen Shengli 1993, Vol. 3, 486–507.
85 See section 7.3 (below) for the discussion of other financial problems.
86 ZJSN 1993, 53–56.
87 Guangdong sheng jihua shengyu tiaoli, 18 September 1998; Guangdong sheng nongcun dusheng zinü fumu he chunsheng er nü jiezha fufu yanglao baoxian shishi banfa, 1998; Shanghai shi jihua shengyu tiaoli, 4 April 2000. See also Cai Fang 2000, 106, 107.
88 ZJSQ 1997, 76–77, 717–718, 918–923.
89 Xie Cheng 1988.
90 Mosher 1983, 242.
91 Greenhalgh 1993, 238–239.
92 Yu Jingyuan *et al.* 1990; Yang Zhuquan 1995, 233–235.
93 Field research; Davis 1989; Krieg and Schädler 1994.
94 Interview 1390.
95 See also Krieg and Schädler 1994.
96 On different forms of preferential treatment see also Xie Cheng 1988.
97 ZJSQ 1997, 80–81, 733–734; Zhongguo jihua shengyu zhixing xiaoguo yanjiu ketizu 1996, 35; Scharping 2000a and 2000b.
98 Song Zexing 1987, 330–331; ZJSQ 1997, 291–292.
99 For descriptions of the sanctions used in the 1970s see Parish and Whyte 1978, 142–144; Whyte and Parish 1984, 160–161.
100 Such fines for non-contraception are laid down in the present birth-planning regulations of Jiangxi, Hubei and Liaoning provinces. For a discussion of contextual violations of birth planning norms punishable under criminal or administrative law see section 10 below.
101 Mosher 1983, 225–261.
102 Potter and Potter 1988, 241.
103 White 1985, 351.
104 Huang Shu-min 1989, 176; Interview 2486.
105 Kaufman, Zhang Zhirong *et al.* 1989, 714–721; Greenhalgh 1993, 239–242.
106 Ibid. For a later field report on developments in this area between 1988 and 1993 see Greenhalgh *et al.* 1994.
107 Li Jiali 1995, 579–581.
108 Cheng Changbin and Deng Jianming 1994.
109 Field research.
110 Chan *et al.* 1992, 319.
111 Aird 1990, 71–72.
112 Zhonggong Beijing shiwei 1992, 510.
113 For a documentation of Zhejiang and Liaoning regulations see Scharping 2000a, 37–87, and Scharping 2000b, 5–56.

114 Shanghai regulations from 1992 and Jiangsu regulations from 1990 in ZRGFFQ 1994, 942–947 (German translation of the Jiangsu document in Scharping and Heuser 1995, 370–379). The sums have been left unchanged in more recent versions of the regulations. A catalogue of additional fines not contained in the provincial birth-planning regulations is also available from Qingtian county in Zhejiang; see Scharping 2000a, 95–99.

115 Interviews 4190, 4593; field research. For averages of local fines in 1995 ranging from 0.1 to 4.5 annual per capita incomes see also Zhongguo jihua shengyu zhixing xiaoguo yanjiu ketizu 1996, 35–36.

116 ZJSN 1996, 76; ZJSN 1997, 175–176.

117 Own calculations from census figures and annual household survey data. For the figure from the nationwide survey on fertility and household economics see Tian Xueyuan 1993, 337.

118 Zhang Weidong and Zhang Sulin 1990.

119 Ibid.; Yu Jingyuan et al. 1990; *Guowuyuan gongbao*, 24 April 1995; ZJSQ 1997, 81.

120 Such clauses are contained in regulations from Jilin, Shaanxi, Ningxia, Anhui, Hebei, Inner Mongolia and Beijing promulgated in 1989 to 1994. See ZRGDFH 1995, 445–448, 1838–1841, 1945–1948; ZRGZQ 1995, 515–524.

121 Cai Fang 2000, 192.

122 *RR*, 8 May 2000.

123 The ruling of the Supreme Court is dated 13 August 1990. See also Mosher 1983,252; Shi Chengli 1988, 192.

124 Ibid.; ZJSN 1986, 110.

125 Scharping 2000b, 93; *CND*, 26 November 2000.

126 Kuang Ke 1989. See also *Zhongguo qingnian bao*, 30 August 2000.

127 Zhongguo jihua shengyu zhixing xiaoguo yanjiu ketizu 1996, 38.

128 *South China Morning Post*, 20 December 2000; *CND*, 22 December 2000.

129 Chen Shengli and Zhao Shi 1991, 276.

130 ZJSN 1994, 270, 301.

131 Shi Chengli 1988, 196; ZJSQ 1997, 185.

132 *Henan ribao*, 10 May 1990.

133 *Shaanxi ribao*, 8 October 1993.

134 *RZ*, No. 3/1991, 17–20.

135 ZRGDFH 1995, Vol.2, 591; *Nanfang ribao*, 1 May 1998, 27 February 2000.

136 The Heilongjiang regulations of 1989 can be found in Scharping and Heuser 1995, 351–359.

137 *RR*, 3 April 1993.

138 ZRN 1985, 27–29.

139 Shi Chengli 1988, 215–217; Xu Xifa 1995, 189.

140 ZRN 1985, 45–48.

141 For conference volumes and specialized overviews of birth planning among China's national minorities see also Qinghai sheng renkou xuehui 1984; Yunnan sheng renkou xuehui 1984; Yang Yixing 1984; Yu Jinshuan et al. 1985; Xu Xifa 1995; Deng Hongbi 1998. See also the provincial synopses in ZJSQ 1997.

142 Xu Xifa 1995, 190; ZJSN 1993, 51–93.

143 Field research. 1988 regulations in Scharping and Heuser 1995, 344–350; 1990 amendments in ZRGFFQ 1994, 929–931.

144 Field research. 1989 Heilongjiang regulations in Scharping and Heuser 1995, 351–359 (the relevant articles have been unchanged in the revised Heilongjiang regulations of 1994 and 1999); 1993 Jilin regulations in: ZRGFFQ 1994, 936–939. See also Scharping 2000c and the Liaoning documents in Scharping 2000a, 113,118; Scharping 2000b, 17, 26–27.

145 Scharping and Heuser 1995, 304–312, 322–336.

146 For birth planning in Tibet see also: Xu Xifa 1995, 179, 230–240; ZJSN 1996, 232–235; *RY*, No.1/1996, 41–48; ZJSQ 1997, 1361–1365; and the translations of

Tibet birth-planning documents in Scharping 2000b, 57–99. For Tibetan birth-control organisation and fertility levels see also sections 6.5, 7.1.2, 7.2 and 12.8 below.

147 http://www.tibet.com/WhitePaper/white8.html. This document cites an extremely low number of married women in childbearing age, which is far exceeded by census figures. But since it can be reconciled with population data for Lhasa and Shigatse, it probably refers to the 1987 situation in both cities only. For the census results in Tibet see Sheng renkou pucha bangongshi 1992–1993 (with the reference: Xizang zizhiqu 1990 nian renkou pucha ziliao, Vol. 3, Lhasa 1992, pp. 3–5). For contraceptive rates from Tibet in 1999 see Table 3. Some further discussion of birth planning in Tibet is available in Hoppe 1997, 69–84, and Goldstein and Beall 1991.

148 *RY*, No.1/1996, 46; Zhang Kewu 1996, 107–108, 111–112.

149 The 1990 regulations from Ningxia and the 1991 regulations from Xinjiang are available in Xu Xifa 1995, 211–230.

150 Rules for the declaration of nationality status are reprinted in Guojia jihua shengyu weiyuanhui 1992, 177–178, 892–893. For the reclassification issue in the Northeast see also Scharping 2000a, 118; Scharping 2000c. For a perceptive discussion of ethnicity in Xinjiang see Hoppe 1995, 23–40.

151 Scharping 1993, 1997.

152 Ibid.; Song Jianhua 1994; *RR*, 9 July 1995.

153 These are Beijing, Tianjin, Shanghai, Zhejiang, Fujian, Jiangxi, Shandong, Guangdong, Guizhou, Yunnan and Qinghai. See, in the order of mentioning, ZJSN 1987, 34–41; ZJSN 1989, 64–66; Shanghai shi wailai liudong renyuan jihua shengyu guanli banfa, 20 June 2000; ZJSN 1991, 270–275, 284–291; ZJSN 1992, 494–496; *Xinhua*, 26 January 1988.

154 For the text of the national procedures and an official interpretation see ZRGFFQ 1994, 913–914; ZJSQ 1997, 727–732. A German translation of the document is available in Scharping and Heuser 1995, 380–383. The continuous tightening of birth-planning regulations for the migrant population may also be studied in the various stages of relevant regulations from Zhejiang, Liaoning and Tibet; see Scharping 2000a, 65–66, 79–81, 92–94; Scharping 2000b, 39–40, 46, 56, 65, 73–74, 78, 81, 89, 97–98.

155 ZJSN 1998, 82.

156 Interview 1292,1193,2593. See also: *Renkou*, 1/1986,57–58; Liao Xuebin 1988; Chen Shengli and Zhao Shi 1991; Gui Shixun 1992; Lin Jinfeng 1992,72–73; Wu Cangping 1996, 138–144; ZJSQ 1997, 727–732; *CND*, 23 September 1998; ZJSN 1998, 228.

157 *Xinhua*, 5 August 1993; ZJSQ 1997, 715; *ZRB*, 5 September 1994, 15 May 1995.

158 Shi Chengli 1988, 241; *RR*, 23 August 1982.

159 ZJSN 1986, 37–38; ZJSQ 1997, 700.

160 ZJSQ 1997, 733.

7 Problems of organization

1 Shi Chengli 1988, 172. See also *RR*, 9 July 1978.

2 Ibid., 175; ZJSQ 1997, 13–14. The same directive was repeated three years later in a leading article of the Party organ: *RR*. 27 January 1981.

3 Shi Chengli 1988, 214, 221–222, 248–249.

4 ZJSN 1989, 27–28; ZJSN 1990, 67; Ma Bin 1990; ZJSQ 1997, 472–480.

5 *RR*, 3 April 1993.

6 ZJSN 1995, 6. See also section 7.1.4 below.

7 Information for the preceding paragraphs comes from ZJSQ 1997, 12–14, 437–438, *passim*. On organizational arrangements during 1963–78 see also Peng Xizhe 1991, 30, 36–37.

8 Shi Chengli 1988, 177; Jihua shengyu guanlixue 1992, 30; ZJSQ 1997, 14.
9 ZRN 1985, 32; ZJSN 1995, 177; Chang Chongxuan 1992, 45; ZJSQ 1997, 438, 454–455; RY, No.1/1996, 42.
10 ZJSN 1992, 264; ZJSN 1999, 131; ZJSQ 1997, 439–446.
11 Shi Chengli 1988, 217; ZJSQ 1997, 439–446.
12 Scharping 2000b, 100–101. Cf. also section 6.1 above.
13 ZJSN 1986, 57–58; ZJSN 1992, 267–268; ZJSN 1993, 192–194; White 1985, 273–301; Chang Chongxuan 1992, 51; ZJSQ 1997, 454–455, 1159–1175.
14 ZJSQ 1997, 1390–1403.
15 ZJSN 1986, 60–62; ZJSN 1993, 192–194; Chang Chongxuan 1992, 52–57; ZJSQ 1997, 447–460, 1159–1175.
16 Chang Chongxuan 1992, 46–47.
17 See also the list contained in the decision of the Central Committee and the State Council on birth planning from 2 March 2000 in RR, 8 May 2000.
18 UNFPA 1984b; Xinhua, 30 July 1988; Pan Yunkang 1988; Li Jinfeng 1992, 53; ZJSN 1994, 124–125; ZJSQ 1997, 771–772.
19 White 1985, 213–215; Guojia jihua shengyu weiyuanhui weishengbu guanyu peihe zuohao jihua shengyu muying baojian gongzuo de tongzhi, 16 January 1995.
20 Wu Cangping 1996, 140–141; ZJSQ 1997, 747–748.
21 ZJSN 1990, 4–8; Wu Cangping 1996, 140–141; Wei Jinsheng and Wang Shengling 1996, 408–409, 418–419; ZJSQ 1997, 171–173.
22 ZJSQ 1997, 477–480, 484–494.
23 ZJSN 1993, 17–18; ZJSQ 1997, 462–465.
24 White 1985, 213; Chang Chongxuan 1992, 51. For the organizational set-up in Beijing municipal region during the early 1980s see Croll et al. 1985, 197, 201–209. Cf. also section 7.2 below.
25 RR, 7 February 1975; Croll et al. 1985, 219–229; White 1985, 243–267, 273–301; ZJSN 1993, 192–194. For a grass-roots report on rural birth-planning propaganda in 1962 see Myrdal 1963,292.
26 Ibid., 295; ZJSN 1995, 77; ZJSQ 1997, 301, 1211.
27 Chang Chongxuan 1992, 51; Li Jinfeng 1992, 46–47.
28 White 1985, 243–267, 273–301; Li Jinfeng 1992, 54–58; ZJSN 1993, 192–194; ZJSN 1994, 209; Wang Xiuyin 1998. Figures for the Birth-Planning Association from ZJSQ 1997, 1211, and Xinhua, 13 December 1999; total for women of reproductive age according to the 1994 population sample survey.
29 For a discussion of birth planning within the context of village self-administration see Alpermann 2001. See also the case study on birth planning in a Northern Chinese village in Zhang Weiguo 1999.
30 Good descriptions of such responsibility systems and evaluation criteria may be found in Li Jinfeng 1992, 121–131; Chen Jian 1993; RZ, No. 3/1993, 17–20; ZJSN 1994, 209. For the economic sanctions implied by such systems see also section 6.8 above.
31 ZJSQ 1997, 852–854.
32 See Hebei sheng renkou diaocha dui 1996, 51–62; Wang Xiuyin 1998.
33 Jia Tongjin and Sai Yin 1995.
34 Peng Xizhe and Dai Xingyi 1996, 311.
35 ZJSN 1996, 324–325; Jiaozhou jihua shengyu weiyuanhui 1997.
36 Zhu Guoping 1997; Scharping 2000b, 49, 53.
37 Zhongguo jihua shengyu zhixing xiaoguo yanjiu ketizu 1996, 33; Zhang Weiguo 1999.
38 ZWN 1993.
39 RR, 26 June 1974, 7 February 1975, 10 December 1975. Cf. also Lampton 1977 and Davis 1989.
40 For earlier references to malpractices in birth planning documents of 1964–78 see ZJSQ 1997, 898–899, 900–901, 905; 1983 and 1989 Standards for Diagnosis of Concomitant Ailments After Birth Control Surgeries as well as Administrative Procedures

for the Handling and Certification of Concomitant Ailments After Birth Control Surgery are documented in ibid., 914–915, 949–954.

41 ZJSQ 1997, 895–897; UNFPA 1984, 65–67; Guojia jihua shengyu weiyuanhui 1992, 842–846; ZWN 1993, 1996; ZTN 1998; ZFTZ 1991, 484.

42 UNFPA 1984a; Jihua shengyu guanlixue 1992, 301; Jiang Zhenghua 1995, 282–286.

43 Chang Chongxuan 1992, 58; ZJSN 1992, 138–144, 267–268; ZJSN 1993, 17–25; Jihua shengyu guanlixue 1992, 296–305; RY, No. 2/1998, 72–75; ZJSN 1998, 50; ZJSQ 1997, 973.

44 Chang Chongxuan 1991, 151; Zhongguo jihua shengyu zhixing xiaoguo yanjiu ketizu 1996, 34.

45 *RR*, 26 March 1957; ZJSQ 1997, 890–891.

46 Orleans 1960, 67; Chang Chongxuan 1992, 230–237; ZJSQ 1997, 62, 293–296, 895–898, 983, 1035, 1061. Cf. also section 6.5 above.

47 See the research plans and reports in ZJSQ 1997, 10, 901–902, 909, 926, 930, 938. For a list of some traditional prescriptions see also Kane 1987, 67, 144–151.

48 Zhao Shengli 1987; Sun Muhan 1987, 213–215.

49 ZJSQ 1997, 1452–1453; Chang Chongxuan 1992, 57. For an assortment of products and production figures see ibid., 230–237; ZJSN 1994, 107–108.

50 Zhao Shengli 1987; Chang Chongxuan 1992, 57, 239–244; ZJSN 1993, 343; *RYJ* No. 6/1987, 11–13; Sun Muhan 1987, 213–215; Jihua shengyu guanlixue 1992, 310–343; Guojia jihua shengyu weiyuanhui 1992, 563–569; ZJSQ 1997, 458.

51 ZJSN 1993, 343; ZJSQ 1997, 78; ZJSN 1998, 122.

52 Guangzhou shimin shouce 1992, 179–180; Interview 1292.

53 Shi Chengli 1988, 171; Chang Chongxuan 1992, 60; ZJSQ 1997, 1448–1450.

54 ZJSN 1990, 315–317; ZJSN 1993, 319; ZJSN 1996, 15, 33; *RR*, 11 January 1993; ZJSQ 1997, 451, 459, 1175–1217; Chang Chongxuan 1992, 335–348. See also section 7.1.4 above.

55 Chang Chongxuan 1992, 59; ZJSN 1994, 178; ZJSQ 1997, 451–452, 1232–1252.

56 Chang Chongxuan 1992, 51–52; ZJSQ 1997, 1077. On the situation in two large-scale Beijing enterprises during the early 1980's see Croll *et al.* 1985, 209–218.

57 All following data on personnel according to ZJSN 1986, 57–58; ZJSN 1993, 126, 192–194; Li Jinfeng 1992, 35; Chang Chongxuan 1992, 43; ZJSQ 1997, 712 and *passim*. Cf. also White 1985, 243–267.

58 Interview 2190; ZJSN 1990, 211; ZJSN 1992, 37; ZJSQ 1997, 304.

59 Chang Chongxuan 1992, 58; ZJSN 1993, 192–194; ZJSQ 1997, 447–449.

60 ZJSN 1998, 192. For the assessment of workload see Peng Xizhe and Dai Xingyi 1996, 311.

61 ZJSQ 1997, 800–802, 1085–1089; ZJSN 1998, 51, 192.

62 Sun Muhan 1987, 215–216; ZWN 1984, 125–126; ZWN 1985, 125–127; ZWN 1986, 70–72; UNFPA 1984a, 81–982; ZJSN 1994; ZJSN 1998, 184; ZJSQ 1997, 807, 1085–1086.

63 Interview 2190; Chen Jian 1993; *RY*, No. 1/1996, 44; ibid., No.2/1998, 74.

64 Calculations according to price indices for urban consumer prices and data for average wages in the health sector in ZTN 1997; ZLTN 1997. The average wage for the health sector includes non-medical personnel.

65 ZJSN 1992, 267–268; Zhou Changhong 1995; ZJSQ 1997, 90–91.

66 *RR*, 14 January 1988.

67 Field research; Zhou Changhong 1995; Zhongguo jihua shengyu zhixing xiaoguo yanjiu ketizu 1996, 39.

68 ZJSQ 1997, 61, 997–998, 1025; Peng Xizhe 1991, 32; Interview 1286.

69 For the contributors to social expenditures between 1971 and 1993 see Gao Ersheng *et al.* 1997, 23.

70 Own calculations according to data in Table 16, budgetary data and the general retail price index in ZTN 1997.

71 Own calculations according to national budget data in ZTN 2000.

72 ZJSN 1992, 138–144; ZJSN 1995, 78; ZJSN 1997, 173–174; ZJSN 1999, 131, 134. Interviews 1286, 1386, 1486, 1292, 1492.
73 Chang Chongxuan 1992, 286; ZJSN 1994, 115; ZJSN 1997, 175; ZJSQ 1997, 1023. For a survey of seventy-seven birth-planning stations in townships and towns see *RY*, No.2/1988, 73.
74 ZJSQ 1997, 999–1000, 1020–1024.
75 For general principles of budgetary management in birth planning see: Jihua shengyu guanlixue 1992, 344–371.
76 *RY*, No. 1/1996, 44.
77 For a field report on such a situation in an Anhui township see Peng Xizhe and Dai Xingyi 1996, 228–314.
78 Chang Chongxuan 1992, 276–279; ZJSN 1992, 138–144; ZJSQ 1997, 1041.
79 ZJSN 1994, 113; ZJSN 1995, 165; ZJSQ 1997, 1029–1030. For references to funding arrangements in Tibet see the Autonomous Region's 'Provisional Measures for Birth-Planning Management' of May 1992 in Scharping 2000b, 97–98.
80 Calculations on the basis of crude figures and information in ZJSN 1996, 18, 76; ZJSN 1997, 174–175. See also section 6.8 above.
81 Greenhalgh 1990, 228.
82 ZJSN 1996, 18; ZJSQ 1997, 851–852; Cai Fang 2000, 14.
83 *RYJ*, No. 4/1987, 12; White 1985, 271; Guojia jihua shengyu weiyuanhui 1992, 570–571; ZJSQ 1997, 1042. 1993 figures according to Gao Ersheng *et al.* 1997, 23–24.
84 For privately financed contraceptives see also section 7.1.6 above; for present problems of financing and future plans see Gao Ersheng *et al.* 1997; ZJSN 1999, 134.

8 Planning and evaluation

1 Cf. Orleans 1979.
2 Song Jian *et al.* 1985, 29.
3 If no separate information is given, all following data hail from Chen Shengli and Zhao Shi 1991, 226–229, 259–284; Li Jinfeng 1992, 12–22; Jihua shengyu guanlixue 1992. The Provisional Rules for the Formulation of Population Plans are available in ZJSQ 1997, 841–842, 855–856.
4 Wang Jiye and Hull 1991, 78–82.
5 UNFPA 1989.
6 ZJSQ 1997, 841.
7 ZJSN 1991, 96–100; ZJSN 1992, 188–189; Jihua shengyu guanlixue 1992,51–54; ZRGFFQ 1994,194–195.
8 Interviews 1192, 1292; Jihua shengyu guanlixue 1992, 41–45, 200–205; Song Jianhua 1994.
9 Song Jianhua 1994; Li Jinfeng 1992, 128.
10 Interviews 1186, 3186, 1286.
11 Interview 1492; ZRGFFQ 1994, 917–918.
12 Ibid.; interview 2486.
13 ZJSN 1992, 189–191; ZJSQ 1997, 841.
14 Jihua shengyu guanlixue 1992, 47–59; Li Jinfeng 1992, 128–129.
15 Cf. section 6.7 and Table 9 above. For the definition of birth planning indicators cf. Sichuan yixueyuan 1978; Yuan Fang 1988; Chen Shengli and Zhao Shi 1991; Jihua shengyu guanlixue 1992, 200–205.
16 On the household registration system after 1949 see Aird 1968, 218–239. The 1958 regulations on household registration continue to be in force and are reprinted in ZRN 1985, 83–85. On records of the health system see also Merli 1998.
17 Sun Muhan 1987, 218–221; Chang Chongxuan 1992, 123.
18 Sun Muhan 1987, 222.
19 Chang Chongxuan 1992, 128–135; ZJSQ 1997, 834–837.

20 Ibid., 223. For recommended data sheets and filing cards at the grass-roots level see also Jihua shengyu guanlixue 1992, 387–395; ZJSN 1993, 292–293; Hebei sheng renkou diaocha dui 1996, 34–40.
21 Interview 2286; ZJSN 1992, 499; ZJSN 1993, 47–50, 70–72; Chen Jian 1993; ZJSN 1994, 73; ZJSN 1996, 32; ZJSQ 1997, 72–73; Jia Tongjin and Sai Yin 1995; *RYJ*, No.4/1998, 28; *Sichuan ribao*, 13 July 2000. For a more detailed discussion and documentation of all following data cf. also section 12 above.
22 ZJSN 1989, 15–21. The 1997 birth total and birth rate as obtained by the birth-planning reports amounted to 13.88 million and 11.53‰; the rival figures from the annual sample survey of the Statistical Bureau were 20.38 million or 16.57‰ respectively. Cf. ZJSN 1998, 435–436, and ZRTN 1998, 3, 360. For falsification of birth reports and regional figures see also section 10, Chart 1 and Table 21 below.
23 Interview 1194; *PDR*, No. 2/1993; Nygren and Hoem 1993; State Family Planning Commission 1997, 23–25; Zeng Yi 1995; Zhang Weimin *et al.* 1997, 46. See also Merli and Raftery 2000.
24 Field research.
25 ZJSN 1999, 87–90; Nygren and Hoem 1993; Zeng Yi 1995; Cai Fang 2000, 7.
26 ZJSN 1993, 73–74.
27 Coale 1984, 27–31.
28 *Zhongguo tongji xinxi bao*, 2 January 1989; *RX*, No. 6/1993, 50–55. See also Chart 3 in section 12.1 below.
29 The 1996 year-end total from the registers was 1195.46 million, to which 3.2 million from the military have to be added. The year-end total from the annual sample survey was 1223.89 million. Data are taken from ZRTN 1999.
30 Jiang Zhenghua 1995, 125, 130; Zeng Yi 1995.
31 Jia Tongjin and Sai Yin 1995. See also the description of survey practices in section 7.1.4 below.
32 Survival rates by own calculations from census and micro-census materials. On census data quality see also Zha Ruichuan *et al.* 1996, Vol. I, 47–108, 221–227, who employ a wide range of different methods for evaluating the 1990 census. Their calculations for persons born in 1989 and 1990 result in an under-reporting of approximately 4 per cent. Zhang Weimin *et al.* (1997, 40–42, 65) end up with an average excess of 6 percent for cohorts born between 1979 and 1989 by adjusting the sampling ratio of the 1995 micro-census to produce population totals that conform to the 1995 annual sample survey. But there is no way to prove the reliability of the latter either. For the continuous revision of the 1990 birth rate see ZJSN 1997, 134–135.
33 Zhang Weimin *et al.* 1997, 46–47; ZJSN 1996, 17–18.
34 For data problems with regard to contraceptive surgery and abortions cf. also sections 6.5 and 6.6 above.
35 Cf. information in sections 6.8 and 7.1.4 above.
36 Guojia jihua shengyu weiyuanhui 1992, 673–675; ZJSQ 1997, 1088–1119; ZJSN 1996, 191–192.
37 Ibid.
38 For further information on petition sections or complaint bureaus see Shi Tianjian 1997, 60–64, 94.

9 Gender roles, family size and sex preferences

1 CD, 2 May 1988; *Xinhua*, 6 November 1994, 23 January 1995.
2 State Statistical Bureau 1986,Vol.1, 86–100; State Statistical Bureau 1989, Vol.1, 153–181; Feng Xiaotian 1991; Wang Feng 1996; ZRN 1997, 257–260. On different survey outcomes resulting from different wording of the questionnaire and on urban family-size preferences see also Milwertz 1997, 93–85,120–149,160–182.

3 Zhang Ziyi *et al.* 1982; Guo Shenyang 1985; Zhong Sheng 1986; Wang Feng 1996; Peng Xizhe and Dai Xingyi 1996, 150–156. For the argument that a son preference realized has also been instrumental for reducing the number of higher-order births see the analysis of the 1982 fertility survey for peasant women born in 1914–30: Zhao Zhongwei 1997.
4 See sources in ibid. Also Whyte and Gu 1987; Wei Jinsheng and Wang Shengling 1996, 337, 343–344; Zhongguo jihua shengyu zhixing xiaoguo yanjiu ketizu 1996, 33; Zhao Zhongwei 1997, 740; Johnson, Huang and Wang 1998, 476–478, 489.
5 Arnold and Liu Zhaoxiang 1986.
6 A few special survey results for the usually high family-size preferences of national minorities are available in Deng Hongbi 1998, 97–103.
7 Tian Xueyuan 1993, 336. For some local survey results from Liaoning, Heilongjiang, Shaanxi and Sichuan see Wei Jinsheng and Wang Shengling 1996, 297–346; Wang Ling 1997. For motivational aspects of childbearing of city women in Beijing and Shenyang see Milwertz 1997, 160–182.
8 See also Wang Dongfeng 1982; Lu Li 1990; Lü Hongping 1991; Cao Jingzhuang 1990; Zhang Yuanping 1991; Peng Xizhe and Dai Xingyi 1996. For a good summary discussion with historical depth see Greenhalgh 1988.
9 Data on income sources hail from the 1987 sample survey of the aged population. See Tian Xueyuan 1989; Tian Xueyuan 1991, 147–185. For the census figure see Peng Xizhe and Dai Xingyi 1996, 66.
10 For a good field report on prevailing practices see Zhang Xiaoquan 2000.
11 Peng Xizhe and Dai Xingyi 1996. See also Zhang Feng 1997; *RY*, No. 1/1997, 71–72. For another good general discussion of peasant fertility motivation see Wei Jinsheng and Wang Shengling 1996, 183–296.
12 Whyte and Gu 1987, 483–486.
13 Lü Hongping 1991.
14 Lu Li 1990.
15 This is reported by Gates (1993) for business women in Chengdu and by Cao Jingzhuang (1990) in his study of wealthy peasants in a Liaoning district. For the balance of childrearing costs versus utility see Tian Xueyuan 1993; Peng Xizhe and Daixingyi 1996, 56–72; Wang Ling 1997.
16 Zhang Ziyi *et al.* 1982; Liu Xian 1985; Guo Shenyang 1985; Wei Jinsheng and Wang Shengling 1996, 300, 329–331, 339–346.
17 ZRZS 1983, 17; *RR*, 22 February 1985.
18 Cao Jingzhuang 1990. Cf. also Wei Jinsheng and Wang Shengling 1996, 297–314.
19 Liu Xian 1985.
20 *RY*, No. 6/1992, 20–23.
21 For further discussion of gender discrimination see section 10 below; for an analysis of its consequences for fertility differentials, sex structure at birth and underlying factors see sections 12.3 and 13.1 below.

10 Strategies and evidences of non-compliance

1 ZJSQ 1997, 701, 744–745, 939, 959–960. See *inter alia* the birth-planning regulations from Zhejiang and Liaoning in Scharping 2000a, 45–47, 69–72, 84–86, 95–99; Scharping 2000b, 45, 53–54, 97, plus further regulations from Fujian, Hubei, Guangdong and Shaanxi in ZRGFFQ 1994, 956–960, 969–972, 975–979; *Shaanxi ribao*, 10 August 1994.
2 See the cases culled from Chinese press reports in Bianco and Hua Chang-ming 1988. Other descriptions of strategies for thwarting birth control are available in Zhou 1996, 176–205; Zhang Weiguo 1999.
3 Zhou 1996, 180; Shi Chengli 1988, 248–249.
4 Zhong Weiqiao 1987; Chen Jian 1993; Zeng Yi 1994, 26–27. Rates for women aged 10 to 19 between 1944 and 1988 in Chang Chongxuan 1991, 100. For an

investigation report on the reasons for the resurgence of early marriage see ZRN 1994, 532–543.

5 *RZ*, No. 3/1991, 21–23; ZJSQ 1997, 89–90, 92–93; Scharping 2000a; Qingtian xian shishi Zhejiang sheng jihua shengyu tiaoli banfa, 15 May 1996.

6 ZJSN 1989, 11; ZJSN 1992, 387; Guojia jihua shengyu weiyuanhui 1992, 584, 649, 657–658; Zhongguo jihua shengyu zhixing xiaoguo yanjiu ketizu 1996, 35; field research.

7 *CND*, 7 September 1997, 11 September 1997; *Ming Bao*, Hongkong, 8 September 1997.

8 Zeng Yi *et al.* 1993, 291–294.

9 *Xinhua*, 6 May 1996, 29 December 2001; ZJSQ 1997, 984; *CND*, 30 December 1998, 12 April 2000.

10 For a survey with questions on cadre attitudes towards sex-specific abortions see Zhongguo jihua shengyu zhixing xiaoguo yanjiu ketizu 1996, 32, 36.

11 Ji Yi 1989.

12 Ji Yi 1989; *CND*, 3 February 1999.

13 Johansson and Nygren 1991, 44–45; Johansson 1995.

14 ZTN 1986.

15 Adoption law in ZRN 1992, 35–38. ZTN (1998) gives a number of c. 26,000 to 21,000 notarial documents for child adoptions in 1996 and 1997. Other sources from 1996 refer to some 8000 to 10,000 cases per year: Johnson 1996; Johnson *et al.* 1998, 482, 492. For the legal background see Heuser 1999, 363 367. On the 1999 amendment of adoption rules, first in Guangdong then at national level, see *CND*, 5 April 1999, 31 May 1999.

16 *RR*, 7 April 1983; *Xinhua*, 17 April 1983; Bianco and Hua Chang-ming 1988, 157–158; ZJSQ 1997, 23; Zeng Yi *et al.* 1993. For details on the sex proportion at birth see section 13.1 below.

17 For the methodology employed in this estimate and further details see section 13.1 below.

18 Chen Jian 1993; Yang Zhuquan 1995, 254; Human Rights Watch 1996, 77–136; Johnson 1996; Johnson *et al.* 1998, 473–481.

19 ZJSQ 1997, 735–736; ZRGFFQ 1994, 933–935.

20 Yang Zhuquan 1993, 239–240. For details cf. section 12 below.

21 *RX*, No. 6/1993, 50–55; Zha Ruichuan *et al.* 1996, Vol. I, 95–96.

22 Qian Zhenchao 1997.

23 Chang Chongxuan 1992, 409–410.

24 Wang Hean 1998.

25 ZRN 1985, 18–19.

26 Sha Jicai 1994, 486–487.

27 The figures are based on a comparison of original and revised total fertility rates from the 1995 micro-census as reported in ZRTN 1997 and ZJSN 1997. Cf. also section 12.5 below.

28 ZJSN 1993, 71–72.

29 Field research.

11 Female marriage trends

1 This may also be seen in the discussion of total age-specific marriage rates in Peng Xizhe 1991, 123–125, and Blayo 1997, 229–232. On marriage cohorts see also section 13.2 below.

2 A good synopsis of historical nuptiality trends is available in Lee and Wang Feng 1999, 63–82. Data for 1930 come from later adjustments of the large rural survey of J.L. Buck and from Dingxian in Hebei; contemporaneous local data from Jiangsu and Taiwan are higher by about 2 years. Data for 1949 to 1979 hail from the 1982 fertility

survey. See Barclay *et al.* 1976; Gamble 1968, 39–44; Ch'iao Ch'i-ming *et al.* 1938, 36; Wolf and Huang 1980, 133–142; Quanguo 1% renkou shengyulü chouyang diaocha fenxi 1983, 98–129. All following statements on historical trends are based on these sources. For more detailed discussions of marriage trends up until 1987 see Peng Xizhe 1991, 119–128, 177–185, 231–245; Coale *et al.* 1991; Zhou Qing 1992; Blayo 1997, 205–244.

3 *CND*, 28 May 1999; ZJSN 1998, 122; '98 Zhongguo renkou, 15.

4 Cf. Yu Xuejun *et al.* 1994.

5 Late-marriage rates for 1949 to 1978 from ZSTZ 1990, 37; later data from ZJSN 1995 and Jiang Zhenghua 1995.

12 Fertility levels

1 On underregistration see Coale 1984, 2, 28; Calot 1984; Banister 1987, 235, 353. On the general background see Aird 1961; Scharping 1985 to 1986, Vol. II. A reinterpretation of the disputed Buck survey from 1929 to 1931 resulted in a birth rate of 41‰, but is itself disputed. Smaller local samples from Hebei, Jiangsu and Yunnan between 1926 to 1939 ranged between 20‰ and 45‰. See Barclay *et al.* 1976; contributions from Arthur Wolf and Ansley Coale in Hanley and Wolf 1985, 154–195; Chen Ta 1946, 81–126; Ch'iao Ch'i-ming *et al.* 1938; Gamble 1968, 21–62. The birth rates for 1949 to 1979 come from a reconstruction by Judith Banister; for a rival adjustment from China with notably lower rates for 1953–57 see Yuan Yongxi 1991, 617. The official time series is reproduced in all government compendiums, among them editions of ZRTN and the authoritative LTZH 1990, 2.

2 See also section 13.2 below.

3 Age-specific fertility rates from the birth-planning reports can be found in ZJSN 1986, 1990 and 1991.

4 For 1987 to 1992 data see Jiang Zhenghua 1995. For 1994 to 1997 see ZRTN 1995 to 1998. For the 1950s and 1960s see Chen Shengli and Coale 1993; Quanguo 1% renkou shengyulü chouyang diaocha fenxi 1983, 152–154; Banister 1987, 230; Peng Xizhe 1991, 129–133, 185–195, 245–253. For the 1920s and 1930s see Ch'iao Ch'i-ming *et al.* 1938; Barclay *et al.* 1976; Coale 1984; Wolf 1984. For discussions of the contentious historical record and painstaking reconstructions from genealogical data see Harrell 1995; Lee and Campbell 1997, 90–101; Lee and Wang Feng 1999, 84–88.

5 For a fuller treatment of TAFR and TDFR see Fang Fang 1987; Coale and Chen Shengli 1987; Coale *et al.* 1991; Peng Xizhe 1991,146–147; Chen Shengli and Coale 1993; Lin Fude 1994; for the discussion of TPPR see Feeney and Yu Jingyuan 1987; Luther *et al.* 1990; Feeney and Wang Feng 1993.

6 For a time series and cohort rates see Chen Shengli and Coale 1993; Quan guo 1% renkou shengyulü chouyang diaocha fenxi 1983, 42–44; Peng Xizhe 1991, 140–144. For 1929 to 1931 figures see Barclay *et al.* 1976; Wolf 1985; Coale 1985; for historical fertility trends see Harrell 1995.

7 See the discussions in Chen Jian 1993; Feeney and Yuan Jianhua 1994; Zeng Yi 1995. Cf. also section 8.2 above. An instructive discussion of Chinese fertility in the 1990s is also available in Attané 2000.

8 Own calculations from the increment of cohort parities between the 1990 census and the 1995 micro-census result in a TAFR of 1.51 for 1993.

9 For survey and census results see ZJSN 1986; ZRTN 1992; Liang Jimin and Chen Shengli 1993, Vol. 3; Jiang Zhenghua 1995. For results from the birth-planning reports see ZJSN 1990. For an analysis of TAFRs and TDFRs by birth order see Wang Feng *et al.* 1990; Coale *et al.* 1991; Peng Xizhe 1991,137ff.

10 For parity progression ratios from 1955 to 1992 and further discussion, see Feeney and Yu Jingyuan 1987; Luther *et al.* 1990; Feeney *et al.* 1992; Feeney and Wang Feng 1993; Feeney 1996; State Family Planning Commission 1997, 59–98.

11 Zhao Zhongwei 1997. Cf. also Wang Feng 1988. On historical precedences see Lee and Campbell 1997.
12 Kim Choe Minja *et al.* 1992; Qian Zhenchao 1997; Hao Hongsheng and Gao Ling in State Family Planning Commission 1997, 59–98. For the sex ratio at birth see section 13.1 below.
13 Lee and Campbell 1997; Coale *et al.* 1988.
14 International Statistical Institute 1991, 274–291; Wang Feng and Yang Quanhe 1996.
15 The 1945 to 1979 time series from the 1982 survey is reproduced in Blayo 1997, 298. Divergent time series for the 1980s in Chang Chongxuan 1991, 128–132; Feeney and Wang Feng 1993; Zeng Yi 1994, 28. For a distribution by years elapsed see also Luther *et al.* 1990, 346.
16 ZJSN 1998, 1. For an illuminating field report on changing policies towards marriage age and birth spacing in rural areas of Beijing municipal region see also Zeng Yi 1994, 40–49.
17 Total fertility rates in this and the following sections always signify the conventional summation of age-specific fertility rates, i.e. TAFRs.
18 Cf. the different figures for 1978 to 1989 in ZRTN 1988; Kua shiji de Zhongguo renkou 1994; and Yuan Yongxi 1996. For unadjusted provincial fertility rates of the 1995 micro-census see ZRTN 1997; for an adjustment differing from the one used in Table 29 see Gao Ling *et al.* 1997, 27.
19 For extended discussions of regional fertility trends see, among others, Banister 1987, 251–296; Li Bohua 1990; Gu Baochang 1991; Peng Xizhe 1991, 157–176, 218–226, 245–263; Feeney *et al.* 1993; Kim Choe Minja *et al.* 1993; Kua shiji de Zhongguo renkou 1994; Lin Fude 1994; Chen Wei 1995; Yuan Yongxi 1996; Zha Ruichuan *et al.* 1996, Vol. 1, 254–258. For Peng Peiyun's official categorization of provinces by fertility level see ZJSN 1996, 16–20. More detailed population data for the county level are available in Guowuyuan renkou pucha bangongshi 1987; Wang Ming 1996.
20 In the following paragraphs all figures for the four fertility areas are mean values weighted by provincial population shares. Population data come from the 1990 census and the surveys of 1982, 1988, 1992 and 1995. Summary statements for other economic and social indicators refer to the 1989 to 1999 period.
21 For a fuller treatment of urban–rural fertility trends from 1950 to 1986 see also Peng Xizhe 1991, 155–275. A 1976 to 1990 time series of reconstructed age-specific fertility rates for either cities, towns and countryside is available in Feeney *et al.* 1992, 42. On the background of urban development since 1949 see Kirkby 1985; Chan Kam Wing 1994. For a multivariate analysis of the 1987 in-depth fertility survey in Beijing, Liaoning, Shandong, Guangdong, Gansu and Guizhou see Kim Choe Minja *et al.* 1992. For retrospective analysis of a subsample from the 1982 fertility survey see Wang Feng 1988.
22 The discussion here is based on the recalculation of retrospective figures from the 1982 fertility survey in Chen Shengli and Coale 1993, which differs notably from the earlier tabulation in Quanguo 1% renkou shengyulü chouyang diaocha fenxi 1983. The latter is used in most Western works published to date. Cf. also Banister 1987, 243–248.
23 Wang Feng *et al.* 1990, Figure 9.
24 Feeney and Yu Jingyuan 1987, 82–85.
25 Raw data are contained in the statistical compendiums introduced in section 3 above. Extracts from these and some earlier analyses are available in the following works: For the 1982 data, Quanguo 1% renkou shengyulü chouyang diaocha fenxi 1983, 80–85; Lavely and Freedman 1990; Peng Xizhe 1991, 66–85; for the 1987 data, Feeney *et al.* 1989, 311–313; Wang Jiye and Hull 1991, 168; for the 1992 data, State Family Planning Commission 1997, 99–107. No information is available from the 1995 micro-census.
26 For a deeper analysis of education and fertility in the period 1952 to 1982 see Wang Feng 1988; Lavely and Freedman 1990.

27 Figures calculated from census information and data in State Family Planning Commission 1997, 106.
28 Peng Xizhe 1991, 68–70.
29 See e.g. Peng Xizhe and Dai Xingyi 1996, 144–183; Qian Zhenchao 1997, 225–226.
30 On the nexus between marriage, fertility, wealth and social status in traditional China see Buck 1937, 381–386; Gamble 1954, 39–45, 84; Yang 1959, 17–19, and various contributions to the volumes edited by Hanley and Wolf 1985 and Harrell 1995.
31 An extract of the figures in chart form is reproduced in Ma Xia 1994, 133. The information on the situation for different age groups comes from own analysis of the data records.
32 Wei Jinsheng and Wang Shengling 1996, 325–331; Qian Zhenchao 1997.
33 On migration see Scharping 1997; Scharping 1999; Pieke and Mallee 1999; Solinger 1999.
34 Interview 3490. The Shanghai, Chongqing and Xi'an figures are from Gui Shixun 1992. See also *R*, No.1/1986, 75–58; Liao Xuebin 1988; *RR*, 30 June 1988; *Xinhua*, 3 March 1989; ZJSN 1996, 32; Wang Jianmin and Hu Qi 1996, 131–148; ZJSN 1998, 82; Bu Xinmin 1998, 195–207.
35 In the 1986 survey figures (used in Tan Xiaoqing 1990, Yang Zihui 1991 and Ma Xia 1994, 117–135) floating population from the countryside was barely covered. More than 50 percent of the migrants canvassed hailed from other urban places; 90 percent had obtained official permission for a change of residence, and even among rural–urban migrants of the years 1980 to 1986 that percentage still amounted to more than 80 percent (own calculations from the data records). In the migration-specific fertility figures of the 1988 survey (quoted in Chang Chongxuan 1991, 237–247), place of birth served as a proxy for place of out-migration, and place of household registration substituted place of in-migration.
36 Hoy 1999.
37 For overviews of minority population developments see Yang Yixing *et al.* 1988; Zhang Tianlu 1989; Kua shiji de Zhongguo (Zonghe juan) 1994, 273–320; Yang Kuifu 1995. For a good specialised study on Guizhou see Yan Tianhua 1996; for a broader study of extra-demographic factors in population development of the Northeast see Scharping 2000c.
38 Peng Xizhe 1991, 113–115.
39 Zhongguo renkou qingbao yanjiu zhongxin 1989, 21–29; Liang Jimin and Chen Shengli 1993, Vol. 3; Gao Ersheng and Yuan Wei 1997, 32.
40 China Financial and Economic Publishing House 1988, 27–29; Zhang Tianlu and Huang Rongqing 1996, 301–334. On Xinjiang fertility rates see also Anderson and Silver 1995.
41 Correlation coefficients are based on own calculations from ethno-specific data of the 1990 census.
42 For ethno-specific abortion rates and contraceptive rates see Gao Ersheng and Yuan Wei 1997, 39–103.
43 Zhang Fengyu 1998. One methodical reservation concerns the low level of statistical values for the explanatory power of the models. Another is the (seemingly unavoidable) practice of substituting ethno-specific analysis of the population with area-specific analysis of autonomous areas, most of which accommodate a Han-Chinese majority.

13 Changes in sex and age structure

1 Own calculations from census figures and 1991 to 1998 data of the annual sample survey on population dynamics.

2 For a first report on the problem in the central Party daily see *RR*, 7 April 1984. Cf. also the report on the first national conference on the sex ratio at birth, which was convened in June 1986 by the State Birth-Planning Commission: ZJSN 1987, 32–33.

3 For a Chinese report with clearly exaggerated figures see the translation from the Liaoning journal *Lilun yu shijian* in *SWB*, 4 April 1997. Conference reports and contributions in: ZJSN 1993, 138–139; ZJSN 1995, 109–111; Tu Ping in ZJSQ 1997, 662–664, 1434; Tu Ping 1993; Zeng Yi *et al.* 1993; Gao Ling 1995. See also section 10 above on regulations against infanticide and prenatal sex determination.

4 For retrospective sex ratios with gliding averages from the 1982 survey see Coale and Banister 1994; for retrospective sex ratios at birth from the 1988 survey see Liang Jimin and Chen Shengli 1993, Vol.II, 17.

5 See Johansson and Nygren 1991, 42, with data from the 1988 fertility survey.

6 Similar data from the 1988 fertility survey are available in *RYJ*, No.5/1997, 52–58. For the analysis of 1990 census data see Yuan Jianhua and Skinner 2000. Cf. also the analysis of Beijing data from the 1995 micro-census in Gao Ling *et al.* 1997.

7 Tu Ping 1993, 8; Gao Ling 1995, 107–111; Anderson and Silver 1995.

8 For a more detailed report on the sex ratio in Guangxi see *Zhongguo tongxun she*, 12 October 1993.

9 For an intriguing analysis of sex ratios along the urban–rural continuum in the Lower Yangzi Macro-region see Yuan Jianhua and Skinner 2000; for an analysis of the 1995 micro-census data see Gao Ling *et al.* 1997.

10 Data for the above statements may be found in Tu Ping 1993, 8; Gao Ling 1995, 105–107.

11 For a detailed derivation of these calculations and the arguments on under-registration, see the following two standard works: Zeng Yi *et al.* 1993; Gao Ling 1995. Some Chinese studies set the normal sex ratio of births at 1070. The figures presented above also take alternative values of 1055 or 1060 into consideration. For doubts as to the representativeness of the hospital sample see Coale and Banister 1994.

12 Johansson and Nygren 1991; Johansson 1995; Gao Ling 1995; Johnson *et al.* 1998.

13 In 1990, sex ratios at birth for South Korea and Taiwan amounted to 1125 and 1118 respectively; in Hongkong and among the Chinese population of Singapore sex ratios for the age group 0 stood at 1097 and 1077. See also Park Chai Bin and Cho Nam-Hoon 1995; Goodkind 1996.

14 Gu Baochang and Roy 1996.

15 Wu Cangping 1988b. On traditional practices of sex-specific screening and neglect of new-born children see Lang 1946, 150–152; Lee 1981; Linck 1988, 66; Leutner 1989, 35–36, 43, 61–74; for village studies with brief reference to infanticide and neglect in traditional China see Fei Hsiao-tung 1939, 32–34; Yang 1959, 15, 19; for two of the few more precise assessments of the demographic importance of infanticide and fatal neglect in traditional China see Wolf and Huang 1980, 230–241; Lee and Campbell 1997, 58–82.

16 See Coale and Banister (1994) for the data and arguments against the adoption factor. For a retrospective analysis of 1990 census data see Yuan Jianhua and Skinner 2000.

17 The 1992 fertility survey resulted in infant mortality rates of 30.7‰ for males and 41.8‰ for females; the 1995 micro-census in mortality rates for age group 0 of 28.0‰ for males and 37.5‰ for females. The expected rates for females would be 23.6‰ and 21.5‰, respectively. For recorded and adjusted infant mortality rates between 1981 and 1995 see Kua shiji de Zhongguo renkou (zonghe juan) 1994, 186–191; Yuan Yongxi 1996, 67–69; Zha Ruichuan *et al.* 1996, Vol.I, 88–102; Gao Ersheng *et al.* 1997; 1995 nian quanguo 1% renkou chouyang diaocha ziliao.

18 The calculation rests on adjusted infant mortality rates of 32.19‰ for males and 36.83‰ for females and on a standard value for the proportion of male versus female infant mortality equal to 1.3. For infant mortality rates from the 1992 fertility survey see the above note. For enumerated and calculated birth data from the 1990 census see Gao Ling, 111; Wu Cangping 1996, 203–204; for an earlier calculation from a

1 per cent sample of the 1990 census see Tu Ping in ZJSQ 1997, 662–663. For the historical estimate see Eastman 1988, 21. See also Merli and Raftery 2000, 113.

19 An excellent discussion of cohort effects in Chinese fertility dynamics is contained in Feeney *et al.* 1992. Defects of the 1995 data are visible in the chart. Due to mortality effects, all individual birth cohorts should become smaller with the passage of time. In the chart some get bigger, however.

20 For a calculation of working-age population by legal definitions see Yuan Yongxi 1996, 136–140.

21 Figures in this and the following paragraphs come from own calculations and the more detailed discussion in Zha Ruichuan *et al.* 1996, 110–153.

14 Looking back: causal structures and policy impact

1 Li Rongshi 1986; Jiang Zhenghua 1986; Poston and Gu Baochang 1987; Poston and Jia Zhongke 1989; Peng Xizhe and Huang Juan 1993; Sun Wensheng and Jin Guanghua 1994. The most ambitious attempts at measuring are Wei Jinsheng and Wang Shengling 1996, Zhang Fengyu 1997.

2 Wei Jinsheng and Wang Shengling 1996, 97–124; Lin Fude and Zhai Zhenwu 1996, 8–9; Qian Zhenzhao 1997, 225; Zhang Fengyu 1997, 76–98.

3 Zeng Yi *et al.* 1991; Wei Jinsheng and Wang Shengling 1996, 80–96.

4 For the latest relevant summaries of the official news media see *Xinhua*, 26 August 1999, 27 September 1999; *RR*, 14 October 1999; for earlier statements with different figures see *GR*, 4 September 1980; *ZRB*, 2 January 1989; for more elaborate recent evaluations see Wu Zhongguan and Xiao Lijin 1994; Wei Jinsheng and Wang Shengling 1996, 24–80. The following commentary is based on the sources from the 1990s.

5 Ibid; Zhongguo weilai renkou fazhan yu shengyu zhengce ketizu 2000.

6 For two recent, detailed Chinese discussions of the effects of population growth on various social and economic sectors see Kua shiji de Zhongguo renkou (Zonghe juan) 1994, 363–422; Lin Fude and Zhai Zhenwu 1996. For a dissenting discussion of the long-range links between demographic and economic developments in China see also Lee and Wang Feng 1999.

7 For a Chinese attempt at cost-benefit analysis see Wu Zhongguan and Xiao Lijin 1994, 549–550. In Western literature, the most detailed attempt to discuss the balance of birth-planning costs and benefits as of the early 1980s can be found in Tien 1991, 215–231.

15 Looking forward: demographic projections and their implications

1 Cf. Chart 19 (above) for projections from the 1980s. For their political background see sections 4.1, 4.2, 5.2, 5.3 and 5.4 above. For Chinese projections from the 1990s see the section 16 and the following sources: ZJSN 1990, 92–94; Kua shiji de Zhongguo renkou (Zonghe juan) 1994, 423–446; Zeng Yi 1994, 31–40, 56–62, 70–79; Chen Wei 1995; Tu Ping 1995; Zha Ruichuan *et al.* 1996, Vol. II, 339–421; Lin Fude and Zhai Zhenwu 1996, 1–63; Yuan Yongxi 1996, 303–316; State Family Planning Commission 1997, 109–115; ZRTN 1997, 489–492; Li Jianxin 1997.

2 See in particular: Zeng Yi 1994 and Zha Ruichuan *et al.* 1996, Vol. II, 339–421.

16 Weighing the options: past experience and new ideas

1 Hu An'gang 1989a, 3–13, 66–69, 75–152. Cf. also the synopsis of Hu's analysis in the Party journal *Liaowang* (Hu An'gang 1989b) and his modified present views in Hu An'gang 2000.

2 Ibid., 232, 239.
3 Ibid., 52, 180–184, 197–219, 235–248.
4 The above views have been condensed from the following sources: *Zhongguo tongxun she*, 11 April 1993; Zou Ping 1993, 23–28; Yang Zhuquan 1995, 132–140; Lin Fude and Zhai Zhenwu 1996, 253, 325–326; RY, No. 2/1997, 30–38; State Family Planning Commission 1997, 112; Wu Cangping and Mu Guangzong 1998; *Xinwen wanbao*, 13 April 2001.
5 See Lin Fude in RY, No. 2/1997, 33; Peng Xizhe in: CND, 26 October 1997; Yang Zhuquan 1995, 227; *Xinhua*, 14 April 2000.
6 For important studies on food consumption and grain production see Carter and Zhong Fu-ning 1988; Zhongguo tudi ziyuan shengchan nengli ji renkou chengzailiang yanjiu 1992; Brown 1995; Smil 1995; Zhu Lilan 1995; Lin Fude and Zhai Zhenwu 1996, 196–269; Huang Jikun et al. 1996; World Bank 1997b; Wang Xianjin 1997; Tian Xueyuan 1997, 34–63; Ash and Edmonds 1998; Aubert 1999; Heilig 1999; Li Chengxun 1999, 92–136. Cf. also fn. 29 for section 4 above.
7 For basic literature on employment problems in the reform period see Taylor and Banister 1988; World Bank 1992b; Hebel and Schucher 1992; Lin Fude and Zhai Zhenwu 1996, 96–107; Wu Cangping 1996, 1–42; Scharping 1997; Tian Xueyuan 1997, 94–116; Li Chengxun 1999, 349–361; Wang Dahai 1999; Hebel and Schucher 1999; Hu An'gang 2000, 49–77.
8 For important studies on trends in ageing and problems of old-age security see Banister 1989; Tian Xueyuan 1991; Krieg and Schädler 1994; Lin Jiang 1994; Du Peng 1994; Krieg and Schädler 1995; Lin Jiang 1995; Tu Ping 1995; Tian Xueyuan 1997, 117–143; Zhang Wenfan 1998; Croll 1999; Li Chengxun 1999, 374–385; Chen Jiagui et al. 2000.
9 Own calculation at comparable prices in 1980 yuan under the assumption of reliable official figures for GDP growth and a year-end population total of c. 1.275 billion in 2000. Lower GDP growth than officially reported in the late 1990s and/or a higher population total would reduce per capita GDP in 2000 to anywhere between 2,000 and 2,100 yuan at 1980 prices.
10 Own calculations at comparable prices in 1995 yuan, with conversion to US$ at the exchange rate of 1993–95. See also the World Bank's World Development Report 1997 and the projections in Ma Hong 1989; Hu An'gang 1989; Hu An'gang 2000.
11 RR, 9 August 1993.
12 The above views have been condensed from the following sources: Zeng Yi et al. 1993; Gu Baochang and Mu Guangzong 1994; Zeng Yi 1994, 19 52, 95–98; Yang Zhuquan 1995, 82–85; Tu Ping 1995; Wu Canping and Mu Guangzong 1995; Lin Fude and Zhai Zhenwu 1996, 326; Zha Ruichuan et al. 1996, 422–424; RY, No. 1/1996, 49–60; Li Jianxin 1997; Ma Yingtong 1997; Liang Zhongtang and Tan Kejian 1997.
13 PDR, No. 2/1993, 401; Wu Canping and Mu Guangzong 1995; Chen Wei 1995; RY, No. 1/1996, 49–60; RY, No. 2/1997, 37; Li Jianxin 1997. For the Peng Peiyun quotation see: ZRB, 16 February 1994; the opinion survey has been reported in CND, 30 November 1997.
14 *Xinhua*, 23 February 1998, 15 April 1998, 10 July 1998. For reports on the research project and the new Yicheng investigation see ZJSN 1999, 130; Zhongguo weilai renkou fazhan yu shengyu zhengce ketizu 2000.
15 RR, 8 May 2000; *Xinhua*, 19 December 2000. Cf. also section 5.5 (above) for developments in population policy during the 1990s.
16 RR, 23 March 1994, 14 March 1999; *South China Morning Post*, 3 March 1999.
17 Huang Shumin 1989, 178.

Bibliography

Aird (1961): Aird, John S., *The Size, Composition, and Growth of the Population of Mainland China*, Washington

Aird (1968): Aird, John S., Population Growth, in: Eckstein, Alexander, et al., ed., *Economic Trends in Communist China*, Chicago, pp. 183–327

Aird (1986): Aird, John S., Coercion in Family Planning: Causes, Methods, and Consequences, in: Joint Economic Committee, ed., *China's Economy Looks Toward the Year 2000, Vol. 1: The Four Modernizations*, Washington, pp. 184–221

Aird (1990): Aird, John S., *Slaughter of the Innocents, Coercive Birth Control in China*, Washington

Alpermann (2001): Alpermann, Björn, *Der Staat im Dorf, Dörfliche Selbstverwaltung in China in den 90er Jahren*, Hamburg

Anderson and Silver (1995): Anderson, Barbara, A., and Brian D. Silver, Ethnic Differences in Fertility and Sex Ratios at Birth in China: Evidence from Xinjiang, *Population Studies*, No. 49, pp. 211–226

Anhui jingji nianjian (1985): *Anhui jingji nianjian* [Anhui Economic Yearbook], Hefei

Arnold and Liu Zhaoxiang (1986): Arnold, Fred, and Liu Zhaoxiang, Sex Preference, Fertility, and Family Planning in China, *PDR*, No. 2, pp. 221–246

Ash and Edmonds (1998): Ash, Robert F., and Richard Louis Edmonds, China's Land Resources, Environment and Agricultural Production, *CQ*, No. 156, London, pp. 836–879

Ashton et al. (1984): Ashton, Basil, Kenneth Hill, Alan Piazza and Robert Zeitz, Famine in China, 1958–61, *PDR*, No. 4, pp. 613–645

Attané (2000): Attané, Isabelle, La fécondité chinoise à l'aube du XXIe siècle: constats et incertitudes, *Population*, No. 2, pp. 233–264

Attané and Sun Minglei (1998): Attané, Isabelle, and Sun Minglei, Natalité et fécondité en Chine, Quel crédit accorder aux données récentes?, *Population*, No. 4, pp. 847–857

Aubert (1999): Aubert, Claude, The 'Grain Problem' in China: A Statistical Illusion?, in: Ash, Robert, and Werner Draguhn, ed., *China's Economic Security*, Richmond, pp. 62–83

Banister (1987): Banister, Judith, *China's Changing Population*, Stanford

Banister (1989): Banister, Judith, The Aging of China's Population, *Problems of Communism*, Washington, November–December, pp. 62–77

Banister (1992): Banister, Judith, China's Population Changes and the Economy, in: Joint Economic Committee, ed., *China's Economic Dilemmas in the 1990s, The Problems of Reforms, Modernization, and Interdependence*, Armonk, pp. 234–251

Banister (1996): Banister, Judith, The PRC: End of Century Population Dynamics, in: Lin Chong-pin, ed., *PRC Tomorrow, Development Under the Ninth Five-Year Plan*, Kaohsiung, pp. 63–83

Banister (1998): Banister, Judith, Population, Public Health and The Environment in China, CQ, No. 156, pp. 986–1015

Banyuetan [Fortnightly Chats], Beijing

Barclay *et al.* (1976): Barclay, George W., et al., A Reassessment of the Demography of Traditional Rural China, *Population Index*, Vol. 42, No. 4, Washington, pp. 605–635

Beijing jingji xueyuan (1977): Beijing jingji xueyuan, *Renkou lilun* [Population Theory], Beijing

Betke (1998): Betke, Dirk, Umweltkrise und Umweltpolitik, in: Herrmann-Pillath, Carsten, and Michael Lackner, ed., *Länderbericht China, Politik, Wirtschaft und Gesellschaft im chinesischen Kulturraum*, Bonn, pp. 325–357

Bian Yanjie (1986): Bian Yanjie, Shixi woguo dusheng zinü jiating shenghuo fangshi di jiben tezheng [Basic Characteristics of the Life Style of One-Child Families in China], ZSK, No. 1, pp. 91–106

Bianco and Hua Chang-ming (1988): Bianco, Lucien and Hua Chang-ming, Implementation and Resistance: The Single-Child Family Policy, in: Feuchtwang, Stephan, et al., ed., *Transforming China's Economy in the Eighties, Vol. I: The Rural Sector, Welfare and Employment*, London, pp. 147–168

Blayo (1997): Blayo, Yves, *Des Politiques Démographiques en Chine*, Paris

Bongaarts and Greenhalgh (1985): Bongaarts, John, and Susan Greenhalgh, An Alternative to the One-Child Policy in China, PDR, No. 4, pp. 585–617

BR: *Beijing Review*, Beijing

Bray (1997): Bray, Francesca, *Technology and Gender, Fabrics of Power in Late Imperial China*, Berkeley

Brown (1995): Brown, Lester R., *Who Will Feed China? – Wake-Up Call For a Small Planet*, New York

Bruk (1959): Bruk, S.I., *Naselenie Kitaja, MNR i Korei*, Moscow

Bu Xinmin (1998): Bu Xinmin, ed., *Guangdong sheng 1995 nian 1% renkou chouyang diaocha youxiu wenji* [A Collection of Outstanding Articles on the 1995 1%-Sampling Survey on Population in Guangdong], Guangzhou

Buck (1937): Buck, John Lossing, *Land Utilization in China, A Study of 16,786 Farms in 168 Localities, and 38,256 Farm Families in Twenty-Two Provinces in China, 1929–1933*, Shanghai

Cai Fang (2000): Cai Fang, ed., *2000 nian: Zhongguo renkou wenti baogao, Nongcun renkou wenti jiqi zhili* [2000: Chinese Demographic Report, Rural Population Problems and Their Handling], Beijing

Calot (1984): Calot, Gérard, Données nouvelles sur l'évolution démographique en Chine, *Population*, No. 4–6, pp. 807–836, 1045–1062

Cao Jingzhuang (1986): Cao Jingzhuang, Nongcun jingji gaige yu jihua shengyu [Economic Reforms in the Countryside and Birth Control], RYJ, No. 4, pp. 7–11, 64

Cao Jingzhuang (1990): Cao Jingzhuang, Shixi nongmin shengyuguan zhuanbian de jingji tiaojian he linjiedian [A Preliminary Analysis of the Economic Conditions and the Critical Threshold for Changes in Peasant Childbearing Preferences], RYJ, No. 3, pp. 19–24

Cao Jingzhuang (1993): Cao Jingzhuang, Gaige kaifang xingshe xia de chengshi jihuashengyu gongzuo [Urban Birth Control Under Conditions of Reform and Opening-Up], *Renkou yu jihua shengyu*, No. 1, Shijiazhuang, pp. 42–49

Carter and Zhong Fu-ning (1988): Carter, Colin A., and Zhong Fu-ning, *China's Grain Production and Trade, An Economic Analysis*, Boulder

Cartier (1984): Cartier, Michel, Les leçons du troisième recensement chinois, *Courrier des Pays de l'Est*, No. 282, Paris, pp. 31–51

CD: *China Daily*, Beijing

Chan et al. (1992): Chan, Anita, Richard Madsen and Jonathan Unger, *Chen Village Under Mao and Deng*, Berkeley

Chan Kam Wing (1994): Chan Kam Wing, *Cities With Invisible Walls, Reinterpreting Urbanization in Post-1949 China*, Oxford

Chandrasekhar (1959): Chandrasekhar, S., *China's Population, Census, and Vital Statistics*, Hongkong

Chang Chongxuan (1991): Chang Chongxuan, ed., *Zhongguo shengyu jieyu chouyang diaocha lunwen ji* [National Sample Survey on Fertility and Contraception, Studies], Beijing

Chang Chongxuan (1992): Chang Chongxuan, ed., *Dangdai Zhongguo de jihua shengyu shiye* [Birth Planning in Contemporary China], Beijing

Chao Kang (1986): Chao Kang, *Man and Land in Chinese History, An Economic History*, Stanford

Chen and Tyler (1982): Chen, Charles H.C., and Carl W. Tyler, Demographic Implications of Family Size Alternatives in the People's Republic of China, CQ, No. 89, pp. 65–73

Chen Changbin and Deng Jianming (1994): Chen Changbin and Deng Jianming, Dangqian jihua shengyu xingzheng zhifa de nandian ji wenti jianxi [A Short Analysis of Implementation Problems of Present Birth-Planning Regulations], RYJ, No. 2, pp. 23–24

Chen Da (1957): Chen Da, Jieyu, wanhun yu xin Zhongguo renkou wenti [Birth Control, Late Marriage and New China's Population Problems], *Xin jianshe*, No. 5, Beijing, pp. 1–15

Chen Gaoyi and Wan Xiuzhen (1991): Chen Gaoyi and Wan Xiuzhen, Shanghai shi 7687 li rengong liuchan qingkuang fenxi [An Analysis of 7867 Cases of Induced Abortions in Shanghai City], *Renkou*, No. 2, Shanghai, pp. 23–29

Chen Jiagui et al. (2000): Chen Jiagui, Hans Jürgen Rösner et al., *Current Social Security Reform in Urban China*, Beijing

Chen Jian (1993): Chen Jian, 1992–1993 nian jihua shengyu zhuangkuang de fenxi yu yuce [Analysis and Forecast of Birth Control 1992–1993], in: Jiang Liu, Lu Xueyi and Da Tianlun, ed., *1992–1993 nian Zhongguo: Shehui xingshe fenxi yu yuce* [China in 1992–1993: Analyses and Forecasts of the Social Situation], Beijing, pp. 212–223

Chen Ta (1946): Chen Ta, *Population in Modern China*, Chicago

Chen Pi-chao (1985): Chen Pi-chao, Birth Control Methods and Organisation in China, in: Croll, Davin and Kane, pp. 135–148

Chen Qi (1988): Chen Qi, ed., *2000 nian Zhongguo de ziran ziyuan* [China's Natural Resources in the Year 2000], Beijing

Chen Shengli and Coale (1993): Chen Shengli, and Ansley Coale, *Zhongguo ge sheng shengyulü shouce 1940–1990* [Handbook of Fertility Rates for all Chinese Provinces 1940–1990], Beijing

Chen Shengli and Zhao Shi (1991): Chen Shengli and Zhao Shi, ed., *Renkou tongji yu jihua* [Population Statistics and Population Planning], Beijing

Chen Wei (1995): Chen Wei, Zhongguo de di shengyu lü [China's Low Fertility Rate], ZSK, No. 2, pp. 75–96

Chen Yuguang and Zhang Zehou (1983): Chen Yuguang and Zhang Zehou, Lun woguo renkou de jiating jiegou [On the Family Structure of China's Population], RYJ, No. 4, pp. 23–29

Chen Yun (1986): *Chen Yun wenxuan 1956–1985* [Selected Works of Chen Yun 1956–1985], Beijing

Ch'iao Ch'i-ming et al. (1938): Ch'iao Ch'i-ming et al., An *Experiment in the Registration of Vital Statistics in China*, Oxford, Ohio

China Financial and Economic Publishing House (1988): China Financial and Economic Publishing House, ed., *New China's Population*, New York

China Population Association (1997a): China Population Association, *Brief Introduction to the Population Research Institutions in China*, Beijing

China Population Association (1997b): China Population Association, ed., *23rd IUSSP General Population Conference, Symposium on Demography of China*, Beijing

CND: *China News Digest*

Coale (1984): Coale, Ansley J., *Rapid Population Change in China, 1952–1982*, Washington

Coale (1985): Coale, Ansley J., Fertility in Rural China: A Reconfirmation of the Barclay Assessment, in: Hanley and Wolf, pp. 186–195

Coale and Banister (1994): Coale, Ansley J., and Judith Banister, Five Decades of Missing Females in China, *Demography*, Vol. 31, No. 3, Madison, pp. 459–478

Coale and Chen Shengli (1987): Coale, Ansley J., and Chen Shengli, *Basic Data on Fertility in the Provinces of China, 1940–82*, Honolulu

Coale and Freedman (1993): Coale, Ansley J., und Ronald Freedman, Similarities in the Fertility Transition in China and Three Other East Asian Populations, in: Leete, Richard, and Iqbal Alam, ed., *The Revolution in Asian Fertility, Dimensions, Causes, and Implications*, Oxford, pp. 208–238

Coale et al. (1988): Coale, Ansley J., et al., *The Distribution of Interbirth Intervals in Rural China, 1940s to 1970s*, (Papers of the East-West Population Institute, No. 109), Honolulu

Coale et al. (1991): Coale, Ansley J., et al., Recent Trends in Fertility and Nuptiality in China, *Science*, Vol. 251, No. 4992, New York, pp. 389–393

Cooney and Li Jiali (1994): Cooney, Rosemary Santana, and Li Jiali, Household Registration Type and Compliance with the 'One Child' Policy in China, 1979–1988, *Demography*, Vol. 31, No. 1, Madison, pp. 21–32

CQ: *China Quarterly*, London

Crane and Finkle (1989): Crane, Barbara B., and Jason L. Finkle, The United States, China, and the United Nations Population Fund: Dynamics of US Policymaking, *PDR*, No. 1, pp. 23–59

Croll (1981): Croll, Elisabeth, *The Politics of Marriage in Contemporary China*, Cambridge

Croll (1985): Croll, Elisabeth, Fertility Norms and Family Size in China, in: Croll, Davin and Kane, pp. 1–36

Croll (1993): Croll, Elisabeth, A Commentary on the New Draft Law on Eugenics and Health Protection, *China Information*, Vol. VIII, No. 3, Leiden, pp. 32–37

Croll (1999): Croll, Elisabeth, Social Welfare Reform: Trends and Tensions, *CQ*, No. 159, London, pp. 684–699

Croll et al. (1985): Croll, Elisabeth, Delia Davin and Penny Kane, ed., *China's One-Child Family Policy*, London

Cui Guangzu (1988): Cui Guangzu, Kongzhi renkou zengzhang guanjian zaiyu chang zhu bu xie [Constancy is the Key to Control of Population Growth], *RY*, No. 3, pp. 53–55

Davin (1985): Davin, Delia, The Single-Child Family Policy in the Countryside, in: Croll, Davin and Kane, pp. 37–82

Davis (1989): Davis, Deborah, Chinese Social Welfare: Policies and Outcomes, *CQ*, No. 119, pp. 577–597

Davis and Harrell (1993): Davis, Deborah, and Stevan Harrell, ed., *Chinese Families in the Post-Mao Era*, Berkeley

Demography, Madison

Deng Hongbi (1998): Deng Hongbi, ed., *Zhongguo shaoshu minzu renkou zhengce yanjiu* [Studies on Population Policies for China's National Minorities], Chongqing

Deng Xiaoping (1983): *Deng Xiaoping wenxuan, 1975–1982* [Selected Works of Deng Xiaoping, 1975–1982], Beijing

Dikötter (1995): Dikötter, Frank, *Sex, Culture, and Modernity: Sexual Identities in the Early Republican Period*, London

Dikötter (1998): Dikötter, Frank, *Imperfect Conceptions: Medical Knowledge, Birth Defects, and Eugenics in China*, London

Domenach and Hua Chang-ming (1987): Domenach, Jean-Luc, and Hua Chang-ming, *Le mariage en Chine*, Paris

Döring (1997): Döring, Ole, *Technischer Fortschritt und kulturelle Werte in China, Humangenetik und Ethik in Taiwan, Hongkong und der Volksrepublik China*, Hamburg

Du Peng (1994): Du Peng, *Zhongguo renkou laolinghua guocheng yanjiu* [Studies on the Aging of China's Population], Beijing

Eastman (1988): Eastman, Lloyd E., *Family, Fields, and Ancestors, Constancy and Change in China's Social and Economic History 1550–1949*, New York

Edmonds (1994): Edmonds, Richard Louis, *Pattern's of China's Lost Harmony: A Survey of the Country's Environmental Degradation and Protection*, London

Elvin (1973): Elvin, Mark, *The Pattern of the Chinese Past, A Social and Economic Interpretation*, Stanford

Evans (1997): Evans, Harriet, *Women and Sexuality in China, Dominant Discourses on Female Sexuality Since 1949*, Cambridge

Falbo (Fan Danni) (1996): Falbo, Toni (Fan Danni), ed., *Zhongguo dusheng zinü yanjiu* [Studies on Single Children in China], Shanghai

Fang Fang (1987): Fang Fang, Woguo sanshi nian lai hunyin se shengyu moshi de zhuanbian [Changes in China's Marriage and Fertility Patterns During the Last Thirty Years], *RYJ*, No. 2, pp. 26–37

FBIS: *Foreign Broadcast Information Service*, Springfield

Feeney (1996): Feeney, Griffith, Fertility in China: Past, Present, Prospects, in: Lutz, Wolfgang, ed., *The Future Population of the World, What Can We Assume Today?*, London, pp. 85–108

Feeney and Wang Feng (1993): Feeney, Griffith, and Wang Feng, Parity Progression and Birth Intervals in China: The Influence of Policy in Hastening Fertility Decline, *PDR*, No. 1, pp. 61–101

Feeney and Yu Jingyuan (1987): Feeney, Griffith, and Yu Jingyuan, Period Parity Progression Measures of Fertility in China, *Population Studies*, No. 41, pp. 77–102

Feeney and Yuan Jianhua (1994): Feeney, Griffith, and Yuan Jianhua, Below Replacement Fertility in China?, A Close Look at Recent Evidence, *Population Studies*, No. 48, pp. 381–394

Feeney et al. (1989): Feeney, Griffith, et al., Recent Fertility Dynamics in China: Results from the 1987 One Percent Population Survey, *PDR*, No. 2, pp. 297–322

Feeney et al. (1992): Feeney, Griffith, et al., *Recent Fertility Trends in China: Results From the 1990 Census*, Paper for the International Seminar on China's 1990 Population Census, Beijing

Feeney et al. (1993): Feeney, Griffith, et al., Provincial Level Fertility Trends in China, Estimates From the 1990 Census, Unpublished Paper, Honolulu

FEER: *Far Eastern Economic Review*, Hongkong

Fei Hsiao-tung (1939): Fei Hsiao-tung, *Peasant Life in China, A Field Study of Country Life in the Yangtze Valley*, London

Feng Litian *et al.* (1987): Feng Litian, Wang Shuxin and Meng Haohan, Weichengnian renkou touzi diaocha yanjiu [A Survey Study on Investments in Children], ZRK, No. 1, pp. 12–17

Feng Xiaotian (1991): Feng Xiaotian, Dusheng zinü fumu de shengyu yiyuan [Childbearing Preferences of One-Child Parents], RY, No. 5, pp. 30–33

Freedman (1970): Freedman, Maurice, ed., *Family and Kinship in Chinese Society*, Stanford

Gamble (1968): Gamble, Sidney D., *Ting Hsien: A North China Rural Community*, Stanford

Gao Ersheng *et al.* (1997): Gao Ersheng *et al.*, Jihua shengyu yaoju shoufei zhengce de tantao [A Discussion of the Policy on Charges for Contraceptive Drugs and Devices], RY, No. 1, pp. 21–26

Gao Ersheng *et al.* (1997): Gao Ersheng, Li Lu and Song Guixiang, *Ying'er siwanglü yanjiu* [Studies on Infant Mortality], Hangzhou

Gao Ersheng and Yuan Wei (1997): Gao Ersheng and Yuan Wei, ed., *Zhongguo shaoshuminzu shengzhe jiankang* [Reproductive Health Of Chinese Minority Nationalities], Beijing

Gao Ling (1995): Gao Ling, Woguo renkou chusheng xingbiebi de tezheng jiqi yingxiang yinsuo [The Characteristics of the Sex Ratio at Birth of the Chinese Population and the Factors Influencing It], ZSK, No. 1, pp. 99–115

Gao Ling *et al.* (1997): Gao Ling, Xia Ping and Liu Xiaolan, Beijing shi renkou chusheng xingbiebi fenxi [An Analysis of the Sex Ratio at Birth in Beijing], RY, No. 5, pp. 25–33

Gates (1993): Gates, Hill, Cultural Support for Birth Limitation among Urban Capital-Owning Women, in: Davis and Harrell, pp. 251–274

GR: *Guangming ribao* [Enlightenment], Beijing

Goldstein and Beall (1991): Goldstein, Melvyn C., and Cynthia Beall, China's Birth Control Policy in the Tibet Autonomous Region, *Asian Survey*, Vol. 31, No. 3, Berkeley, pp. 285–303

Gongyuan 2000 nian de Zhongguo (1984): *Gongyuan 2000 nian de Zhongguo* [China in the Year 2000], Beijing

Goodkind (1991): Goodkind, Daniel, Creating New Traditions in Modern Chinese Populations: Aiming for Birth in the Year of the Dragon, PDR, No. 4, pp. 663–686

Goodkind (1996): Goodkind, Daniel, On Substituting Sex Preference Strategies in East Asia: Does Prenatal Sex Selection Reduce Postnatal Discrimination?, PDR, No. 1, pp. 111–125

Gransow (1992): Gransow, Bettina, *Geschichte der chinesischen Soziologie*, Frankfurt

Greenhalgh (1986): Greenhalgh, Susan, Shifts in China's Population Policy, 1984–86: Views from the Central, Provincial, and Local Levels, PDR, No. 3, pp. 491–515

Greenhalgh (1988): Greenhalgh, Susan, Fertility as Mobility: Sinic Transitions, PDR, No. 4, pp. 629–674

Greenhalgh (1990): Greenhalgh, Susan, The Evolution of the One-Child Policy in Shaanxi, 1979–88, CQ, No. 122, pp. 191–229

Greenhalgh (1992): Greenhalgh, Susan, State-Society Links: Political Dimensions of Population Policies and Programmes, with Special Reference to China, in: Philipps and Ross, pp. 276–298

Greenhalgh (1993): Greenhalgh, Susan, The Peasantization of One-Child Policy, in: Davis and Harrell, pp. 219–250

Greenhalgh and Bongarts (1987): Greenhalgh, Susan, and John Bongaarts, Fertility Policy in China: Future Options, *Science*, Vol. 235, New York, pp. 1167–1172

Greenhalgh *et al.* (1994): Greenhalgh, Susan, Zhu Chuzhu and Li Nan, Restraining Population Growth in Three Chinese Villages, 1988–93, *PDR*, No. 2, pp. 365–395

Gu Baochang (1991): Gu Baochang, Cong 2‰ shengyu diaocha kan 80 niandai woguo nongcun shengyu qushe [Trends in Chinese Rural Fertility As Viewed From the 2‰ Fertility Survey], *RD*, No. 1, pp. 10–18

Gu Baochang and Mu Guangzong (1994): Gu Baochang and Mu Guangzong, Chongxin renshi Zhongguo renkou wenti [A Reconsideration of China's Population Problem], *RY*, No. 5, pp. 2–10

Gu Baochang and Roy (1996): Gu Baochang and Krishna Roy, Zhongguo dalu, Zhongguo Taiwan sheng he Hanguo chusheng ying'er xingbiebi shitiao de bijiao fenxi [A Comparative Analysis of the Imbalances of the Sex Ratio at Birth on the Chinese Mainland, in China's Taiwan Province and in South Korea], *RY*, No. 5, pp. 1–16

Gu Shengzu and Jian Xinhua (1994): Gu Shengzu and Jian Xinhua, *Dangdai Zhongguo renkou liudong yu chengzhenhua* [Population Mobility and Urbanisation in Contemporary China], Wuhan

Gu Shengzu and Xu Yunhao (1985): Gu Shengzu and Xu Yunhao, Nongcun yuling funü dui jihua shengyu de zhishi, taidu yu shijian chutan [A Preliminary Study of Birth-Planning Knowledge, Attitudes and Experience Among Peasant Women in Reproductive Age], *Tongji*, No. 6, Beijing, pp. 19–21

Guangdong sheng jihua shengyu tiaoli [Guangdong Provincial Birth-Planning Regulations], 18 September 1988

Guangdong sheng nongcun dusheng zinü fumu he chunsheng er nü jiezha fufu yanglao baoxian shishi banfa [Guangdong Provincial Implementation Procedures Concerning Old-Age Insurance for Rural Parents of Single Children and Couples With Sterilization After the Birth of Two Daughters], 1998

Guangdong sheng renkou pucha bangongshi (1990): Guangdong sheng renkou pucha bangongshi, ed., *Guangdong renkou fenxi xuanbian* [Selected Analyses on Population in Guangdong], Guangzhou

Guangzhou shimin shouce (1992): *Guangzhou shimin shouce* [Citizen Handbook for Guangzhou], Guangzhou

Gui Shixun (1992): Gui Shixun, Guanyu qieshi jiaqiang liudong renkou jihua shengyu guanli di jige wenti [Some Problems in Strengthening Birth Planning for the Migrant Population], *Renkou xinxi*, No. 1, Shanghai, pp. 15–25

Guo Shenyang (1985): Guo Shenyang, Jiating renkou touzi jiqi dui renkou guocheng de yingxiang [Human Investments of Families and Their Influence on Demographic Processes], *Renkou*, No. 1, Shanghai, pp. 20–25

Guojia jihua shengyu weiyuanhui (1992): Guojia jihua shengyu weiyuanhui, ed., *Jihua shengyu wenxian huibian, 1981–1991* [Collected Documents on Birth Planning, 1981–1991], Beijing

Guojia jihua shengyu weiyuanhui (1995): Guojia jihua shengyu weiyuanhui, ed., *Zhongguo jihua shengyu gongzuo gangyao 1995–2000* [China's Birth-Planning Program 1995–2000], Beijing

Guojia jihua shengyu weiyuanhui (1999): Guojia jihua shengyu weiyuanhui, ed., *Deng Xiaoping renkou sixiang xuexi gangyao* [A Study Outline for Deng Xiaoping Thought on Population], Beijing

Guowuyuan gongbao [State Council Bulletin], Beijing

Guowuyuan renkou pucha bangongshi (1987): Guowuyuan renkou pucha bangongshi, Zhongguo kexueyuan dili yanjiusuo, ed., *Zhongguo renkou ditu ji* [Population Atlas of China], Beijing

Han Yi (1986): Han Yi, Zhongguo de xiao huangdi [China's Little Emperors], *Xinhua wenzhai*, No. 7, Beijing, pp. 128–138

Hanley and Wolf (1985): Hanley, Susan B., and Arthur P. Wolf, ed., *Family and Population in East Asian History*, Stanford

Hardee-Cleaveland and Banister (1988): Hardee-Cleaveland, Karen, and Judith Banister, Fertility Policy and Implementation in China, 1986–88, *PDR*, No. 2, pp. 245–286

Harrell (1995): Harrell, Stevan, ed., *Chinese Historical Micro-Demography*, Berkeley

He Bochuan (1990): He Bochuan, *Shan'ao shang de Zhongguo, wenti, kunjing, tongku de xuanze* [China in a Fix: Problems, Difficulties and Bitter Options], Hongkong

He Qinglian (1988): He Qinglian, *Renkou: Zhongguo di xuanjian* [Population: The Sword Hanging Over China], Chengdu

Hebei sheng renkou diaocha dui (1996): Hebei sheng renkou diaocha dui, ed., *Hebei sheng renkou diaocha peixun jiaocai* [Training Materials for Population Surveys in Hebei Province], Shijiazhuang

Hebel and Schucher (1992): Hebel, Jutta, and Günter Schucher, *Zwischen Arbeitsplan und Arbeitsmarkt, Strukturen des Arbeitssystems in der VR China*, Hamburg

Hebel and Schucher (1999): Hebel, Jutta, and Günter Schucher, ed., *Der chinesische Arbeitsmarkt, Strukturen, Probleme, Perspektiven*, Hamburg

Heberer, Taubmann et al. (1998): Heberer, Thomas, Wolfgang Taubmann et al., *Chinas ländliche Gesellschaft, Urbanisierung und sozio-ökonomischer Wandel auf dem Lande*, Opladen

Heilig (1999): Heilig, Gerhard K., *China Food, Can China Feed Itself?* (CD-ROM), Laxenburg

Heilongjiang sheng jihua shengyu tiaoli [Heilongjiang Provincial Birth-Planning Regulations], 18 December 1999

Herrmann-Pillath (1991): Herrmann-Pillath, Carsten, *Transformation und Geschichte in China: Versuch einer theoretischen Interpretation* (Sonderveröffentlichung des Bundesinstituts für ostwissenschaftliche und internationale Studien), Köln

Hershatter (1997): Hershatter, Gail, *Dangerous Pleasure, Prostitution and Modernity in Twentieth-Century China*, Berkeley

Heuser (1999): Heuser, Robert, *Einführung in die chinesische Rechtskultur*, Hamburg

Ho Ping-ti (1959): Ho Ping-ti, *Studies on the Population of China, 1368–1953*, Cambridge, Mass.

Hoppe (1995): Hoppe, Thomas, *Die ethnischen Gruppen Xinjiangs, Kulturunterschiede und interethnische Beziehungen*, Hamburg

Hoppe (1997): Hoppe, Thomas, *Tibet heute – Aspekte einer komplexen Situation*, Hamburg

Hoy (1999): Hoy, Caroline, Issues in the Fertility of Temporary Migrants in Beijing, in: Pieke, Frank, and Hein Mallee, ed., *Internal and International Migration: Chinese Perspectives*, Richmond, pp. 134–155

Hsu (1971): Hsu, Francis L.K., *Under the Ancestors' Shadow – Kinship, Personality, and Social Mobility in China*, Stanford

Hu An'gang (1989a): Hu An'gang, *Renkou yu fazhan – Zhongguo renkou jingji wenti de xitong yanjiu* [Population and Development – A Systematic Study of Chinese Population Economics], Hangzhou

Hu An'gang (1989b): Hu An'gang, Jinnian woguo renkou yuanhe shikong [Why There Was a Loss of Birth Control in Recent Years], *Liaowang*, No. 10, pp. 22–23

Hu An'gang (2000): Hu An'gang, ed., *Zhongguo zuoxiang* [Prospects of China], Beijing

Hu Baosheng et al. (1981): Hu Baosheng et al., Guanyu woguo zong renkou mubiao de queding [The Determination of a Target for China's Total Population], *RYJ*, No. 5, pp. 15–18, 64

Huang Jikun et al. (1996): Huang Jikun, Scott Rozelle and Mark W. Rosegrant, China's Food Economy to the Twenty-First Century: Supply, Demand, and Trade, IFPRI, Washington

Huang Runlong (1994): Huang Runlong, Liudong renkou shengyu yiyuan yu shengyu xingwei diaocha [A Survey on Family Size Preferences and Fertility Among the Floating Population], ZRN, pp. 598–602

Huang Shu-min (1989): Huang Shu-min, The Spiral Road, Change in a Chinese Village Through the Eyes of a Communist Party Leader, Boulder

Hull (1990): Hull, Terence H., Recent Trends in Sex Ratios at Birth in China, PDR, No. 1, pp. 63–83

Human Rights Watch (1996): Human Rights Watch, ed., Death by Default, A Policy of Fatal Neglect in China's State Orphanages, New York

International Statistical Institute (1991): International Statistical Institute, Fertility in China, Proceedings of the International Seminar on China's In-Depth Fertility Survey, Voorburg

Ji Yi (1989): Ji Yi, Zhongguo de hei haizi [China's Black-Market Children], Renshi jian, No. 11, Chengdu, pp. 59–73, 121

Jia Tongjin and Sai Yin (1995): Jia Tongjin and Sai Yin, Renkou biandong qingkuang chouyang diaocha xianzhuang yu wenti fenxi [The Current Situation of the Sample Survey on Population Dynamics and an Analysis of Its Problems], RY, No. 5, pp. 28–31

Jiang Tao (1993): Jiang Tao, Zhongguo jindai renkou shi [Modern Chinese Population History], Hangzhou

Jiang Zhenghua (1986): Jiang Zhenghua, Shehui jingji yinsuo dui Zhongguo shengyulü di yingxiang [The Influence of Socioeconomic Factors on China's Fertility Rate], RY, No. 3, pp. 25–30

Jiang Zhenghua (1995): Jiang Zhenghua, ed., 1992 nian Zhongguo shengyulü chouyang diaocha shuju ji [Statistics of 1992 Fertility Sampling Survey in China], Beijing

Jiang Zhenghua and Chen Songbao (1988): Jiang Zhenghua and Chen Songbao, Zhongguo shengyulü bianhua ji renkou fazhan fenxi [An Analysis of Changes in the Fertility Rate and in the Demographic Development in China], RY, No. 5, pp. 2–7

Jiaozhou jihua shengyu weiyuanhui (1997): Jiaozhou jihua shengyu weiyuanhui, Jihua shengyu sanyiyi gongzuofa keti yanjiu baogao [Investigation Report on the Three-One-One Work Method in Birth Planning], Jiaozhou (Mimeograph)

Jihua shengyu guanlixue [Birth-Planning Administration], Beijing

Jingji ribao [Economic Daily], Beijing

Jingji yanjiu [Economic Studies], Beijing

'98 Zhongguo renkou (1999): Guojia tongjiju, ed., '98 Zhongguo renkou [China's Population in 1998], Beijing

Johansson (1995): Johansson, Sten, Lun xiandai Zhongguo de shouyang [On Adoption in Modern China], RY, No. 6, pp. 20–31

Johansson and Nygren (1991): Johansson, Sten, and Ola Nygren, The Missing Girls of China: A New Demographic Account, PDR, No. 1, pp. 35–51

Johnson (1994): Johnson, D. Gale, Effects of Institutions and Policies on Rural Population Growth With Application to China, PDR, No. 3, pp. 503–531

Johnson (1996): Johnson, Kay, The Politics of the Revival of Infant Abandonment in China, With Special Reference to Hunan, PDR, No. 1, pp. 77–98

Johnson et al. (1998): Johnson, Kay, Huang Banghan and Wang Liyao, Infant Abandonment and Adoption in China, PDR, No. 3, pp. 469–510

Kane (1987): Kane, Penny, The Second Billion, Population and Family Planning in China, Harmondsworth

Kane (1988): Kane, Penny, *Famine in China 1959–61*, London

Kaufman et al. (1989): Kaufman, Joan, Zhang Zhirong et al., Family Planning Policy and Practice in China: A Study of Four Rural Counties, *PDR*, No. 4, pp. 707–729

Kessler (1990): Kessler, Wolfgang, Im gebremsten Galopp ins Jahr des Pferdes: Neues Recht der Geburtenplanung in der VR China, *Verfassung und Recht in Übersee*, Vol. 23/2, Hamburg, pp. 109–126

Kim Choe Minja et al. (1992): Kim Choe Minja, Guo Fei, Wu Jianming and Zhang Ruyue, Progression to Second and Third Births in China: Patterns and Covariates in Six Provinces, *International Family Planning Perspectives*, Vol. 18, No. 4, New York, pp. 130–136

Kirkby (1985): Kirkby, Richard R.J., *Urbanisation in China: Town and Country in a Developing Economy 1949–2000 AD*, London

Krieg and Schädler (1994): Krieg, Renate, and Monika Schädler, ed., *Social Security in the People's Republic of China*, Hamburg

Krieg and Schädler (1995): Krieg, Renate, and Monika Schädler, *Soziale Sicherheit im China der neunziger Jahre*, Hamburg

Kua shiji de Zhongguo renkou [China's Population at the Turn of the Century], 33 Vol., Beijing

Kuang Ke (1989): Kuang Ke, Renkou chusheng lifa chuyi [Suggestions for Population and Childbearing Legislation], *Shehui kexue*, No. 8, Shanghai, pp. 35–37

Lampton (1977): Lampton, David M., The *Politics of Medicine in China: The Policy Process, 1949–1977*, Boulder

Lang (1946): Lang, Olga, *Chinese Family and Society*, New Haven

Lavely and Freedman (1990): Lavely, William, and Ronald Freedman, The Origins of Chinese Fertility Decline, *Demography*, Vol. 27, No. 3, Madison, pp. 357–367

Lee (1981): Lee, Bernice J., Female Infanticide in China, in: Guisso, Richard W., and Stanley Johannessen, ed., *Women in China, Current Directions in Historical Scholarship*, Youngstown, pp. 169–177

Lee and Campbell (1997): Lee, James Z., and Cameron D. Campbell, *Fate and Fortune in Rural China, Social Organization and Population Behavior in Liaoning 1774–1873*, Cambridge

Lee and Wang Feng (1999): Lee, James Z., and Wang Feng, *One Quarter of Humanity, Malthusian Mythology and Chinese Realities, 1700–2000*, Cambridge

Lee Yok-shiu (1988): Lee Yok-shiu, The Urban Housing Problem in China, *CQ*, No. 115, London, pp. 387–407

Legge (1960): Legge, James, *The Chinese Classics*, translated by James Legge, Vol. II: *The Works of Mencius*, Hongkong

Lei Jieqiong (1994): Lei Jieqiong, ed., *Gaige yilai Zhongguo nongcun hunyin jiating de xin bianhua* [The Change of the Marriage and the Family in the Chinese Countryside Since the Reform of the Economic System], Beijing

Leutner (1989): Leutner, Mechthild, Geburt, *Heirat und Tod in Peking, Volkskultur und Elitekultur vom 19. Jahrhundert bis zur Gegenwart*, Berlin

Levy (1949): Levy, Marion J., *The Family Revolution in Modern China*, Cambridge, Mass.

Li Bohua (1990): Li Bohua, Woguo 28 ge sheng, zizhiqu, zhexiashi shengyulü de bianhuia [Changes of the Fertility Rate in the 28 Provinces, Autonomous Regions and Centrally Administered Municipalities of China], *RYJ*, No. 3, pp. 3–12

Li Chengxun (1999): Li Chengxun, ed., *2020 nian de zhongguo, Dui weilai jingji jishu shehui wenhua shengtai huanjing de zhanwang* [China in the Year 2020, Future Prospects for Economy, Technology, Society, Culture and Natural Environment], Beijing

Li Honggui (1990): Li Honggui, Cong shengyu, jieyu chouyang diaocha kan woguo jihua shengyu di chengjiu [The Achievements of Chinese Birth Planning As Seen From the Sample Survey on Fertility and Contraception], *RY*, No. 3, pp. 8–12

Li Honggui and Zhao Shi (1990): Li Honggui and Zhao Shi, ed., *Quanguo shengyu jieyu chouyang diaocha quanguo shuju juan* [National Data Volume of the National Sample Survey on Fertility and Contraception], Beijing

Li Jiali (1995): Li Jiali, China's One-Child Policy: How and How Well Has It Worked? A Case Study of Hebei Province, 1979–88, *PDR*, No. 3, pp. 563–585

Li Jiang (1994): Li Jiang, Parity and Security: A Simulation Study of Old-Age Support in Rural China, *PDR*, No. 2, pp. 423–448

Li Jianxin (1997): Li Jianxin, Butong shengyu zhengce xuanze yu Zhongguo weilai renkou [Different Options for Birth Policies and China's Future Population], *RY*, No. 1, pp. 13–20

Li Jinfeng (1992): Li Jinfeng, ed., *Jihua shengyu guanli* [The Administration of Birth Planning], Beijing

Li Rongshi (1986): Li Rongshi, Shilun jingji shouru dui funü shengyulü de yingxiang [A Preliminary Study on the Influence of Economic Income on Female Fertility], *RY*, No. 6, pp. 19–23

Liang Jimin (1986): Liang Jimin, ed., *Jihua shengyu shouce* [Handbook of Birth Planning], Beijing

Liang Jimin and Chen Shengli (1993): Liang Jimin and Chen Shengli, ed., *Quanguo shengyu jieyu chouyang diaocha fenxi shuju juan* [Analytical Data of the National Sample Survey on Fertility and Contraception], 4 Vol., Beijing

Liang Jimin and Peng Zhiliang (1984): Liang Jimin and Peng Zhiliang, Quanmiande zhengquede liaojie he guanche dang di jihua shengyu zhengce [Correctly Understand and Implement the Party's Birth-Planning Policy], *RY*, No. 3, pp. 11–15

Liang Zhongtang and Tan Kejian (1997): Liang Zhongtang and Tan Kejian, Shanxi-sheng Yicheng-xian 'wanhun wanyu jia jiange' shengyu zhengce shishi xiaoguo de renkouxue fenxi [A Demographic Analysis of the Fertility Policy of 'Late Marriage, Late Birth and Longer Spacing' Pursued in Yicheng County, Shanxi Province], *ZRK*, No. 5, pp. 1–10

Liao Xuebin (1988): Liao Xuebin, Chengxiang liudong renkou jihua wai shengyu di yuanyin ji duice [Above-Quota Births Among the Migrant Population and Remedial Measures], *RX*, No. 2, pp. 43–46

Liaowang [Outlook], Beijing

Lin Fude (1987): Lin Fude, Woguo shengyulü zhuanbian de yinsuo fenxi [Analysis of Factors in the Changes in China's Fertility Rate], *RY*, No. 1, pp. 15–21

Lin Fude (1994): Lin Fude, Qu hunling yingxiang hou de Zhongguo shengyulü zhuanbian xingshe [Changes in the Chinese Fertility Rate After Excluding the Influence of the Marriage Age], *ZRK*, No. 6, pp. 10–20

Lin Fude *et al.* (1991): Lin Fude, Wang Feng and Yan Rui, Zhongguo shengyulü zhuanbian de jinqi taishe [Recent Trends in Chinese Fertility Change], *RY*, No. 5, pp. 2–7

Lin Fude and Zhai Zhenwu (1996): Lin Fude and Zhai Zhenwu, ed., *Zou xiang ershiyi shiji de Zhongguo renkou, huanjing yu fazhan* [China's Population, Environment and Development at the Turn of the Twenty-first Century], Beijing

Lin Jiang (1994): Lin Jiang, Parity and Security: A Simulation Study of Old-Age Support in Rural China, *PDR*, No. 2, pp. 423–448

Lin Jiang (1995): Lin Jiang, Changing Kinship Structure and its Implications for Old-Age Support in Urban and Rural China, *Population Studies*, Vol. 49, London, pp. 127–145

Linck (1988): Linck, Gudula, *Frau und Familie in China*, München

Liu Dalin (1992): Liu Dalin, ed., Zhongguo dangdai xing wenhua, *Zhongguo liangwan li xing wenming diaocha baogao* [Sexual Behaviour in Modern China, A Report on the Nation-Wide 'Sex Civilization' Survey on 20,000 Subjects in China], Shanghai

Liu Feng (1990): Liu Feng, Guanyu dangqian renkou xingshe jiqi duice di ji dian sikao [Some Thoughts on the Present Situation in Population Development and on Remedial Measures], *RY*, No. 3, pp. 6–7

Liu Hongkang (1988): Liu Hongkang, *Renkou shouce* [Population Handbook], Chengdu

Liu Longjian (1990): Liu Longjian, Zhongguo xinan san sheng yuling funü shengyulü zhejie yingxiang yinsuo chutan [A Preliminary Investigation of Direct Influences on the Fertility Rate of Women in Reproductive Age in Three Provinces of Southwest China]; *RY*, No. 1, pp. 32–36

Liu Xian (1985): Liu Xian, Shanghai shi sheng yiyuan he shouru shuiping de neizai jizhi fenxi [An Analys of Childbearing Preferences and Their Internal Relationship to Income Levels], *Renkou*, No. 3, Shanghai, pp. 21–25

Liu Zheng (1988): Liu Zheng, ed., *Zhongguo renkou wenti yanjiu* [Studies on Chinese Population Problems], Beijing

Liu Zheng et al. (1980): Liu Zheng, Wu Cangping and Lin Fude, Dui kongzhi woguo renkou zengzhang de wu dian jianyi [Five Proposals on Controlling Population Growth in Our Country], *RY*, No. 1, pp. 1–5

Liu Zheng et al. (1981): Liu Zheng, Song Jian et al., *China's Population: Problems and Prospects*, Beijing

LTZH (1990): Guojia tongjiju, ed., *Quanguo ge sheng, zizhiqu, zhixiashi lishi tongji ziliao huibian 1949–1989* [A Collection of Historical Statistics from All Provinces, Autonomous Regions and Centrally Administered Municipalities in China 1949–1989], Beijing

Lü Hongping (1991): Lü Hongping, Lun zinü de chengben – shouyi guanxi yu jiating shengyu juece [On the Cost-Benefit Structure of Childbearing and Family Fertility Decisions], *RYJ*, No. 3, pp. 22–26

Lu Li (1990): Lu Li, Xiangdi haizi xiaoyong yu xiangdi nongcun shengyulü [Lowering Childbearing Utility and Lowering the Rural Fertility Rate], *RYJ*, No. 3, pp. 13–18

Luther et al. (1990): Luther, Norman Y., Griffith Feeney and Zhang Weimin, One-Child Families or a Baby Boom? Evidence from China's 1987 One-per-Hundred Survey, *Population Studies*, No. 44, London, pp. 341–357

Ma Bin (1990): Ma Bin, Qiwu renkou shikong, wenti zheng shi chu zai 12 yi zuoyou he kai xiao kouzi [The Problem of Loss of Control in Population Development Is Grounded in the 'ca 1.2 Billion' and the 'Opening of a Small Hole'], in: Zhongguo renkou xuehui, ed., *Di wu ci quanguo renkou kexue taolunhui lunwen xuan* [Contributions to the Fifth National Symposium on Population Science], Beijing, pp. 55–58

Ma Hong (1989): Ma Hong, ed., *2000 nian de Zhongguo* [China in the Year 2000], Beijing

Ma Xia (1994): Ma Xia, ed., *Zhongguo chengzhen renkou qianyi* [Migration in China's Urban Places], Beijing

Ma Yinchu (1979): Ma Yinchu, *Xin renkou lun* [New Population Theory], Beijing

Ma Yingtong (1988): Ma Yingtong, 1986 yu 1981 nian di liang ci renkou huisheng bijiao yanjiu [A Comparative Analysis of the Two Renewed Upsurges of Population in 1981 and 1986], *ZRK*, No. 5, pp. 27–31

Ma Yingtong (1997): Ma Yingtong, Ruogan renkou kongzhi wenti zai-fenxi yu ruogan xueshu guandian zhouyi [A Further Analysis of Some Problems of Population Control With Some of My Personal Academic Viewpoints], *RYJ*, No. 1, 9–17

Mao Zedong (1961): Mao Zedong, *Selected Works*, 4 Volumes, Beijing

Mao Zhifeng (1995): Mao Zhifeng, *Shidu renkou yu kongzhi* [Optimum Population and Control], Xi'an

Merli (1998): Merli, Giovanna M., Underreporting of Births and Infant Deaths in Rural China: Evidence from Field Research in One County in Northern China, CQ, No. 155, London, pp. 637–655

Merli and Raftery (2000): Merli, Giovanna M., and Adrian E. Raftery, Are Births Under reported in Rural China? Manipulation of Statistical Records in Response to China's Population Policies, *Demography*, Vol. 37, No. 1, pp. 109–126

Milwertz (1997): Milwertz, Cecilia Nathansen, *Accepting Population Control, Urban Chinese Women and the One-Child Policy*, Richmond

Mingbao, Hongkong

Mosher (1982): Mosher, Steven W., Birth Control: A View from a Chinese Village, *Asian Survey*, Vol. 22, No. 4, Berkeley, pp. 356–368

Mosher (1983): Mosher, Steven W., *Broken Earth: The Rural Chinese*, New York

Mosher (1993): Mosher, Steven W., *A Mother's Ordeal: One Woman's Fight Against China's One-Child Policy*, New York

Myrdal (1963): Myrdal, Jan, *Report From a Chinese Village*, Harmondsworth

Nan Zhongji (1993): Nan Zhongji, Zhanwang 90 niandai Zhongguo de shengyu zhuanbian [A Perspective of Fertility Changes in China During the 1990s], RY, No. 3, pp. 14–19

Ni Jia (1987): Ni Jia, Zhiding yu xiada niandu renkou chusheng kongzhi zhibiao di jiben yuanze he fangfa [Basic Principles and Methods For Determining and Promulgating Birth Control Quotas], RYJ, No. 5, pp. 48–51

Nygren and Hoem (1993): Nygren, Ola, and Britta Hoem, *Recent Trends in Fertility and Contraceptive Use in China: Results from a Sample Survey* (unpublished manuscript), Stockholm

Orleans (1966): Orleans, Leo A., Birth Control: Reversal or Postponement?, CQ, No. 3, London, pp. 59–73

Orleans (1972): Orleans, Leo A., *Every Fifth Child: The Population of China*, Stanford

Orleans (1979): Orleans, Leo A., ed., *Chinese Approaches to Family Planning*, White Plains

Pan Yunkang (1988): Pan Yunkang, Xing geming he xing jiaose geming [Sexual Revolution and the Revolution of Gender Roles], *Shehui*, No. 6, Shanghai, pp. 24–26

Parish and Whyte (1978): Parish, William L., and Martin K. Whyte, *Village and Family in Contemporary China*, Chicago

Park Chai Bin and Cho Nam-Hoon (1995): Park Chai Bin and Cho Nam-Hoon, Consequences of Son Preference in a Low-Fertility Society: Imbalance of the Sex Ratio at Birth in Korea, *PDR*, No. 1, pp. 59–84

PDR: *Population and Development Review*, New York

Peng Xizhe (1987): Peng Xizhe, Demographic Consequences of the Great Leap Forward, *PDR*, Vol. 13, pp. 639–670

Peng Xizhe (1989): Peng Xizhe, Major Determinants of China's Fertility Transition, CQ, No. 117, pp. 1–37

Peng Xizhe (1991): Peng Xizhe, *Demographic Transition in China, Fertility Trends since the 1950s*, Oxford

Peng Xizhe (1993): Peng Xizhe, Regional Differentials in China's Fertility Transition, in: Leete, Richard, and Iqbal Alam, ed., *The Revolution in Asian Fertility, Dimensions, Causes, and Implications*, Oxford, pp. 99–127

Peng Xizhe and Huang Juan (1993): Peng Xizhe and Huang Juan, Shilun jingji fazhan zai Zhongguo shengyulü zhuanbian guocheng zhong de zuoyong [A Preliminary Study on the Role of Economic Development in Chinese Fertility Transition], RYJ, No. 1, pp. 25–30

Peng Xizhe and Dai Xingyi (1996): Peng Xizhe and Dai Xingyi, *Zhongguo nongcun shequ shengyu wenhua* [The Fertility Culture of Chinese Rural Communities], Shanghai

Peng Zhiliang (1987): Peng Zhiliang, Jihua shengyu yinggai lifa [We Need Birth-Planning Legislation], *RY*, No. 4, pp. 36–37

Perkins (1969): Perkins, Dwight H., *Agricultural Development in China, 1368–1968*, Edinburgh

Phillips and Ross (1992): Phillips, J.F., and J.A. Ross, ed., *Family Planning Programmes and Fertility*, Oxford

Pieke and Mallee (1999): Pieke, Frank, and Hein Mallee, ed., *Internal and International Migration, Chinese Perspectives*, Richmond

Population, Paris

Population Studies, London

Poston (1997): Poston, Dudley L., Cultural, Social, and Economic Determinants of Family Size Norms in China, With Special Attention to Son Preference, in: *International Population Conference*, Beijing, Vol. 3, Beijing

Poston and Gu Baochang (1987): Poston, Dudley L., and Gu Baochang, Socio-Economic Development, Family Planning, and Fertility in China, *Demography*, Vol. 24, No. 4, Madison, pp. 531–551

Poston and Jia Zhongke (1989): Poston, Dudley L., and Jia Zhongke, Socioeconomic Structure and Fertility in China: A County-Level Investigation, Paper at the XXIst International Population Conference of the IUSSP, New Delhi

Poston and Yaukey (1992): Poston, Dudley L., and David Yaukey, ed., *The Population of Modern China*, New York

Potter and Potter (1990): Potter, Sulamith Heins, and Jack M. Potter, *China's Peasants, The Anthropology of a Revolution*, Cambridge

Qian Zhenchao (1997): Qian Zhenchao, Progression to Second Birth in China: A Study of Four Rural Counties, *Population Studies*, No. 51, pp. 221–228

Qiao Duanbo (1991): Qiao Duanbo, Nongcun zaolian zaohun zaoyu yuanyin fenxi jiqi duice yanjiu [A Study on the Reasons for Early Love, Early Marriage and Early Birth in the Villages and on Remedial Measures], *RZ*, No. 3, pp. 21–23

Qinghai sheng renkou xuehui (1984): Qinghai sheng renkou xuehui, ed., *Qinghai minzu renkou wenti tantao* [Contributions on the Population Problems of National Minorities in Qinghai], Xining

Qingtian xian shishi Zhejiang sheng jihua shengyu tiaoli banfa [Qingtian County Implementation Rules for the Zhejiang Birth-Planning Regulations], 15 May 1996

Qiu Shuhua et al. (1994): Qiu Shuhua, Liu Yunrong, Gao Ersheng and Zhang Liying, ed., Biyun fangfa shiyong donglixue, *Zhongguo nongcun xianchang diaocha baogao* [Dynamics of Contraceptive Use in Rural China], Beijing

Qu Geping and Li Jinchang (1994): Qu Geping and Li Jinchang, *Population and the Environment in China*, Boulder

Qu Yibin (1988): Qu Yibin, Woguo renkou chushenglü mingxian huisheng di yuanyin ji duice tantao [A Discussion of the Renewed Upsurge of the Birth Rate in China and of Remedial Measures], *RY*, No. 2, pp. 53–56

Quanguo 1‰ renkou shengyulü chouyang diaocha fenxi (1983): Renkou yu jingji bianjibu, ed., *Quanguo 1‰ renkou shengyulü chouyang diaocha fenxi* [Analyses of the 1‰ Sample Survey on Fertility in China], Beijing

RD: *Renkou dongtai* [Population Trends], Beijing

Renkou [Population], Shanghai

RR: *Renmin ribao* [People's Daily], Beijing

RX: *Renkou xuekan* [Demographic Journal], Changchun

RY: *Renkou yanjiu* [Population Studies], Beijing

RYJ: *Renkou yu jingji* [Population and Economics], Beijing

RYJS: *Renkou yu jihua shengyu* [Population and Birth Planning], Beijing

RZ: *Renkou zhanxian* [Demographic Frontline], Shijiazhuang

Saith (1981): Saith, Ashwani, Economic Incentives for the One-Child Family in Rural China, CQ, No. 87, pp. 493–500

Scharping (1981): Scharping, Thomas, *Umsiedlungsprogramme für Chinas Jugend 1955–1980, Probleme der Stadt-Land-Beziehungen in der chinesischen Entwicklungspolitik*, Hamburg

Scharping (1985–86): Scharping, Thomas, *Chinas Bevölkerung 1953–1982*, Vol. I–IV (Berichte des Bundesinstituts für ostwissenschaftliche und internationale Studien), Köln

Scharping (1997): Scharping, Thomas, ed., *Floating Population and Migration in China, The Impact of Economic Reforms*, Hamburg

Scharping (1999): Scharping, Thomas, Selectivity, Migration Reasons and Backward Linkages of Rural-Urban Migrants: A Sample Survey of Migrants to Foshan and Shenzhen in Comparative Perspective, in: Pieke, Frank, and Hein Mallee, ed., *Internal and International Migration: Chinese Perspectives*, Richmond, pp. 73–102

Scharping (2000a): Scharping, Thomas, ed., *The Evolution of Regional Birth-Planning Norms, 1954–97* (I), (*Chinese Sociology and Anthropology*, Vol. 32, No. 3), Armonk

Scharping (2000b): Scharping, Thomas, ed., *The Evolution of Regional Birth-Planning Norms, 1954–97* (II), (*Chinese Sociology and Anthropology*, Vol. 32, No. 4), Armonk

Scharping (2000c): Scharping, Thomas, The Integration of Manchuria: Political Change, Demographic Development and Ethnic Structure From the Early Qing Period to Present Times (1610–1993), in: Bieg, Lutz, and Erling von Mende, ed., *Ad Seres et Tungusos, Festschrift für Martin Gimm*, Wiesbaden, pp. 343–376

Scharping and Heuser (1995): Scharping, Thomas, and Robert Heuser, ed., *Geburtenplanung in China, Analysen, Daten, Dokumente*, Hamburg

Scharping and Sun Huaiyang (1997): Scharping, Thomas, and Sun Huaiyang, ed., *Migration in Chinas Guangdong Province, Major Results of a 1993 Sample Survey on Migrants and Floating Population in Shenzhen and Foshan*, Hamburg

Schoenhals (1987): Schoenhals, Michael, *Saltationist Socialism, Mao Zedong and the Great Leap Forward*, Stockholm

Schran (1978): Schran, Peter, China's Demographic Evolution 1850–1953 Reconsidered, CQ, No. 75, London, pp. 639–646

Sha Jicai (1994): Sha Jicai, ed., *Gaige kaifang zhong de renkou wenti yanjiu* [Studies on Population Problems in the Period of Reforms and Opening Up], Beijing

Shanghai shi jihua shengyu tiaoli [Shanghai Municipal Birth-Planning Regulations], 4 April 2000

Shanghai shi wailai liudong renyuan jihua shengyu guanli banfa [Shanghai Municipal Administrative Procedures for Birth Planning Among In-Migrants from Outside], 20 June 2000

Sheng renkou pucha bangongshi (1992–93): Sheng renkou pucha bangongshi, ed., *Sheng 1990 nian renkou pucha ziliao* [Provincial Tabulations of the 1990 Population Census], 85 vol., various places

Shi Chengli (1980): Shi Chengli, Jianguo yilai jihua shengyu gongzuo gaikuang [An Outline of Birth Planning Since the Founding of the People's Republic of China], XR, No. 2, Lanzhou, pp. 33–48

Shi Chengli (1988): Shi Chengli, *Zhongguo jihua shengyu huodong shi* [A History of Birth Planning in China], Urumqi

Shi Tianjian (1997): Shi Tianjian, *Political Participation in Beijing*, Cambridge, Mass.

Sichuan yixueyuan (1978): Sichuan yixueyuan, ed., *Weisheng tongjixue* [Health Statistics], Beijing

Skinner (1987): Skinner, G. William, Sichuan's Population in the Nineteenth Century: Lessons From Disaggregated Data, *Late Imperial China*, Vol. 8, No. 1, Pasadena, pp. 1–79

Smil (1993): Smil, Vaclav, *China's Environmental Crisis, An Inquiry into the Limits of National Development*, Armonk

Smil (1995): Smil, Vaclav, Who Will Feed China?, CQ, No. 143, pp. 801–813

Snow (1973): Snow, Edgar, *The Long Revolution*, London

Solinger (1999): Solinger, Dorothy, *Contesting Citizenship in Urban China: Peasant Migrants, the State, and the Logic of the Market*, Berkeley

Song Duanyu et al. (1981): Song Duanyu et al., Renkou yuce moshi he quanguo renkou yuce [Population Projection Models and the Projection of the National Population], *Ziran zazhi*, No. 4, Shanghai, pp. 249–252

Song Jian and Li Guangyuan (1980): Song Jian and Li Guangyuan, Renkou fazhan de dingliang yanjiu [A Quantitative Study of Population Development], *Jingji Yanjiu*, Beijing, No. 2, pp. 60–67

Song Jian and Yu Jingyuan (1985): Song Jian and Yu Jingyuan, *Renkou kongzhi lun* [On Population Control], Beijing

Song Jian et al. (1982): Song Jian, Tian Xueyuan, Yu Jingyuan and Li Guangyuan, *Renkou yuce he renkou kongzhi* [Projection and Control of Population], Beijing

Song Jian et al. (1985): Song Jian, Tuan Chi-hsien and Yu Jing-yuan, *Population Control in China, Theory and Applications*, New York

Song Jianhua (1994): Song Jianhua, Renkou jihua guanli de sikao [Thoughts on the Implementation of Population Plans], RYJ, No. 2, pp. 25–27

Song Zexing (1987): Song Zexing, ed., *Zhongguo renkou: Liaoning fence* [Encyclopedia of Chinese Population: Liaoning], Beijing

South China Morning Post, Hongkong

State Family Planning Commission (1997): State Family Planning Commission, ed., *1992 National Fertility and Family Planning Survey, China, Selected Research Papers in English*, Beijing

State Statistical Bureau (1986): State Statistical Bureau, ed., *China In-Depth Fertility Survey, Phase I*, 2 Vol., Beijing

State Statistical Bureau (1989): State Statistical Bureau, ed., *China In-Depth Fertility Survey, Phase II*, 2 Vol., Beijing

SWB: *Summary of World Broadcasts, Part III: The Far East*, Reading

Sun Jingxin (1993): Sun Jingxin, Renzhen guanche zhixing jiben guoce cujinshehui jingji xietiao fazhan [Implement the Basic State Policy and Promote Balanced Socio-Economic Development], *Renkou yu jihua jingji*, No. 1, Shijiazhuang; pp. 23–26

Sun Jingxin (1994): Sun Jingxin, ed., *Zhongguo zangzu renkou yanjiu xilie* [Series on China's Tibetan Population], 5 Vol., Beijing

Sun Jingzhi (1957): Sun Jingzhi, *Shiwu laiyuan yu renkou zengzhang* [Food Resources and Population Growth), Beijing

Sun Muhan (1987): Sun Muhan, *Zhongguo jihua shengyu shigao* [A Preliminary History of Birth Planning in China), Beijing

Sun Wensheng and Jin Guanghua (1994): Sun Wensheng and Jin Guanghua, Shehui jingji fazhan de shengyulü xiaoying yanjiu [A Study of the Effects of Socio-Economic Development on the Fertility Rate], RY, No. 6, pp. 10–21

Tan Xiaoqing (1990): Tan Xiaoqing, Zhongguo nongcun qianyi funü de shengyulü bianhua [Changes of Fertility Rates Among Women Migrants From the Villages], RYJ, No. 4, pp. 13–15, 6

Taylor (1988): Taylor, Jeffrey R., Rural Employment Trends and the Legacy of Surplus Labour, 1978–1986, CQ, No. 116, pp. 736–766

Taylor and Banister (1988): Taylor, Jeffrey R., and Judith Banister, *China: The Problem of Employing Surplus Rural Labor*, U.S. Bureau of the Census, Washington

Tian Xueyuan (1984): Tian Xueyuan, *Zhongguo renkou kongzhi he fazhan qushe yanjiu* [A Study on Population Control and Demographic Trends in China], Beijing

Tian Xueyuan (1989): Tian Xueyuan, 1987 nian Zhongguo laonian renkou chouyang diaocha baogao [Report on the 1987 Sample Survey of the Aged Population in China], *ZRN*, pp. 299–319

Tian Xueyuan (1990): Tian Xueyuan, San ci renkou langchao di congji he xiangying di hongguan juece yanjiu [A Study of the Three Waves of Population and Macro-Level Responses], *ZRK*, No. 1, pp. 1–7

Tian Xueyuan (1991): Tian Xueyuan, *Zhongguo laonian renkou jingji* [Population Economics for the Aged in China], Beijing

Tian Xueyuan (1994): Tian Xueyuan, Zhongguo 1992 nian jiating jingji yu shengyu 10 shengshi chouyang diaocha baogao [Report on a 1992 Sample Survey of Family Economics and Fertility in Ten Chinese Provinces and Municipalities], *ZRN*, pp. 334–340

Tian Xueyuan (1997): Tian Xueyuan, *Da guo zhi nan: Dangdai Zhongguo renkou wenti* [The Hardships of Greatness: Population Problems of Contemporary China], Beijing

Tien (1973): Tien, H. Yuan, *China's Population Struggle, Demographic Decisions of the People's Republic, 1949–1969*, Columbus

Tien (1980): Tien, H. Yuan, ed., *Population Theory in China*, White Plains

Tien (1983): Tien, H. Yuan, Age at Marriage in the People's Republic of China, *CQ*, No. 93, pp. 90–107

Tien (1987): Tien, H. Yuan, Abortion in China, Incidence and Implications, *Modern China*, Vol. XIII, No. 4, New York, pp. 441–468

Tien (1991): Tien, H. Yuan, *China's Strategic Demographic Initiative*, New York

Tu Ping (1993): Tu Ping, Woguo chusheng ying'er xingbiebi wenti tantao [A Discussion of the Sex Ratio at Birth in China], *RY*, No. 1, pp. 6–13

Tu Ping (1995): Tu Ping, Zhongguo renkou laolinghua yu renkou kongzhi [The Aging of the Chinese Population and Population Control], *ZSK*, No. 6, pp. 61–70

UNFPA (1984a): United Nations Fund for Population Activities, *China, Report of Mission on Needs Assessment for Population Assistance*, Report No. 67, New York

UNFPA (1984b): United Nations Fund for Population Activities, *Report on the Evaluation of CPR/80/P14: Population Education in the Secondary Schools and Teachers Training of the People's Republic of China*, New York

UNFPA (1989): United Nations Population Fund, *Comparative Evaluation of UNFPA Support to Population and Development Planning, Asia and the Pacific Region*, New York

UNFPA (1997): United Nations Population Fund, *Executive Board Document on the China Programme CPR/98/P01*, New York

United Nations Population Devision (2000): United Nations Population Devision, ed., *Long-range World Population Projections: Based on the 1998 Revision*, New York

United Nations Population Devision (2001): United Nations Population Devision, ed., *World Population Prospects: The 1999 Revision*, Washington

United States Census Bureau (2000): United States Census Bureau, IDB Summary Demographic Data for China, www.census.govcgi-bin/ipc

Wang Dahai (1999): Wang Dahai, *Shiye de Zhongguo* [Unemployed China], Beijing

Wang Dongfeng (1982): Wang Dongfeng, Yongji xian Wanjiagou shengchandui renkou chushenglü huisheng qingkuang de diaocha [A Study on the Reincrease of the Birth Rate in Wanjiagou Production Brigade, Yongji County], *RX*, No. 2, 49–50

Wang Feng (1988): Wang Feng, The Roles of Individual's Socioeconomic Characteristics and The Government Family Planning Program in China's Fertility, *Population Research and Policy Review*, Vol. 7, No. 3, Dordrecht, pp. 255–276

Wang Feng (1996): Wang Feng, A Decade of the One-Child Policy: Achievements and Implications, in: Goldstein, Alice, and Wang Feng, ed., *China: The Many Facets of Demographic Change*, Boulder, pp. 97–120

Wang Feng and Yang Quanhe (1996): Wang Feng and Yang Quanhe, Age at Marriage and the First Birth Interval: The Emerging Change in Sexual Behavior Among Young Couples in China, *PDR*, No. 2, pp. 299–320

Wang Feng et al. (1990): Wang Feng, Nancy E. Riley and Lin Fude, China's Continuing Demographic Transition in the 1980s, Paper for the 1990 Population Association of America Annual Meeting, Toronto

Wang Haito et al. (1997): Wang Haito, Maurice D. van Arsdol and David M. Heer, Socio-Economic Determinants of Fertility in Rural China, in: *International Population Conference*, Beijing, Vol. 3, Beijing, pp. 1387–1403

Wang Hean (1998): Wang Hean, Dangqian jihua shengyu gongzuo xin nandian ji duice [New Difficulties in Present Birth-Control Work and Remedial Measures], *RY*, No. 5, pp. 60–62

Wang Jianmin and Hu Qi (1996): Wang Jianmin and Hu Qi, *Zhongguo liudong renkou* [China's Floating Population], Shanghai

Wang Jiye and Hull (1991): Wang Jiye and Terence H. Hull, ed., *Population and Development Planning in China*, North Sydney

Wang Ling (1997): Wang Ling, Lun ren de jiating shengyang jiazhe de zhuanbian [On Changes in the Value of Child Raising], *Jingji tizhi gaige*, Vol. 1, Chengdu, p. 13–33

Wang Ming (1996): Wang Ming, ed., *Zhongguo fenxian zhuyao renkou shuju ji* [Main Population Data of China by County], Beijing

Wang Xianjin (1997): Wang Xianjin, ed., *Zhongguo quanwei renshi lun Zhongguo ziyang yanghuo yanghao zhongguoren* [Authorities in China Give Their Opinions on How the Chinese Government Could Get Enough Food For Her People], Beijing

Wang Xiuyin (1998): Wang Xiuyin, Guanyu jihua shengyu cunmin zizhi de ji ge wenti [Some Problems of Village Self-Administration in Birth Planning], *RY*, No. 4, pp. 67–70

Wei Jinsheng (1988): Wei Jinsheng, Jin shi nian lai Zhongguo renkou zengzhang kongzhi di jige jiben wenti di sikao [Thoughts on Some Basic Problems of Controlling Population Growth in China During the Last Decade], *RYJ*, No. 6, pp. 16–21

Wei Jinsheng and Wang Shengling (1996): Wei Jinsheng and Wang Shengling, ed., *Zhongguo renkou kongzhi pinggu yu duice* [Evaluations and Suggestions on Birth Control in China], Beijing

Wenhui bao [Gazette], Shanghai

White (1985): White, Tyrene, *Population Policy and Rural Reform in China, 1977–1984: Policy Implementation and Interdependency at the Local Level* (unpublished dissertation), Columbus

White (1987): White, Tyrene, Implementing the One-Child-per-Couple Population Program in Rural China: National Goals and Local Politics, in: Lampton, David, M., ed., *Policy Implementation in Post-Mao China*, Berkeley, pp. 284–317

White (1992): White, Tyrene, ed., *Family Planning in China*, (*Chinese Sociology and Anthropology*, Vol. 24, No. 3), Armonk

White (1994): White, Tyrene, The Origins of China's Birth-Planning Policy, in: Gilmartin, Christina, et al., *Engendering China, Women, Culture, and the State*, Cambridge, Mass., pp. 250–278

Whyte and Gu (1987): Whyte, Martin K., and Gu Shengzu, Popular Response to China's Fertility Transition, PDR, No. 13, pp. 471–498

Whyte and Parish (1984): Whyte, Martin King, and William L. Parish, Urban Life in Contemporary China, Chicago

Wolf (1985): Wolf, Arthur P., Fertility in Prerevolutionary Rural China, in: Hanley and Wolf, pp. 154–185

Wolf (1986): Wolf, Arthur P., The Preeminent Role of Government Intervention in China's Family Revolution, PDR, No. 1, pp. 101–116

Wolf and Huang (1980): Wolf, Arthur P., and Huang Chieh-shan, Marriage and Adoption in China, 1845–1945, Stanford

Wong Siu-lun (1984): Wong Siu-lun, Consequences of China's New Population Policy, CQ, No. 98, pp. 220–240

World Bank (1979–): World Bank, World Development Report, Washington

World Bank (1985): World Bank, ed., China: Long-Term Issues and Options, The Main Report, Washington

World Bank (1992a): World Bank, ed., China – Implementation Options for Urban Housing Reform, Washington

World Bank (1992b): World Bank, ed., China Strategies for Reducing Poverty in the 1990s, Washington

World Bank (1997a): World Bank, ed., China 2020, Development Challenges in the New Century, Washington

World Bank (1997b): World Bank, ed., At China's Table, Food Security Options, Washington

World Bank (1997c): World Bank, ed., Old Age Security, Pension Reform in China, Washington

World Bank (2000): World Bank, ed., World Development Indicators Database, www.worldbank.org/data

Wu Cangping (1988a): Wu Cangping, Lun woguo renkou fazhan zhanlue mubiao [On the Strategic Goals of Population Development in China], in: Liu Zheng, pp. 1–31

Wu Cangping (1988b): Wu Cangping, Zhongguo renkou xingbiebi de yanjiu [A Study on the Sex Ratio of the Chinese Population], in: Liu Zheng, pp. 110–148

Wu Cangping (1996): Wu Cangping, ed., Gaige kaifang zhong chuxian de zui xin renkou wenti [Recent Population Problems in the Period of Reform and Opening-Up], Beijing

Wu Cangping and Mu Guangzong (1995): Wu Cangping and Mu Guangzong, Di shengyu yanjiu [A Study of Low Fertility], ZSK, No. 1, pp. 83–98

Wu Jieping and Xiao Bilian (1985): Wu Jieping and Xiao Bilian, Family Planning in China, Paper for the International Symposium on Fertility Regulation Research, Beijing

Wu Zhongguan and Xiao Lijian (1994): Wu Zhongguan and Xiao Lijian, Zhongguo 1971–1990 nian jihua shengyu touru chanchu xiaoyi pinggu yanjiu [A Cost-Benefit Evaluation of Chinese Birth Planning 1971–1990], ZRN, pp. 544–552

Xiao Jiabao (1989): Xiao Jiabao, Woguo jiang yudao de si da weiji jiqi duice [Four Major Crises in China's Future and Ways to Meet Them], Liaowang, No. 10, pp. 24–25; No. 11, pp. 14–15

Xie Cheng (1988): Xie Cheng, Youguan youdai dusheng zinü jiqi jiating zhengce wenti di tantao he jianyi [Contributions and Suggestions on Preferential Policies for Single Children and Their Families], RYJ, No. 1, pp. 20–22

XR: Xibei renkou [Population in Northwest China], Lanzhou

Xinan si sheng (qu) renkou fazhan zhanlüe yantaohui (1986): Xinan si sheng (qu) renkou fazhan zhanlüe yantaohui, ed., Renkou fazhan zhanlüe yanjiu [Studies on the Strategy of Population Development], Chengdu

Xu Xifa (1995): Xu Xifa, *Zhongguo shaoshu minzu jihua shengyu gailun* [An Outline of Birth Planning Among the National Minorities of China], Urumqi

Yan Tianhua (1996): Yan Tianhua, *Guizhou shaoshu minzu renkou fazhan yu wenti yanjiu* [Studies on Population Development and Problems of Guizhou's National Minorities], Beijing

Yang (1959): Yang, C.K., *A Chinese Village in Early Communist Transition*, Cambridge, Mass.

Yang Kuifu (1995): Yang Kuifu, ed., *Zhongguo shaoshuminzu renkou* [The Population of China's National Minorities], Beijing

Yang Yixing (1984): Yang Yixing, Shaoshuminzu di renkou xianzhuang he jihua shengyu [The Present Demographic Situation of National Minorities and Birth Planning], RY, No. 4, pp. 37–41

Yang Yixing et al. (1988): Yang Yixing, Zhang Tianlu and Xiong Yu, *Zhongguo shaoshu minzu renkou yanjiu* [Studies on the Population of China's National Minorities], Beijing

Yang Zhuquan (1995): Yang Zhuquan, *Zhongguo renkou falü zhidu yanjiu* [Studies on the System of Population Law in China], Beijing

Yang Zihui (1991): Yang Zihui, Lun liudong renkou de shengyu xingwei [The Fertility of Migrants], RYJ, No. 3, pp. 3–13

1995 nian quanguo 1% renkou chouyang diaocha ziliao: Quanguo renkou chouyang diaocha bangongshi, ed., *1995 nian quanguo 1% renkou chouyang diaocha ziliao* [Materials of the 1995 1%-Sampling Survey on Population in China], Beijing

Yu Jingyuan et al. (1990): Yu Jingyuan, Zou Ping and Liu Jianping, Zhongguo xian jieduan de renkou kongzhi he duice [The Present Phase of Chinese Population Control and Remedial Measures], in: Zhongguo renkou xuehui, ed., *Di wu ci quanguo renkou kexue taolunhui lunwen xuan* [Contributions to the Fifth National Symposium on Population Science], Beijing, pp. 65–69

Yu Jinshun et al. (1985): Yu Jinshun et al., Zhengque jiejue shaoshuminzu diqu de renkou wenti [Correctly Solve the Population Problems of China's Minority Areas], *Minzu yanjiu*, No. 4, Beijing, pp. 1–6

Yu Xuejun et al. (1994): Yu Xuejun, Wang Zhichun and Yang Xun, Zhongguo 80 niandai de zaohun zaoyu zhuangkuang jiqi dui renkou kongzhi di yingxiang [The Influence of Early Marriage and Early Birth on Birth Control in China During the 80s], RY, No. 1, pp. 26–30

Yuan Fang (1988): Yuan Fang, ed., *Shehui tongjixue* [Social Statistics], Beijing

Yuan Jianhua and Skinner (2000): Yuan Jianhua and G. William Skinner, Shaping the Gender Configuration of Offspring Sets: The Spatial Patterning of Reproductive Strategizing in Contemporary China, Paper for the Annual Meeting of the Association of Asian Studies, San Diego

Yuan Yongxi (1991): Yuan Yongxi, ed., *Zhongguo renkou, Zonglun* [China's Population, General Volume], Beijing

Yuan Yongxi (1996): Yuan Yongxi, *80 niandai Zhongguo renkou biandong fenxi* [Analysis of China's Population Dynamics in the 80s], Beijing

Yunnan sheng renkou pucha bangongshi (1989): Yunnan sheng renkou pucha bangongshi, ed., *Zhongguo xinanbu renkou xianzhuang yanjiu* [Studies on the Demographic Situation in Southwest China], Kunming

Yunnan sheng renkou xuehui (1984): Yunnan sheng renkou xuehui, ed., *Xinan shaoshuminzu renkou taolunhui lunwen diaocha baogao* [Contributions and Survey Reports for the Symposium on the Minority Population of Southwest China], Kunming

Zeng Yi (1987): Zeng Yi, Shilun renkou chengzhenhua dui kongzhi woguo renkou zengzhang di yingxiang [A Preliminary Study of the Influence of Urbanisation on the Control of Population Growth in China], *RYJ*, No. 6, pp. 30–36

Zeng Yi (1988): Zeng Yi, Is the Chinese Family Planning Program 'Tightening Up'?, *PDR*, No. 2, New York, pp. 333–338

Zeng Yi (1994): Zeng Yi, *Zhongguo renkou fazhan taishe ji duice tantao* [A Discussion of the Chinese Demographic Situation and Remedial Measures], Beijing

Zeng Yi (1995): Zeng Yi, Woguo 1991–1992 nian shengyulü shifou dada di yu tidai shuiping? [Is China's Fertility Rate in 1991–1992 Greatly Below the Replacement Level?], *RY*, No. 3, pp. 7–14

Zeng Yi (1997): Zeng Yi, Dilemmas of Family Size Norms in China, in: *International Population Conference*, Beijing 1997, Vol. 3, Beijing, pp. 1405–1418

Zeng Yi and Schultz (1998): Zeng Yi and T. Paul Schultz, Nongcun jiating chengbao zirenzhi dui shengyulü de yingxiang [The Impact of Rural Family-Contracting Systems on the Fertility Rate], *ZSK*, No. 1, pp. 129–144

Zeng Yi et al. (1991): Zeng Yi et al., A Demographic Decomposition of the Recent Increase in Crude Birth Rates in China, *PDR*, No. 3, pp. 435–458

Zeng Yi et al. (1993): Zeng Yi et al., Causes and Implications of the Recent Increase in the Reported Sex Ratio at Birth in China, *PDR*, No. 2, pp. 283–302

ZFTZ (1991): Zhonghua quanguo funü lianhehui, ed., *Zhongguo funü tongji ziliao 1949–1989* [Statistics on Chinese Women 1949–1989], Beijing

Zha Ruichuan et al. (1996): Zha Ruichuan, Zeng Yi and Guo Zhigang, ed., *Zhongguo disi ci quanguo renkou pucha ziliao fenxi* [An Analysis of the Fourth National Population Census], 2 Vol., Beijing

Zhai Shengming (1994): Zhai Shengming, Nongcun renkou kongzhi: 80 niandai de huigu he 90 niandai de duice [Population Control in the Villages: A Review of the 80s and Remedial Measures for the 90s], *Nongcun jingji yu shehui*, No. 1, Beijing, pp. 52–56, 47

Zhang Feng (1997): Zhang Feng, The Influences of Local Tradition on Population Control: A Case Study of a Poor Rural Community in Guangdong Province, China (Paper for the 23rd IUSSP Conference), Beijing

Zhang Fengyu (1997): Zhang Fengyu, *Zhongguo shengyu he biyun shiyong de duocengci yanjiu* [A Multi-Level Exploration of Fertility and Contraceptice Use in China], Beijing

Zhang Fengyu (1998): Zhang Fengyu, Jiushi niandai Zhongguo shengyu he renkou ziran zengzhang shuiping yanjiu [A Study on the Level of Chinese Fertility and Natural Population Increase in the Nineties], *ZSK*, No. 4, pp. 97–112

Zhang Guangzhao and Yang Zhiheng (1988): Zhang Guangzhao and Yang Zhiheng, *Zhongguo renkou jingji sixiang shi* [A History of Thinking on Population Economics in China], Chengdu

Zhang Huaiyu (1981): Zhang Huaiyu, Lun renkou yu jingji jianji dangqian nongcun renkou kongzhi wenti [On Population and Economics and on the Problem of Population Control in Rural Areas], *Jingji yanjiu*, No. 12, Beijing, pp. 32–37, 60

Zhang Kaimin (1989): Zhang Kaimin, *Shanghai laonian renkou* [Shanghai's Aged Population], Shanghai

Zhang Kaimin (1990): Zhang Kaimin, *Shanghai renkou qianjing zhanwang* [The Future Outlook for Shanghai's Population], Shanghai

Zhang Kewu (1996): Zhang Kewu, *Renkou minzuxue jianlun* [A Short Outline of Ethno-Demography], Beijing

Zhang Tianlu (1989): Zhang Tianlu, *Minzu renkouxue* [Ethno-Demography], Beijing

Zhang Tianlu (1993): Zhang Tianlu, ed., *Zhongguo shaoshuminzu shequ renkou yanjiu* [Demographic Studies on Minority Communities in China], Beijing

Zhang Tianlu and Huang Rongqing (1996): Zhang Tianlu and Huang Rongqing, ed., *Zhongguo shaoshuminzu renkou diaocha yanjiu* [Surveys on the Population of China's National Minorities], Beijing

Zhang Weidong and Zhang Sulin (1990): Zhang Weidong and Zhang Sulin, Kongzhi renkou yu tudi zhidu [Population Control and the System of Land Holdings], RY, No. 2, pp. 40–43

Zhang Weiguo (1999): Zhang Weiguo, Implementation of State Family Planning Programmes in a Northern Chinese Village, CQ, No. 157, pp. 202–230

Zhang Weimin *et al.* (1997): Zhang Weimin, Yu Hongwen and Cui Hongyan, Current Changes of China's Population, A Brief Analysis on the Population Data of China's 1995 1% Population Sample Survey, in: 23rd IUSSP General Population Conference, *Symposium on Demography of China*, Beijing, pp. 36–71

Zhang Wenfan (1998): Zhang Wenfa, Zhongguo renkou laolinghua yu zhanlüexing de xuanze [The Aging of the Chinese Population and Strategic Choices], RYJ, No. 1, pp. 55–59

Zhang Xiaoquan (2000): Zhang Xiaoquan, Gender Difference in Inheritance Rights: Observations from a Chinese Village, Paper Prepared for ECARDC VI Conference in Leiden

Zhang Xibo and Han Tinglong (1987): Zhang Xibo and Han Tinglong, ed., *Zhongguo geming fazhi shi* [The History of Revolutionary Law in China, 1921–1949], Vol. I, Beijing

Zhang Xinxia (1987): Zhang Xinxia, Shixi woguo qiwu qijian de renkou zengzhang xingshe [A First Analysis of Chinese Population Increase During the Period of the 7th Five-Year Plan], RY, No. 6, pp. 36–39

Zhang Yuanping (1991): Zhang Yuanping, Woguo nongcun renkou shengyu shikong de shehui xinli fenxi [A Social and Psychological Analysis of the Loss of Control of Childbearing in Chinese Rural Areas], RY, No. 5, pp. 54–58

Zhang Zehou and Chen Yuguang (1981): Zhang Zehou and Chen Yuguang, Shilun woguo renkou jiegou yu guomin jingji fazhan de guanxi [A Preliminary Study of the Relationship Between China's Population Structure and National Economic Development], ZSK, No. 4, pp. 29–46

Zhang Ziyi *et al.* (1982): Zhang Ziyi *et al.*, *Zhongguo qingnian de shengyu yiyuan – Beijing, Sichuan liang di chengxiang diaocha baogao* [Childbearing Preferences of Chinese Youth – Survey Reports from Cities and Villages of Beijing and Sichuan], Tianjin

Zhao Wenlin and Xie Shujun (1988): Zhao Wenlin and Xie Shujun, *Zhongguo renkou shi* [The Population History of China], Beijing

Zhao Zhongwei (1997): Zhao Zhongwei, Deliberate Birth Control Under a High-Fertility Regime: Reproductive Behavior in China Before 1970, PDR, No. 4, pp. 729–767

Zhong Sheng (1986): Shengchan zerenzhi hou funü de shengyi yiyuan [Childbearing Preferences of Women After the Introduction of the Responsibility System for Economic Production], RX, No. 2, pp. 28–31, 36

Zhong Weiqiao (1987): Zhong Weiqiao, Premarital Sex Among Young People in Langjun District, Yingcheng County, *Qingnian yanjiu*, February 1987, pp. 40–44, translated in: *Chinese Sociology and Anthropology*, Vol. 21, No. 3 (Chinese Women, VI; Guest Editor: Stanley Rosen], Armonk, pp. 70–77

Zhonggong Beijing shiwei (1992): Zhonggong Beijing shiwei, ed., *Beijing banshi shouce* [Handbook for Bureaucratic Formalities in Beijing], Beijing

Zhonggong dangshi ziliao (1993): Zonggong zhongyang dangshi yanjiu shi, ed., *Zhonggong dangshi ziliao* [Materials on the History of the Chinese Communist Party], Vol. 47, Beijing

Zhongguo chengshi jiating (1985): *Zhongguo chengshi jiating, Wu chengshi jiating diaocha baogao ji ziliao huibian* [China's Urban Families, Report and Materials from a Family Survey in Five Cities], Ji'nan

Zhongguo 21 shiji yicheng (1994): *Zhongguo 21 shiji yicheng, Zhongguo 21 shiji renkou, huanjing yu fazhan baipishu* [China's Agenda for the 21st Century, White Book on China's Population, Environment and Population in the 21st Century], Beijing

Zhongguo funü bao [Chinese Women Daily], Beijing

Zhongguo jihua shengyu gongzuo gangyao (1995): Guojia jihua shengyu weiyuanhui, ed., *Zhongguo jihua shengyu gongzuo gangyao 1995–2000* [A Program for Birth Planning in China 1995–2000], Beijing

Zhongguo jihua shengyu zhixing xiaoguo yanjiu ketizu (1996): Zhongguo jihua shengyu jixing xiaoguo yanjiu ketizu, Jiceng nongcun jihua shengyu zhixing qingkuang de diaocha yu fenxi [A Survey and Analysis of Birth-Planning Implementation in the Grassroots Villages], *RY*, No. 1, pp. 30–40

Zhongguo keji bao [Chinese Science and Technology Daily], Beijing

Zhongguo qingnian bao [Chinese Youth News], Beijing

Zhongguo renkou congshu (1987–93): *Zhongguo renkou congshu* [Encyclopedia of Chinese Population], 32 Vol., Beijing

Zhongguo renkou qingbao yanjiu zhongxin (1989): Zhongguo renkou qingbao yanjiu zhongxin, ed., *Ba ge shaoshuminzu funü hunyu qingkuang chouyang diaocha shuju huibian* [Monograph of Sampling Survey Data on Women's Marriage and Fertility of Eight Minority Nationalities of China], Beijing

Zhongguo tongxun she, Hongkong

Zhongguo tudi ziyuan shengchan nengli ji renkou chengzailiang yanjiu [A Study of the Productive Potential and the Carrying Capacity of China's Land Resources], Beijing

Zhongguo weilai renkou fazhan yu shengyu zhengce ketizu (2000): Guojia jihua shengyu weiyuanhui Zhongguo weilai renkou fazhan yu shengyu zhengce ketizu, Zhongguo weilai renkou fazhan yu shengyu zhengce yanjiu [A Study of China's Future Population Development and Birth Policy], *RY*, No. 3, pp. 18–34

Zhongguo 1982 nian renkou pucha ziliao: Guojia tongjiju renkou tongjisi, ed., *Zhongguo 1982 nian renkou pucha ziliao* [Materials of the 1982 Population Census of China], Beijing

Zhongguo 1987 nian 1% renkou chouyang diaocha ziliao: Guojia tongjiju renkou tongjisi, ed., *Zhongguo 1987 nian 1% renkou chouyang diaocha ziliao* [Materials of the 1987 1%-Sampling Survey on Population in China], 3 Vol., Beijing

Zhongguo 1990 nian renkou pucha ziliao: Guojia tongjiju renkou tongjisi, ed., *Zhongguo 1990 nian renkou pucha ziliao* [Materials of the 1990 Population Census of China], 4 Vol., Beijing

Zhou (1996): Zhou, Kate Xiao, How the Farmers Changed China, Power of the People, Boulder

Zhou Changhong (1995): Zhou Changhong, Woguo xianji jihua shengyu gongzuo renyuan shiqi zhuangkuang ji pingjia [An Appraisal of Morale Among County-Level Birth-Planning Personnel in China], *RX*, No. 2, pp. 49–53

Zhou Qing (1992): Zhou Qing, ed., *Dangdai Zhongguo hunyin jiating yu renkou fazhan* [Marriage, Family and Population Development in Present-Day China], Beijing

Zhou Shujun (1984): Zhou Shujun, China's Population Development Until the Year 2000, *BR*, No. 14, pp. 21–23

Zhu Guoping (1997): Zhu Guoping, Jiaqiang cunji jihua shengyu gongzuo zhitan [Random Remarks on the Strengthening of Birth Control on the Village Level], *RYJ*, No. 4, pp. 26–29

Zhu Lilan (1995): Zhu Lilan, ed., Kejiao *xingguo, Zhongguo mai xiang 21 shiji de zhongda zhanlüe juece* [Science and Education for a Prosperous China Important Strategic Decisions on China's March Toward the 21st Century], Beijing

ZJSN (1986–): Zhongguo jihua shengyu weiyuanhui, ed., *Zhongguo jihua shengyu nianjian* [Yearbook of Chinese Birth Planning], Beijing

ZJSQ (1997): Peng Peiyun, ed., *Zhongguo jihua shengyu quanshu* [Encyclopedia of Birth Planning in China], Beijing

ZLTN (1997): Guojia tongjiju, ed., *Zhongguo laodong tongji nianjian* [China Labour Statistical Yearbook], Beijing

ZMT (1991): Guojia minwei, ed., *Zhonghua minzu tongji 1949–1990* [Statistics on Chinese Nationalities 1949–1990], Beijing

Zou Ping (1985): Zou Ping, Beijing shi bufen weihun qingnian rengong liuchan qingkuang de diaocha [A Survey of Abortions Among Some Unmarried Youth in Beijing], *Qingnian yanjiu*, No. 10, Beijing, pp. 57–61

Zou Ping (1988a): Zou Ping, Renkou lifa gongzuo di zhanlüe yanjiu [The Strategy of Legislation on Population Matters], *RYJ*, No. 2, pp. 11–15

Zou Ping (1988b): Zou Ping, Woguo jihua shengyu difang fagui jianshe zongshu [The Establishment of Regional Birth-Planning Regulations in China], *RYJ*, No. 6, pp. 6–9

Zou Ping (1993): Zou Ping, *Zhongguo renkou faxue* [Chinese Population Law], Beijing

ZQ: *Zhongguo qingnian* [Chinese Youth], Beijing

ZRB: *Zhongguo renkou bao* [China Population Daily], Beijing

ZRGDFH (1995): *Zhonghua renmin gongheguo difangxing fagui huibian* [Collected Local Laws and Regulations of the People's Republic of China], 2 Vol., Beijing

ZRGFFQ (1994, 1996): Zhongguo renda changweihui fazhi gongzuo weiyuanhui, ed., *Zhonghua renmin gongheguo falü fagui quanshu* [Collected Laws and Regulations of the People's Republic of China], Vol. 10, Vol. 12, Beijing

ZRGZQ (1995): Quanguo renda changweihui fazhi gongzuo weiyuanhui, ed., *Zhonghua renmin gongheguo zhongcaifa quanshu* [Encyclopedia of Mediation Law in the People's Republic of China], Beijing

ZRK: *Zhongguo renkou kexue* [Population Science of China], Beijing

ZRN (1985–): Zhongguo shehui kexueyuan renkou yanjiusuo, ed., *Zhongguo renkou nianjian* [Chinese Population Yearbook], Beijing

ZRTN (1988–): Guojia tongjiju renkou tongjisi, ed., *Zhongguo renkou tongji nianjian* [China Population Statistics Yearbook], Beijing

ZRZS (1983–): Zhongguo renkou qingbao ziliao zhongxin, ed., *Zhongguo renkou ziliao shouce* [Handbook of Chinese Population Materials], Beijing

ZSK: *Zhongguo shehui kexue* [Chinese Social Sciences], Beijing

ZSTZ (1985–): Guojia tongjiju shehui tongjisi, ed., *Zhongguo shehui tongji ziliao* [Statististical Materials on Chinese Society], Beijing

ZTN (1981–): Guojia tongjiju, ed., *Zhongguo tongji nianjian* [China Statistical Yearbook], Beijing

ZWN (1984–): Guojia weishengbu, ed., *Zhongguo weisheng nianjian* [China Yearbook of Health], Beijing

Index

Aba 89
Abortion 7, 12, 17, 22, 46, 48, 54, 56, 78,
  105, 107, 117–25, 171, 178, 180–81,
  202, 226, 230, 312, 314, 321, 339
  ban 30, 44–45, 47, 120, 310
  compulsory 16, 52, 54–55, 76, 109,
    118–20
  costs 49, 117–118, 193, 312, 320
  misreporting 122
  pills 120
  rate 120–25, 217
  rules 30, 45, 120, 312
  sex-specific 120, 226–28, 291, 294, 296,
    321
  timing 52, 57, 89, 119–20
Administration for Housing and Real
  Estate 167
Administration for Industry and
  Commerce 128, 157, 167
Administration for Land Management and
  Resources 167
Adoption 76, 88, 97, 217, 225, 227–28,
  261, 295, 365 n 15
Age structure See Population: age structure
Aird, J.S. 7
Ancestor worship 11, 12, 104, 218, 220,
  307
Anhui 46, 85, 99, 102, 104–5, 110, 112,
  115, 119, 123–24, 127, 131, 134–35,
  139, 180, 192, 206, 215, 217, 224,
  227–28, 234, 243, 246–47, 266–68,
  282, 293–94, 297, 362 n 77
Arable land See Cultivated land
Army 30, 49, 71, 153, 161–62, 164, 166,
  168, 183, 186, 208, 213
Association for Population Studies 51,
  53–54, 58, 74, 184

Banister, J. 249, 366 n 1
Barefoot doctors See Doctors

Beijing 16, 30, 46, 92, 94, 98, 102, 104,
  110, 123–24, 126–27, 130, 135, 138,
  143, 151, 156, 165, 213–15, 217,
  233–34, 243, 246–47, 266–68,
  282–83, 293, 334, 367 n 16
Beijing University 47
Birth 249–53
  absolute numbers 36, 65, 67, 105, 199,
    201–2, 205, 249–51, 299, 321, 326
  averted 315–16, 330
  deliveries 95, 109, 145, 176, 227, 295
  illegitimate 92, 95, 118, 122, 137, 144,
    227, 253, 320
  intervals See Birth: spacing
  late birth 15, 17, 58, 62, 93–95, 201,
    264, 315, 338, 341
  limits 48, 51–54, 56, 59, 61, 62, 96, 209,
    311, 354 n 22
  orders 17, 59–63, 66–67, 69, 102,
    200–1, 203, 251–53, 263, 274, 276,
    279, 290, 292, 312–13, 341
  outside plan See Birth: unauthorized
  permits 50, 55, 94–96
  rash birth 137, 144
  rate 174, 199–202, 249–51, 256–57,
    314, 363 n 22
  sex ratio 15, 20, 79, 206, 217, 263, 283,
    288–98, 301, 321, 325, 338, 369 n 13
  spacing 12, 15, 17, 47, 49, 59–64, 66,
    70, 80, 93, 102–3, 260, 263–65, 283,
    314–15, 320, 338, 367 n 16
  unauthorized 3, 22, 65, 68, 72, 128, 137,
    199, 202, 204–5, 227, 231–34, 282,
    291, 332
Birth planning
  administration 16, 48, 50–51, 55, 60,
    77, 89, 168–69, 176, 186, 331–32
  budget 49, 56, 67, 72–74, 77, 133–34,
    156, 161, 166, 178, 189–96, 201,
    230, 235, 331–32

commissions 18–19, 67, 72–73, 86–89, 159–65, 167–68, 183, 185–88, 193–94, 203
conference 33, 35, 47, 49–50, 52, 56–57, 59, 61–62, 65–67, 72, 78, 80, 86, 97, 149–50, 158–60, 162–63, 168–69, 195, 350 n 16–17
contracts 52, 54, 56, 65, 90, 144, 172
cost-benefit analysis 317
deposits 93, 95, 108, 157
implementation rules 86, 89–90, 109
incentives *See* Incentives
insurance 171
law 52, 76, 84, 109, 227, 356 n 54
medical certificates 66, 75, 166, 179, 226
offences 22, 137, 224–35
rate 174, 199–202, 231
regulations 16–17, 21, 52, 56, 60, 62, 64, 66, 74–77, 83–91, 98–101, 107, 120, 130–32, 155, 157, 163, 198, 201, 203, 224, 226, 268, 331–32, 334, 342
report system 110, 156 57, 163, 207–9, 225, 231, 245, 249, 260
responsibility systems 8, 56, 75, 78, 149, 166, 175, 183, 196, 227, 231
sanctions *See* Sanctions
stations 75, 77, 163, 171, 179–81, 187, 193–94, 332, 362 n 73
suits 85–86
Birth-Planning Association 74, 77, 79, 157, 171, 176, 184–85
Birth out of plan *See* Birth: unauthorized
Bo Yibo 222, 340
Breast-feeding 116–17, 264, 320
Brothers 103
Brown, L. 334
Buck, J.L. 257, 365 n 2, 366 n 1
Buddhists 153

Cadres 3, 7, 17, 43, 56, 61, 64, 67, 70, 72–76, 78, 136–37, 147–48, 166, 169–72, 185–89, 191, 194, 205, 227, 235, 280, 302, 312, 331, 338
evaluations 74, 78, 149, 172–74, 198, 332
manipulation 206, 229, 231, 233
punishment 54, 78, 148–49, 229, 233
responsibility systems *See* Birth planning: responsibility systems
training 19, 87, 163–64, 187, 189, 194, 201
violence against cadres 72, 225
Carrying capacity 9, 38, 54, 317

Censorship 21–22, 44, 59, 69, 83, 147, 226, 296
Census 22, 199, 202, 204, 206, 258, 297
of 1953 43, 289, 302, 304, 318, 344
of 1964 51, 289, 302, 304, 344
of 1982 13, 33, 36, 58, 197, 206, 275, 284, 289, 292, 299, 304, 313, 344
of 1990 75, 80, 206, 249, 266, 275, 288, 292, 294, 296, 299, 302, 304, 313, 323, 344
of 2000 323, 340, 342, 343–45
Central Committee 31, 39, 45, 47–48, 51, 53, 56, 57, 73, 76–77, 146, 162, 164, 168, 208
circular 52, 59–60, 64, 69, 85, 87, 146, 150, 185
directive 44, 48, 50, 56, 75, 97, 145, 150, 159, 339
Disciplinary Commission 54, 146, 148, 161, 166, 206, 350 n 35
Open Letter 54, 74, 84, 96, 150
Organization Department 78
Propaganda Department 72, 161
Secretariat 51–52, 56, 58–59, 84, 159–60, 163
United Front Department 150
Chang Chongxuan 63, 67, 77
Changping 92
Chen Boda 31
Chen Changheng 46
Chen Da 46
Chen Muhua 51–53, 55–56, 107, 162
Chen Yun 35, 48, 51, 53, 96, 222, 340, 347 n 15
Chengdu 16, 53, 61, 165
Chiang Kaishek 30, 47
Chief Procuracy 76
Children
abandonment 228–30, 288
child-raising costs 221–22, 278, 316–17
sale of children 227
single children 20, 59, 103, 105, 125, 129, 135, 166, 325, 334, 339
twins 88, 230
China Council for the Promotion of Population Culture 185
China United Rubber (Group) Corporation 182
Chinese Communist Party *See* Party
Chinese Medical Association 184
Chongqing 100, 131, 140, 282
Cities 193, 308, 311, 314, 326, 332
abortion 225
age structure 270
birth limits 51

birth-planning administration 164, 169, 186
child-raising costs 221
contraceptives 44, 46, 105
family 12
family-size preferences 213, 214–16, 314, 321
hospitals 176
implementation rules 89
incentives 125, 133, 135
late marriage 241, 271
manpower need 338
old-age support 220
population ageing 328, 334, 338
population plan 199–200
retirement 302
sanctions 136
second-child permits 89, 94
son preference 217, 223, 291, 294
statistics 203
two-child policy 334, 338
Civil war 30, 258, 264, 299
Clinics *See* Hospitals
Coale, A.J. 249
Coercion 7–8, 16–17, 52, 55–61, 64, 74, 108, 136, 147, 226
Cohabitation 72, 79, 92, 119, 143, 230
Collectivization 258
Communist Youth League 54, 160–61, 166, 170–71, 185
Constitution 50, 56
Consumption 34, 198, 278, 309–10, 313, 316, 333, 337
Contraception 105–17, 137, 310, 315
compulsory 89, 312, 356 n 51, 356 n 54, 357 n 100
sterilization *See* Sterilization
traditional 11, 105, 264
Contraceptives 43, 44, 45, 74, 75, 332
anti-baby pills 95, 105, 107–8, 110–11, 113–14, 166, 182–83
choice 8, 54, 61, 95, 109, 183
condoms 107, 108, 110–11, 113–14, 166, 181–83
costs 49, 183, 189, 191, 194, 196, 320
diaphragms 110–11, 113, 181
distribution 164, 166, 170, 175, 179, 183, 191, 201
failure 17, 107, 125
implants 110–11, 113, 182
imports 45, 181, 182
injections 110–11, 114, 182
IUD 54, 57, 74, 78, 95, 108, 106–11, 113–15, 121, 160, 166, 178, 181–82, 226, 230, 320

non-use 116–17
prevalence 105, 110–17, 121, 174, 203, 268, 310, 314, 320
production 44, 49, 105, 161, 163, 181–83, 201, 202
regulations 181, 350 n 17
sale 44, 181, 183, 196
supply 46, 48, 56, 105, 182, 197
suppositories 114, 181
traditional 182
Corruption 22, 76, 122, 226, 230, 331, 352 n 115
Corvee labour 134
Counties
birth permits 96
birth-planning administration 51, 164–65, 176, 186
birth-planning budget 73, 193
cadres 187
hospitals 176
implementation rules 89
population plan 199–201
sanctions 144
second-child permits 89–90, 94
statistics 203
wages 188
Countryside *See* Peasants *or* Villages
Courts 54, 74, 76, 167
Crimes 30, 55, 76, 92, 107, 118, 136, 147, 224, 228
Critics 8, 15, 46, 53, 58, 61, 64, 68–71, 74, 79, 337–339
Cultivated land 9, 35, 38, 40, 47, 316, 333, 335, 348 n 29
Cultural Revolution 32–33, 39, 49, 105, 120, 136, 154, 159, 161–62, 169–70, 176–78, 184, 189, 197, 239, 258, 266, 271–72, 299, 311–12, 348 n 45

Dalian 74, 216, 218
Danjiang County 219
Datong 70
Daughters 11–12, 56, 59–60, 63, 65, 67, 69–73, 78, 97, 102–3, 109, 224, 229, 231, 263, 321
Death rate *See* Population: death rate
Decollectivization 36, 55, 61, 64, 68, 160, 316, 331
Demography *See* Population Studies
Deng Xiaoping 31, 33, 35, 43, 45, 51, 53–54, 61, 159, 340
Deng Yingchao 43
Departments of Traffic and Transportation 167

Dependency ratio *See* Population: dependency ratio
Dingxian 365 *n* 2, 366 *n* 1
Disabledness 75–76, 88, 97, 102–3, 230, 334
Dissidents *See* Critics
Divorce 12, 79, 91, 224, 230, 241, 320
Doctors 30, 50, 57, 166–67, 170, 176–81, 188, 194, 226, 312
Dongguan 108

Ecology 7, 9, 35, 37, 316
Education 31, 44, 316
and family-size preferences 221
and fertility 275–79, 309–13, 338
and marriage age 243
and sex preference 217
and sex ratio 294–95
illiteracy 267, 269, 277, 322, 334, 343
school enrolment 37, 302, 322, 326
sex education 167
Employment 31–32, 35–36, 38, 40, 198, 302, 304, 309, 312, 316, 326, 335–36, 340
participation rate 328
underemployment 36, 172, 333, 335–36
unemployment 36, 47, 126, 128, 157, 230, 316, 333, 335–36, 340
Enterprises 51, 60, 78, 128–29, 133, 135, 148–49, 157, 162, 169, 183, 190–91, 194, 203
foreign 87, 149, 157, 185
private 79, 146, 156–57, 169, 185, 194, 218, 335
state 79, 183, 186, 189, 336, 361 *n* 56
stock companies 149
township and town 103, 190–91, 208, 213, 218, 220–21, 280, 335, 336
Entrepreneurs 24, 145, 218
Environment *See* Ecology
Ethics 11–12, 307
Eugenics 22, 53, 74, 76, 94–95
Euthanasia 76
Experimental spots 59–60, 63, 70–71, 73, 101–2

Family 6, 10–12, 30, 46, 61, 104, 220, 307–8, 320, 347 *n* 10
Family-size preferences 16, 58, 208, 213–23, 308
Fees 87, 90, 103, 134–35, 156–57, 195, 341
social-support fees 143
Fei Xiaotong 46
Fengyang County 115

Fertility 66, 249–87
age-specific 254–56, 272, 275–77
and sex preference 263
by birth orders 261, 272
by ethnic group 24, 283–87
by occupation 279–80
by regions 6, 78, 104, 265–70, 310–12
by social characteristics 24, 274–83
by urban-rural residence 270–74
duration-specific 256–57, 259
measurement 24, 253–54, 314
parity progression ratios 24, 199, 256–57, 259, 261 63, 268 69, 273
total fertility rate 10, 40, 50, 53, 62, 65, 72, 79–80, 104, 199, 204, 207, 256–61, 267, 271, 273, 276, 278–79, 285–86, 325, 341
Fishermen 103, 216
Five-year plan 49–50, 57, 63–64, 72–73, 80, 150, 188, 193, 197, 199, 201–2, 350 *n* 16, 352 *n* 80
Food 29, 31–35, 44, 310, 333–35
Foundation for Population and Welfare Activities 185
Fujian 17, 46, 99, 102, 104, 110, 112, 123–24, 127, 131, 135, 137, 139, 142, 151, 180, 192, 201, 226, 229, 233–34, 243, 245–47, 266–68, 269, 294
Fushan County 47

Gansu 46, 52, 63, 78, 97, 100, 102–3, 109, 111, 118, 124, 127, 132, 140, 152, 180, 192, 204, 215–16, 227–28, 234, 243, 246–47, 266–68, 293
Gaozhou 226
Garzi 89
Gender 6, 11, 21, 214, 217, 223, 308, 320
Grain production 35, 38, 40, 199, 316, 333–34, 337
Great Leap Forward 31, 33–34, 39, 47–48, 161, 176–177, 184, 225, 239, 251, 256, 258, 261, 264–65, 270, 290, 299–300, 302, 310–11
Greenhalgh, S. 93, 133, 142, 195
Gross domestic product 266, 268–69, 316, 320, 337
Gross national product 34
Guangdong 16–17, 46, 49, 52, 55, 63, 78, 85, 87, 97–104, 106, 108, 111–12, 124, 127–29, 131, 135, 137, 139, 141, 143, 148–49, 151, 154, 160, 172, 180, 192, 215–16, 224, 226–28, 233–34, 243, 246 47, 266 69, 282, 293–94, 297, 309, 341

Guangxi 46, 63, 97, 99, 102–4, 109,
  111–12, 123–24, 127–28, 131,
  139–40, 143, 148, 151, 192, 201,
  204, 234, 243, 246–47, 266–67,
  269–70, 283, 293–94, 297
Guangzhou 94
Guizhou 46, 61, 78, 93, 100, 102–4, 109,
  111, 117, 124, 127, 132, 135, 140,
  151, 154, 180, 192, 204, 215–16,
  234, 243, 246–47, 267, 269, 270,
  283, 293
Guomindang 29–30, 38, 44, 91, 165, 299

Hainan 46, 91, 100, 102–4, 111–12, 119,
  124, 127, 129, 131, 140, 154, 192,
  201, 204, 233–34, 243, 246–47, 267,
  269–70, 293–94
Haishan 257
Hami 153
Harbin 92, 214, 216
He Bochuan 5, 41
Health 31–32, 44, 48, 316, 322
Hebei 17, 46, 49, 87, 97–98, 102–4, 107,
  109–10, 124, 127, 129–30, 137–38,
  142–43, 149, 160, 192, 204, 215–16,
  233–34, 243, 246–47, 266–68, 281,
  293, 348 n 30
Hefei 216
Heilongjiang 17, 46, 98, 102–4, 106, 110,
  124, 127, 129–30, 138, 142–43,
  148–49, 151, 180, 192, 215, 234,
  243, 246–47, 266–68, 281, 293
Henan 46, 97, 99, 102–4, 106, 110, 119,
  123–24, 127, 131, 139, 143, 148,
  151, 154, 179–80, 192, 215, 226,
  234, 243, 246–47, 266–68, 293–94,
  297
Hongkong 101, 158, 320–21, 333, 340,
  369 n 13
Hospitals 46, 50, 95, 135, 166–67, 176–81,
  183, 195, 202, 227, 295, 312
Household registration 88, 146, 155, 166,
  171, 188, 202–5, 207, 230, 249–50
Housing 36–37, 316, 337
Hu An'gang 332
Hu Qiaomu 35, 55, 107, 159–60, 224,
  340
Hu Yaobang 58, 63, 67, 71, 159–60, 340
Hua Guofeng 33, 50–51, 159, 161
Hubei 16, 46, 99, 110, 102, 104, 124,
  126–27, 131, 139, 148, 154, 180,
  192, 196, 204, 215–17, 219, 234,
  243, 246–47, 266–69, 293–94
Huiyang 55
Human rights 3, 8–10, 12, 14, 16, 308

Hunan 46, 49, 99, 103–4, 111, 123–24,
  127–28, 131, 137, 139, 142, 154,
  161, 180, 192, 204, 215, 217, 234,
  243, 246–47, 267–69, 282–83, 293
Hundred-Flowers Campaign 31, 38,
  46–47, 348 n 45

Ili 153
Incentives 52–54, 74–75, 87–89, 125–36,
  167, 331–32, 337
  collective incentives 135
  housing allocation 74, 125, 135
  insurance 75, 77, 129, 185, 194, 225
  kindergarten and school 135
  land allotment 74, 134
  medical care 135
  one-child bonus 128–34, 157, 194
  prolonged maternity leave 133
  pro-natalist 150, 165
  retirement 134, 189
  work allocation 125, 166
Income 332, 337
  and family-size preferences 221–23
  and fertility 280–81, 313, 338
  and marriage age 225, 320
Industrialization 268–69, 335
Infant mortality *See* Mortality: infants
Infanticide 11, 22, 79, 228–29, 288, 294,
  296–98, 307
Informants 74–75, 135, 157, 203, 226
Inner Mongolia 46, 97–98, 104, 109–10,
  119, 124, 127, 130, 133, 138, 145,
  150–51, 192, 233–34, 243, 246–47,
  267–68, 283, 293–94
Intra-uterine devices *See* Contraceptives:
  IUD

Japan 123, 182, 320, 328
Jiang Zemin 79–80, 160, 340
Jiangsu 16, 23, 46, 49, 91–93, 97, 99,
  102–5, 110, 123–24, 126–30, 137,
  139, 143, 160, 176, 180, 192, 213,
  215–16, 234, 243, 245–47, 258,
  266–68, 293–94, 356 n 55, 365 n 2,
  366 n 1
Jiangxi 46, 78, 93, 97, 99, 102, 104, 110,
  112, 118, 124, 127–28, 131, 139,
  176, 180, 192, 233–34, 243, 245–47,
  266–68, 293
Jiangyin County 258
Jieyang 149
Jilin 46, 98, 102–5, 110, 124, 127, 129–30,
  138, 143, 151, 154, 180, 192, 215,
  233–34, 243, 246–47, 266–67, 281,
  283, 293

Ji'nan 205
Joint ventures *See* Enterprises: foreign

Karamay 153
Kunming 57, 142, 366 n 1

Labour Union *See* Trade Union
Land adjustments 145, 220
Land reform 258, 310
Land-use contracts 146
Laws 30, 44, 52–53, 74, 75–77, 85, 94,
    226, 228, 255, 332
Leading Group for Birth Planning 49–51,
    55, 161–62, 168–69, 184
Lee Kuan Yew 334
Lenin, V.I. 30, 44
Lhasa 152
Li Guangyuan 53
Li Jinghan 46
Li Peng 70, 72–73, 79–80, 160, 168
Li Tieying 168
Li Xiannian 31, 35, 51, 53, 57, 67, 340
Liangshan 89
Liaoning 3, 46, 49, 86, 92, 97–98, 102–5,
    110, 119, 123–24, , 127, 129–30,
    134–35, 138, 143, 148, 151, 154,
    160, 176, 192, 214–16, 218, 222,
    228–29, 234, 243, 246–47, 266–67,
    283, 293–94, 350 n 17, 354 n 22
Linzhi 188
Liu Shaoqi 31, 44, 47, 49, 347 n 7

Ma Yinchu 46, 48, 51
Malthus, T.R. 9, 13, 29–30, 38, 48, 337
Managers 78, 149
Manpower need 12, 48, 59, 61, 97, 102,
    104, 218 19, 331
Mao Zedong 29–32, 36, 38, 44–47, 182,
    310, 312, 348 n 45
Marriage 55, 239–48, 320
    age 55, 64, 66, 68, 77, 91–93, 199,
        241–44, 253, 258, 260, 261, 268,
        272, 310–14, 319, 331
    and fertility 255
    early marriage 67, 91, 137, 153, 174,
        205, 224–25, 244–46, 270
    generation-specific 240
    illegal 55, 67, 72, 76, 224
    late marriage 17, 46, 47, 49, 62–63, 70,
        77, 91–93, 102, 174, 201, 239,
        246–48, 264, 315, 319, 338, 341, 367
        n 16
    law 30, 55, 65, 77, 91, 225, 255
    marital status 240–41
    mixed marriage 154

    numbers 55, 65, 200, 203
    registration 66, 74, 91, 94, 166, 171,
        207
    regulations 91, 224, 271
    remarriage 97, 103
    singles 11, 214, 241, 320
    uxorilocal 103, 220
Marx, K. 9
Maternity courses 95
Maternity leave 133, 136, 145
Mencius 11
Mian County 60
Midwives 174, 177 79, 227, 229
Migrants *See* Migration
Migration 24, 36, 42, 48, 62, 65, 76, 79,
    198, 200, 208, 216, 218, 283, 311,
    329, 331, 334–35, 338, 343
    administration 167
    and fertility 216, 270, 281–83, 310
    birth-planning contracts 172
    income 143
    pregnancy tests 107
    regulations 74, 88, 155–56
    statistics 203, 207
    unauthorized births 66, 72, 74, 230
Military *See* Army
Mill, J.S. 38
Miners 103, 218
Ministry of Aeronautics 65
Ministry of Agriculture 77, 145, 146, 166
Ministry of Chemical Industry 166, 182
Ministry of Civil Administration 68, 77,
    129, 166, 171, 207
Ministry of Commerce 44, 49
Ministry of Culture 166
Ministry of Education 167
Ministry of Finance 65, 166, 183, 189
Ministry of Foreign Economic Relations
    and Trade 167
Ministry of Foreign Trade 44
Ministry of Forestry 77
Ministry of Fuels and Chemical Industry
    49
Ministry of Health 31, 39, 43–45, 47–49,
    57, 88, 106, 120, 122, 160–61,
    166–67, 177, 179, 181, 183–84, 186,
    189, 207, 226, 348 n 46, 349 n 5–6,
    350 n 13–14, 355 n 36
    report system 202
Ministry of Justice 68, 107
Ministry of Labour 88, 134, 166
Ministry of Light Industry 44, 181
Ministry of Machine Building 166, 182
Ministry of Personnel 78, 88, 134, 166
Ministry of Public Security 166, 205, 207

Ministry of Radio, Film and Television 167
Ministry of Supervision 167, 206
Ministry of Urban Construction 167
Ministry of Water Conservancy 77
Mobility *See* Migration
Mortality 310–11
    female 289
    infants 203, 206–7, 229, 269, 289, 296,
        297–98, 311, 322
    life expectancy 267–69, 309, 316,
        322–23
Mosher, S. 52, 133, 141
Mountainous areas 102, 218
Muslims 112–13, 153–54, 245, 270, 286,
    292

Nanjing 164
Nanjing Academy for Birth Planning 187
National Association of Journalism
    Workers 185
National Bureau of Statistics *See* State
    Statistical Bureau
National Corporation for Medical
    Appliance Industries 166, 182
National minorities 24, 54, 56–57, 59, 63,
    66, 77, 88, 96, 101, 113, 123,
    150–55, 166, 191, 199, 203, 216,
    218, 253, 268, 269, 283–87, 309,
    312–13
    Blang 285, 292
    Dagur 151, 153, 285
    education 284
    Evenki 151, 285
    Hani 284–85, 292
    Hui 151, 153–54, 284, 286–87
    Kirgiz 284, 286
    Koreans 151, 284–85
    Manchus 151, 154–55, 284–85, 287,
        292
    Miao 284–85
    mixed marriage 154, 226
    Mongols 151, 154–55, 284–85, 287
    Mulam 285, 292
    Oroqon 151, 285
    preferences 154
    Pumi 285, 292
    reclassification 154–55, 226, 283
    Russians 153, 284, 286
    sex ratios 292
    Tajiks 153, 286
    Tatars 153, 286
    Thai 284–85
    Tibetans 24, 77, 152, 284–85, 287, 292
    Tujia 155, 285, 287, 292
    urbanization 284

Uygur 284, 286–87
Uzbeks 153, 286
Xibe 151, 153, 284–85
Yao 285, 292
Yi 284–85, 287
Zhuang 151, 284–85, 292
National People's Congress 32, 44, 50, 55,
    67, 70, 72–73, 162, 168, 198, 208
National Study Association for Politico-
    Ideological Work Among Birth-
    Planning Personnel 185
Natural increase *See* Population: natural
    increase
Neighbourhood committees 74, 95, 157,
    169–70, 183, 188, 203
Ningxia 46, 63, 97, 100–2, 104, 111, 124,
    127, 132, 140, 152–54, 192–93, 204,
    234, 243, 246–47, 267, 269, 283,
    293–94
Notaries 227, 365 *n* 15
Notestein, F. 29

Occupation
    and fertility 279–80, 309–10
    and sex ratio 294
Officials *See* Cadres
Old-age support 5, 10, 12, 40, 53, 74, 104,
    129, 134, 218–19, 317, 322, 328,
    336, 338
One-child certificates 55, 88, 126–28, 201,
    203, 217
One-child policy 4, 42, 51–54, 59, 65, 68,
    96, 277, 294, 300, 313–14, 316, 330,
    333–34, 338
Opposition *See* Critics
Optimum population *See* Population:
    optimum
Orphanages 229
Overseas Chinese 101, 103–04, 158

Pan Guangdan 46
Party 4, 30, 45, 83, 159–60, 164, 330, 331,
    333
    Central Committee *See* Central
        Committee
    committees 84–85, 87, 159, 161, 168,
        171–72, 208
    congress 45
    members 54, 96, 148
    Politburo *See* Politburo
    secretaries 65, 78, 159–60
Peasants 17, 36, 45, 47–49, 53, 66, 67, 70,
    74, 88, 101, 103, 126, 129, 134, 137,
    185, 195, 218, 221, 270, 280, 326,
    328, 331, 338–39, 341

family-size preferences 215–16, 218–22, 314
old-age support 219, 302
resistance 3, 46, 55, 224–33, 332
rich peasants 24, 208, 222, 230
son preference 217
Penalties *See* Sanctions
Peng Peiyun 4, 68–69, 71–73, 76–77, 79–80, 86, 150, 233, 339
Peng Zhen 68
Pensions 302, 336, 340
People's Bank 88, 167
People's Communes 47, 50–52, 55, 61, 133–34, 137, 162, 170, 177, 190, 194, 245
Petitions 208
Politburo 32–33, 39, 47, 51, 79, 163, 198, 228, 347 *n* 15
  Standing Committee 32, 57, 69–72, 84, 160, 163, 339
Political Consultative Conference 160, 162, 168, 208
Political culture 5–6, 307–8, 330, 342
Population
  age structure 4, 64–67, 69, 75, 79, 93, 198, 202, 245, 249, 251, 253, 298–304, 313–14, 321–22, 325–29, 336, 343
  ageing 4, 10, 42, 53, 58, 268, 304, 328, 333–34, 338, 340
  agricultural 97, 103
  death rate 42, 202, 229
  dependency ratio 198, 304
  economics 9, 20, 30–37, 39–41, 44, 47–48, 221, 309, 311–13, 315–17, 337–39
  history 11, 30, 105, 241, 255, 258, 280, 296, 298–99, 308, 365 *n* 2, 366 *n* 1
  natural increase 48, 50–51, 57, 63, 80, 96, 197, 199, 201–2, 329
  non-agricultural 97, 128, 188
  optimum 38–41, 38–41, 317, 330
  overpopulation 29–31, 38, 48, 152, 308, 333, 337, 339–40
  plan 47, 49, 50, 75, 161, 163, 165, 197–202, 233, 318, 339
  police 74
  rural *See* Peasants
  sex ratios 301
  studies 13, 20, 13–25, 29, 51, 53, 184
  survival rates 206, 295
  targets 40, 47–51, 53–54, 57, 61–64, 68, 72–73, 80, 96, 198, 200–2, 209, 330, 332–33, 335, 339
  urban 44, 48, 198, 268–70, 311, 320, 322, 338, 343
Population Council 17, 62, 70
Potter, S.H. and J.M. 52, 141
Poverty 7, 34, 73, 134–35, 142, 191, 195
Pregnancy
  tests 76, 89, 107, 143, 147, 156, 175–76, 181, 230
  unauthorized 118
Prenatal sex determination *See* Abortion: sex-specific
Press 19, 30, 44, 46–49, 164
Procurement quotas 134
Projections 19–20, 34, 38, 39–41, 43, 53, 58, 62, 64–65, 68, 72, 75, 80, 201, 258, 315, 318–29, 332–33, 337, 339
Propaganda 7, 10, 30–31, 44–45, 47–49, 55, 57, 74, 78, 87, 89, 163–64, 166, 185, 201, 310, 332
  foreign 7, 9, 43
Provincial People's Congresses 85–87

Qian Xinzhong 33, 57, 348 *n* 30
Qinghai 46, 97, 100–2, 104, 111–12, 124, 127, 132, 140, 152, 154, 180, 192, 204, 234, 243, 246–47, 265–67, 269, 283, 293–94
Qingtian County 109, 358 *n* 114

Resettlement 32, 36, 48, 152–53
Retirement 302, 326
Revolutionary Committees 85, 159, 161
Rustication *See* Resettlement

Sanctions 52, 54, 65, 72, 75, 87, 89, 136–49, 167, 331
  cadre punishment 148–49
  collective sanctions 147–48
  demotions 145
  discharge 146
  enrolment 136
  fine collection 22, 75, 137, 142, 156, 171, 175, 201, 281
  fines 17, 52, 68, 88, 90, 93, 118, 137–44, 195, 225, 228, 230, 332, 338, 342
  household registration 146, 156
  housing 145, 338
  illegal sanctions 146–47
  land allotment 145–46
  rations 136
  revocation of licenses 145, 156–57
  wage deductions 118–19, 137–44
  work allocation 146
Second-child permits 4, 15, 49, 54, 56, 59–64, 67–73, 75, 64–76, 78, 90,

96–105, 151–54, 163, 172, 200–1,
209, 227, 229–30, 251, 253, 270,
294, 321, 332, 334, 339, 341
Self-employed 66, 72, 79, 88, 126, 128,
145–46, 156–57, 193, 335
Sexual behaviour 12, 123, 125, 184, 225,
239, 263–64, 320
Shaanxi 17, 46, 60, 63, 78, 92–93, 97, 100,
102–9, 112, 118, 124, 127, 129,
132–33, 135, 140, 142, 148, 180,
192, 195, 215–16, 229, 234, 243,
246–47, 267–68, 281, 293, 353
n 125
Shandong 46–47, 49, 59, 63, 71, 78, 99,
102, 104, 109–10, 112, 123–24,
126–27, 131, 139, 143, 148, 151,
154, 160, 175, 180, 192, 205,
215–16, 221, 226, 233–34, 243,
246–47, 267–68, 281, 293–94
Shanghai 32, 37, 45–46, 48, 49–50, 92,
97–98, 102, 104–7, 110, 117, 120,
123–25, 127, 129–30, 133–35,
137–38, 143, 146, 160, 165, 187,
192–93, 202, 214–16, 217, 222, 234,
243, 246–47, 266–68, 272, 282,
293–94, 299, 311, 323, 328, 338, 349
n 13, 350 n 17
Shanxi 46, 53, 70, 92, 98, 103–5, 110, 124,
127, 128–30, 135, 138, 180, 192,
205, 224, 227, 228, 234, 243,
246–47, 267–68, 293
Shao Lizi 44
Shenyang 16, 165, 216
Shigatse 152
Sichuan 46, 49, 54, 63, 86, 88, 100, 102,
104, 110–12, 123–24, 126–28, 132,
140, 151–52, 154, 179, 192, 204,
215–16, 218, 230, 234, 243, 245–47,
267–68, 282, 293
Singapore 321, 334, 369 n 13
Singles *See* Marriage: singles
Snow, E. 182
Social sciences 29, 47
Social security 11, 41, 53, 77, 128, 135,
157, 188, 331, 336
Socialization 20
Son preference 11–12, 62, 68, 127, 217,
220, 229, 263, 283, 291–92, 296,
298, 307, 321
Song Jian 39–40, 42, 53, 65, 197
Song Ping 79
South Korea 123, 296, 298, 320, 325, 369
n 13
Soviet Union 29–30, 44, 153
Stalin, J. 29–30, 44

State Birth-Planning Commission 49, 57,
59–60, 62–63, 65–66, 68, 72, 75–77,
83, 90, 120, 161–65, 167–68, 184,
186, 189, 198, 200, 202–5, 207–8,
225–26, 230, 266, 282, 339, 341
State Commission for Education 166, 167
State Commission for Nationality Affairs
155, 166
State Commission for Science and
Technology 39, 165
State Corporation for Pharmaceutical
Production 166, 182
State Council 39, 43, 48–51, 55–56, 62,
75, 77, 84–85, 88, 145, 159, 161–64,
166, 168, 184, 198, 208, 225
State Pharmaceutical Administration 166,
182
State Pharmacy Corporation 166, 181–82
State Planning Commission 32, 50, 163,
165, 193, 198
State Pricing Bureau 183
State Statistical Bureau 33, 167, 203–7,
249, 251, 260, 341
Statistics 19, 33, 74–75, 202–7, 331, 355 n
36
falsification 6, 66, 72, 75, 80, 106, 122,
126, 174, 203–4, 229, 231, 233, 260,
269, 296, 298, 315
migration 203, 207
over-reporting 112, 122, 246, 320
random checks 75, 174–75, 203–5, 207,
231, 343
report system 22, 75, 87, 126, 164, 170,
202–3, 231, 309
under-reporting 64, 72, 122, 203–6,
233, 249, 253, 255, 260, 261, 266,
289, 295, 297, 325, 341, 343
Sterilization 3, 7, 17, 46–47, 54, 57, 61, 74,
78, 108–11, 115, 121, 178, 181, 226,
230, 310, 320, 326, 332, 341
ban 45
compulsory 52, 78, 91, 94, 108–9, 119,
269
costs 45, 108, 145, 193, 195, 312
prevalence 113
rules 45, 120, 312
targets 201
tubal ligations 110–11, 114, 121
vasectomies 110–11, 114, 121
Street committees 60, 94, 126, 158, 162,
164, 169, 194, 200, 203
Su Xiuzhen 162
Sun Benwen 38, 46
Sun Jingzhi 47
Sun Yatsen 30

Supreme Court 76, 146, 224
Supreme State Conference 46
Surgery 45, 78, 105, 166, 171, 179, 201–2,
    208, 355 *n* 36
  costs 189, 193–95
  malpractices 22, 178–79, 226, 231, 360
    n 40
Surveys
  abortions 122, 125, 296
  adoption 227, 296
  aged population 364 *n* 9
  annual 23, 66, 174, 203, 205, 207, 249,
    343
  birth planning 204
  birth spacing 264
  birth-planning stations 194
  cadre attitudes 56, 189, 235
  child abandonment 296
  contraception 23, 107, 113–15, 184
  family-size preferences 213–23, 363 *n* 2
  fertility 23–24, 58, 72, 204–6, 231, 260,
    275, 341, 367 *n* 21
  infant mortality 298
  infanticide 296
  marriage age 245, 365 *n* 2
  migration 156, 218, 281, 283, 368 *n* 35
  national minorities 284
  one-child certificates 126
  sex ratio 289, 295
  son preference 217, 263
  two-child policy 339
Suzhou 16

Taian 164
Taiwan 158, 319
  abortions 123, 296
  consumption 333
  family-size preferences 321
  fertility 257, 325
  marriage age 320, 365 *n* 2
  sex ratio 298, 325, 369 *n* 13
Taxation 30, 61, 74, 135, 338
Third-child permits 65, 96, 150, 152–53,
    253
Tian Jiyun 73
Tian Xueyuan 53, 58, 337
Tian'anmen crisis 73, 103
Tianjin 46, 52, 61, 85, 92, 98, 102, 104–5,
    110, 123–24, 127, 130, 135, 138,
    160, 180, 192, 215–16, 217, 224,
    234, 243, 246–47, 266–67, 293–94
Tibet 46, 97, 100, 102–4, 111–13, 118,
    124, 127, 132, 140, 147, 152–54,
    161–62, 188, 192–93, 195, 234, 243,
    246–47, 267, 269, 283, 293

birth-planning regulations 77
population 24
White Paper 152
Townships and towns
  administration 170–72, 175
  birth permits 94–95
  birth-planning administration 60, 77,
    126, 164, 170, 187
  birth-planning budget 190, 194–5
  birth-planning stations 180
  cadres 188
  covenants 89–90
  hospitals 176
  population plan 200
  sanctions 144
  second-child permits 68, 90
  statistics 203
Trade Union 45, 160–61, 166, 185
Trial policies *See* Experimental spots
Twelve-Year Program for Agricultural
    Development 45, 47
Two-child policy 48–50, 56, 58, 61–63, 65,
    70, 96, 104, 312, 316, 323, 325, 332,
    334, 338–39

Ulanfu 150
Ultrasound examinations 175, 226, 296,
    297
Unauthorized births *See* Birth:
    unauthorized
Unemployment *See* Employment:
    unemployment
United Nations 3, 7, 330
  Fund for Population Activities 21, 167,
    351 *n* 65
Urbanization *See* Population: urban
Urban-rural gap 6, 48–50, 115, 122, 123,
    169, 192, 214, 217, 241, 247,
    270–74, 277, 279, 302, 310–12, 314
Urumqi 153
USA 3, 16, 29, 123, 320, 333

Value change 278, 308, 320, 321
Villages 176, 219, 311–12, 326, 332
  birth limits 52
  birth permits 95
  birth-planning administration 170–71,
    175
  cadres 169–70, 188
  child-raising costs 221
  collective liability 65
  committees 171–72
  incentives 125, 133–34, 136
  investigations 174–75
  marriage 225

medical network 180
population plan 200
sanctions 136–37
second-child permits 68, 119
statistics 203
statutes 89

Wages 54, 67, 72, 74, 77, 149, 163, 172, 188–89, 193–94, 230, 333, 336
Wan Li 56
Wang Heshou 350 *n* 35
Wang Renzhong 33, 350 *n* 35
Wang Wei 63, 65, 67–69, 71, 74
Wang Ya'nan 47
Wang Zhen 36, 340, 347 *n* 12
Water resources 37, 40, 316
Weinan 108
West Europe 123, 320, 326, 328
White Book 9, 340, 346 *n* 2
White, T. 142
Women 6–8, 43, 53, 76, 160, 171, 220, 223–24, 229, 240, 278, 289, 301, 310, 312, 320–22, 349 *n* 2, 349 *n* 5
Women's Federation 43–44, 46, 50, 68, 160–61, 166, 170–71, 185, 225, 350 *n* 35
Work Conference on Urban Affairs 39, 48, 136
Workers and staff 50, 69, 89, 96, 126, 136–37
World Bank 34
Wu Guixian 161

Wu Jingchao 46
Wu Wenzao 46
Wuhan 16, 142, 147, 165, 216

Xiamen 17, 142
Xi'an 165, 282
Xinjiang 46, 92, 97, 100–4, 111–12, 124, 127, 132, 140, 152–54, 161, 180, 192, 204, 233–34, 243, 245–47, 265, 267, 269, 283–84, 286, 293–94
Xu Yunbei 348 *n* 46

Yicheng County 70–71, 334, 339
Yu Jingyuan 53
Yunnan 46, 89, 97, 100, 102, 104, 111–12, 124, 127, 132, 140, 142, 151–52, 154, 180, 192, 204, 234, 243, 246–47, 267, 269, 283–84, 293

Zhang Chunqiao 32
Zhao Chengxin 46
Zhao Ziyang 7, 55, 61–63, 65, 67–69, 72–74, 102–3, 160, 340
Zhejiang 45–46, 63, 91, 99, 102–4, 109–10, 124, 127, 129–31, 133, 139, 143, 148, 154, 180, 192, 215–16, 227–28, 233–34, 243, 246–47, 266, 268, 293–94, 296
Zhong Huinan 38
Zhou Enlai 31–32, 43–45, 48–49, 162
Zhou Rongxin 161
Zhu Rongji 168, 205, 332

Printed in the United States
by Baker & Taylor Publisher Services